T0185324

Clinical Topics in Old Age Psychiatry

'Clinical Topics In ... '

Other titles in this series:

Clinical Topics in Personality Disorder (2012)
Jaydip Sarkar & Gwen Adshead
9781908020390

Clinical Topics in Child and Adolescent Psychiatry (2014)
Sarah Huline-Dickens
9781909726178

Clinical Topics in Disorders of Intellectual Development (2015)
Marc Woodbury-Smith
9781909726390

Clinical Topics in Old Age Psychiatry

Edited by

Philippa Lilford
Severn Deanery, Bristol

Julian C Hughes
University of Bristol

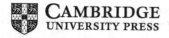
CAMBRIDGE
UNIVERSITY PRESS

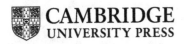
CAMBRIDGE
UNIVERSITY PRESS

Shaftesbury Road, Cambridge CB2 8EA, United Kingdom

One Liberty Plaza, 20th Floor, New York, NY 10006, USA

477 Williamstown Road, Port Melbourne, VIC 3207, Australia

314–321, 3rd Floor, Plot 3, Splendor Forum, Jasola District Centre, New Delhi – 110025, India

103 Penang Road, #05–06/07, Visioncrest Commercial, Singapore 238467

Cambridge University Press is part of Cambridge University Press & Assessment,
a department of the University of Cambridge.

We share the University's mission to contribute to society through the pursuit of
education, learning and research at the highest international levels of excellence.

www.cambridge.org
Information on this title: www.cambridge.org/9781108706148

DOI: 10.1017/9781108594714

First published 2020

A catalogue record for this publication is available from the British Library

Library of Congress Cataloging-in-Publication data
Names: Hughes, Julian C., editor. | Lilford, Philippa, 1989– editor.
Title: Clinical topics in old age psychiatry / edited by Julian Hughes, Philippa Lilford.
Description: Cambridge ; New York, NY : Cambridge University Press, 2021. | Includes
bibliographical references and index.
Identifiers: LCCN 2020022642 (print) | LCCN 2020022643 (ebook) | ISBN 9781108706148
(paperback) | ISBN 9781108594714 (ebook)
Subjects: MESH: Mental Disorders | Alzheimer Disease | Aged | United Kingdom
Classification: LCC RC451.4.A5 (print) | LCC RC451.4.A5 (ebook) | NLM WT 150 |
DDC 618.97/689–dc23
LC record available at https://lccn.loc.gov/2020022642
LC ebook record available at https://lccn.loc.gov/2020022643

ISBN   978-1-108-70614-8   Paperback

....

Philippa dedicates this book to Fergus Hamilton, who during the editing of this book became my husband.

Julian dedicates this book to Matthew Clay, Architect, and Ben Clements, Building Contractor, and his amazing team for designing and building me a study whilst I edited this book.

Contents

Section 4 Law, Ethics and Philosophy

Contributors

Dimitrios Adamis is a consultant psychiatrist in the Sligo-Leitrim Mental Health Services, Sligo, and an honorary member of the University of Limerick Graduate Entry Medical School, Limerick, Ireland.

Niruj Agrawal is a consultant neuropsychiatrist at the Atkinson Morley Regional Neurosciences Centre based at St George's Hospital London and an honorary senior lecturer with St George's, University of London, UK. He is the lead clinician for the regional neuropsychiatry services for South West London and Surrey.

Charlotte L Allan is a consultant old age psychiatrist working for the Northumberland Tyne and Wear NHS Foundation Trust and an honorary clinical senior lecturer, Institute of Neuroscience, Newcastle University, UK.

Martin Atkins is a consultant old age psychiatrist and the clinical lead of the Older Persons Mental Health Service with the Gold Coast Hospital and Health Service, Queensland, Australia.

Vellingiri Raja Badrakalimuthu is a consultant old age and liaison psychiatrist at Parklands Hospital in Southern Health NHS Foundation Trust, UK.

Aileen Beatty is Regional Support Manager at Akari Care, UK, with a lead role in the development and support of services for people with dementia.

Katie Berryman is a research associate in ageing, focusing primarily on the RESPOND trial and falls in Parkinson's disease and their interaction with rivastigmine, University of Bristol, UK.

Nick Brindle is a consultant psychiatrist and an honorary senior lecturer based at The Mount within Leeds and York Partnership Foundation NHS Trust, UK.

Carole Burrell is a senior law lecturer and solicitor at Northumbria Law School, Northumbria University, UK.

Jo Cheffey is a consultant clinical psychologist and strategic lead for older adults psychology, Devon Partnership NHS Trust, UK.

Robert Colgate is a consultant in old age psychiatry based at the Princess of Wales Hospital in Bridgend, South Wales, UK.

Ilana B Crome is an emeritus professor of addiction psychiatry at Keele University and visiting professor at St George's, University of London, UK.

Walter Cullen is a general practitioner and a professor of urban general practice at the University College Dublin School of Medicine, Ireland.

Martin Curtice is a consultant in old age psychiatry at Coventry and Warwickshire Partnership NHS Trust, UK.

Charlotte Emmett is Associate Professor of Law, Northumbria Law School, Northumbria University, UK.

Margaret Esiri is Emeritus Professor of Neuropathology at the University of Oxford, UK.

Olivia Fiertag is a consultant child and adolescent psychiatrist. She is also an honorary researcher at Hertfordshire Partnership University NHS Foundation Trust, UK.

Susham Gupta is a consultant psychiatrist working for EQUIP, City and Hackney Early Intervention Service, East London NHS Foundation Trust, UK.

Helen Greener is a consultant in gender dysphoria and the clinical lead at the Northern Region Gender Dysphoria Service, Cumbria Northumberland Tyne and Wear NHS Foundation Trust, UK.

Katherine Hay is a higher trainee (specialist registrar) in old age psychiatry working for the Northumberland Tyne and Wear NHS Foundation Trust, UK.

Emily J Henderson is an academic geriatrician in ageing and movement disorders working at the University of Bristol and Royal United Hospitals Bath NHS Foundation Trust, UK, with interests in movement disorders, gait, cognition and clinical trials in older adults.

Laura Hill is a consultant in old age psychiatry working for the Devon Partnership NHS Trust, UK.

Julian C Hughes is Honorary Professor, University of Bristol; Visiting Professor, Policy, Ethics and Life Sciences (PEALS) Research Centre, Newcastle University; and Project Partner, The Collaborating Centre for Values-Based Practice in Health and Social Care, St Catherine's College, Oxford.

Kate Jefferies is a consultant in old age psychiatry based in Wokingham Community Mental Health Team for Older People, Berkshire Health Foundation Trust, UK. She has a special interest in young-onset dementias.

David Jolley is a retired consultant psychogeriatrician and some-time professor of old age psychiatry. Currently, he is an honorary reader in psychiatry of old age, University of Manchester, UK, Vice Chair of Christians on Ageing and Associate of Dementia Pathfinders.

Shoned Jones is a higher trainee (specialist registrar) in geriatric medicine training in Wales, UK. She has developed a special interest in movement disorder and Parkinson's, with an emphasis on the use of wearable technology in diagnosis and management.

Alice Jordan is a consultant in palliative medicine at Alice House Hospice Hartlepool and with the Community Specialist Palliative care team as part of North Tees and Hartlepool NHS Trust, UK.

Andrew Kiridoshi is a higher trainee (specialist registrar) in old age psychiatry, Health Education England – North West: Postgraduate Medicine and Dentistry, UK.

Philippa Lilford is a higher trainee (specialist registrar) in general adult and old age psychiatry at Severn Deanery and an honorary research fellow at the University of Bristol.

Stephen J Louw is a consultant physician in the Newcastle upon Tyne Hospitals NHS Foundation Trust, UK.

Biswadeep Majumdar is a consultant in old age psychiatry in Mersey Care NHS Foundation Trust, UK.

David J Meagher is a professor of psychiatry in the Graduate Entry Medical School, University of Limerick, Vice Dean for Postgraduate Training in Psychiatry, Dean of UL–Midwest Deanery, College of Psychiatrists for Ireland, and a consultant psychiatrist, Department of Adult Psychiatry, Midwestern Regional Hospital, Limerick, Ireland.

Alex J Mitchell is a professor of psycho-oncology and liaison psychiatry, Department of Psycho-oncology, Leicestershire Partnership Trust and Department of Cancer and Molecular Medicine, University of Leicester, UK.

Bradley Ng is a consultant psychiatrist with the Gold Coast Hospital and Health Service, Queensland, Australia.

Henry O'Connell is a consultant psychiatrist in the Laois–Offaly Mental Health Services and a clinical tutor and adjunct associate clinical professor in the Graduate Entry Medical School, University of Limerick, Ireland.

Rachel Perkins OBE is a clinical psychologist and senior consultant to Implementing Recovery through Organisational Change (ImROC), and chair of the Disability Advisory Group of the Equality and Human Rights Commission, UK.

Gill Pinner is Vice Dean Clinical Affairs and Professor of Medical Education, University of Nottingham School of Medicine, and an honorary consultant in old age psychiatry, Lincolnshire Partnership NHS Foundation Trust, UK.

Marie Poole is a research associate at the Institute of Health and Society, Newcastle University, UK.

Danika Rafferty is a consultant in old age psychiatry, working in Wales, UK.

Rahul Rao is a consultant old age psychiatrist with South London and Maudsley NHS Foundation Trust and a visiting researcher at the Institute of Psychiatry, Psychology & Neuroscience (IoPPN), King's College London, UK.

Felicity Richards is a consultant in older adult psychiatry at Dorset HealthCare University NHS Foundation Trust, UK.

Anna Richman is a consultant in old age psychiatry in Mersey Care NHS Foundation Trust, UK.

Glenn Roberts is a retired consultant psychiatrist, working and living in Devon, UK, who was previously lead on recovery for the Royal College of Psychiatrists, Academic Secretary to the Faculty of Rehabilitation and Social Psychiatry, and Senior Consultant to Implementing Recovery through Organisational Change (ImROC).

Elizabeth L Sampson is a professor of dementia and palliative care in the Marie Curie Palliative Care Research Department, Division of Psychiatry, University College London, and a consultant in older people's liaison psychiatry at North Middlesex University Hospital, UK.

Lily Scourfield is a medical student at Cardiff University (UK), with an interest in movement disorders and clinical research.

Hugh Series is a consultant in psychiatry of old age, Oxford Health NHS Foundation Trust, UK.

Will Stageman is a consultant old age psychiatrist working for the Northumberland Tyne and Wear NHS Foundation Trust, UK.

Bryan Strange is Director of the Laboratory for Clinical Neuroscience, Centre for Biomedical Technology, Technical University of Madrid, and of the Department of Neuroimaging, Alzheimer's Disease Research Centre, Reina Sofia-CIEN Foundation, Madrid, Spain.

Victoria Sullivan is a consultant forensic psychiatrist, the lead consultant for women's stream and the acting lead consultant for adult forensic services, Edenfield Centre, Prestwich Hospital, Greater Manchester Mental Health NHS Foundation Trust, UK.

Thanakumar Thanulingam is a consultant psychiatrist working for the West London NHS Trust, UK.

Kelli M Torsney is an academic geriatric registrar (a higher trainee) currently undertaking a PhD in clinical neurosciences at Cambridge University, UK. Her research focuses on models of ageing and translation research in Parkinson's disease.

Alison Turner is a state-registered occupational therapist who has worked within the learning disability field and has specialized in older people's mental health services in Wales, UK.

Sobhan Vinjamuri is a lead consultant and professor in nuclear medicine, Royal Liverpool University Hospital, UK.

Christian Walsh is Professional Lead, Leeds Adults and Health, Tribeca House, Leeds, UK.

Ajay Wagle is a consultant general adult psychiatrist in the Norfolk and Suffolk NHS Foundation Trust, UK.

James Warner is a consultant psychiatrist in the Central North West London Foundation Trust, London, UK.

Sarah Wilson is a consultant in old age liaison psychiatry, Nottinghamshire Healthcare NHS Foundation Trust, UK.

Preface

The *Clinical Topics* series brings together papers from one particular area of psychiatry that have been previously published in *Advances in Psychiatric Treatment*, now called *BJPsych – Advances*. This suggests two distinct advantages for the series. First, as the College's Continuing Professional Development (CPD) journal, *Advances* has always reflected topics and issues that are of current importance to the practising consultant psychiatrist. Papers in *Advances* will often contain cutting-edge science and will be written by cutting-edge scientists or academics. But whether or not the papers are written by leaders in the academic field – and it is noteworthy that the papers are often inspired by front-line clinical staff – the issues and topics they cover will be cutting-edge in terms of their clinical and topical relevance.

Second, *Advances* has always had a unique style, which is a little hard to capture. The papers are not reports of new research. They are not systematic reviews of the literature. Yet they contain new research, and they review the literature anyway. But they do so in a style that is accessible and attractive. There are frequently boxes to summarize key points and case histories to illustrate clinical presentations. The content is inclusive, but not exhaustive. It is educational. It is aimed at the 'jobbing' consultant psychiatrist but is read with interest by many who are still in training. These are papers that provide an overview, an up-to-date summary of the field. The style is rigorous but relaxed.

For the current volume we looked back over the last ten years for papers of relevance to old age psychiatry. The initial selection (by PL) contained papers felt to provide a fair spread of topics, which we then grouped under the broad headings of (i) epidemiology and types of disorders, (ii) assessment and investigations, (iii) approaches to management, and, finally, (iv) law, ethics and philosophy. Where there was duplication, we preferred more recent papers, but we also took into con-sideration the content. Needless to say, there were a number of good papers we were sadly unable to include.

Still, in addition, we were encouraged by the helpful reviewers of our proposal to commission some new work. The chapter on epidemiology is new. We had some difficulty finding anyone to write it, so we did so ourselves. We are grateful to the reviewers of that chapter and to one of the anonymous reviewers of the book whose comments undoubtedly improved it. With the book in mind we had previously published the chapter on biomarkers. We encouraged the commissioning of the chapter on mental health in Parkinson's disease and are grateful to Dr Henderson and her team for producing such a useful synopsis. The superb chapter by Carole Burrell and Charlotte Emmett on mental health laws is also new and represents a thorough synthesis of the laws from every part of the United Kingdom (UK). Talking of the legal chapters reminds us to say that whilst the chapter by Nick Brindle and Christian Walsh was based on an earlier paper, it has been rewritten to bring us completely up to date with the law in an area where, nevertheless, things are evolving and changing all the time.

It is important to comment that there is inevitably a parochial bias to some of the chapters that appear in the book. The original articles were written with a UK audience in mind – hence the many references to National Institute for Health and Care Excellence (NICE) guidelines and the like – and some chapters, e.g. reflecting the law, are more relevant solely to England and Wales. This was unavoidable. We hope the Burrell and Emmett chapter mitigates this fault to some degree, at least as far as the law in the United Kingdom is concerned. But we would also plead for indulgence. Abroad, NICE guidelines do not carry the weight they do in the United Kingdom, but they remain *intellectually* authoritative. Other jurisdictions have not been through the palaver caused by deprivation of liberty safeguards in England and Wales, but people are still deprived of their liberty in other countries and the *concerns, concepts and principles*, if not the exact laws, remain applicable.

Like the Brindle and Walsh chapter, many of the chapters that follow have been extensively rewritten since their initial publication. We remain very grateful to all of the authors who squeezed this work into their normal busy schedules. It is invidious to name any particular chapters or authors perhaps, but Alex J Mitchell's chapter on the mini-mental state examination (MMSE) is essentially new; and Andrew Kiridoshi's chapter is more or less a complete rewrite of the earlier paper.

One other point, which gives us some satisfaction, is that a number of the chapters have largely been written by psychiatrists who were still in training at the time of writing. Their chapters sit next to those by internationally known experts. Expertise brings a surety of touch, but it is also good to have a freshness of vision brought to bear on familiar topics.

Inevitably, the range of topics represented here reflects our own inclinations. We make no apology for this. One of us (JCH) has been on the editorial board of *Advances* for some years. In this capacity he has often written for the journal in order to encourage attention to old age psychiatry, so it is not too strange that his work appears here more than the work of others. We hope this does not appear egregious.

But we must apologize that some topics commended to us do not appear in the book. We tried hard to encourage experts in the field to write about genome-wide association studies (GWAS) in connection with Alzheimer's disease (AD), but they were seemingly too busy in their libraries! We had a team of authors working on a chapter on personality disorders in older people – surely a topic worthy of much more attention – but the paper did not come to fruition, although we were grateful to the authors for trying to help us. Another important area we failed to cover was assistive technology.

So, we could have produced a much bigger book. But it is important to recognize that this is not a textbook. It was never the intention that we should cover every topic possible in old age psychiatry (which would be difficult enough even in a large textbook). Rather, the book highlights trends and particular areas of current interest. Elsewhere, there are good and famous textbooks of old age psychiatry which provide a broader account of the field. Even so, there may be topics in this book that you will not find covered in other places; and it is likely that some of them are covered here in a fashion not usually seen. Reflecting its roots, the book is mainly aimed at consultants and trainees in old age psychiatry. However, it may be of interest to all those who work with older people, from old age physicians to mental health nurses, general nurses, social workers, occupational therapists, speech and language therapists, general practitioners and so on. The purpose of this book is not to be a comprehensive review of all topics in old age psychiatry but a closer review of refreshing and noteworthy topics currently relevant to the specialty. We hope to have succeeded in achieving this purpose; and if we have, it is on account of the work of our authors, to whom we again extend our sincere gratitude. If we have not, the fault is solely our own.

On a personal note, we should like to end here by thanking our spouses, Gus and Anne, for their support during the process of editing the book. They are the *sine quibus non*.

Philippa Lilford

Julian C Hughes

Acknowledgement

We should like to thank the authors of the chapters that follow for their patience with us during the gestation of this book. We know how busy clinicians and academics are these days, and we have appreciated the willingness with which the contributors to the book have responded to our requests and nagging with tolerance and even humour.

We particularly wish to thank Anna Whiting (our Editor), Jessica Papworth (Senior Editorial Assistant), Maeve Sinnott (Editorial Assistant) and their colleagues at Cambridge University Press for their kind help, advice, encouragement and sympathy throughout the process of producing the book.

We wish to thank the following for permission to use copyright material: Elsevier for permission to use Figure 12.1, Figure 12.2 and Figure 12.3; John Wiley and Sons for permission to use Figure 15.1; The General Medical Council for permission to use Box 10.2; and Wolters Kluwer Health, Inc. for permission to use Boxes 13.1 and 13.4.

Editors' Note

Any opinions expressed in the book are entirely those of the authors and do not necessarily reflect the views of any organizations with which they are associated. Case histories used in this book are entirely fictional but are based on reality. Every effort has been made to ensure that details about drugs, their indications and their dosages are accurate, but prescribers are urged to check local, contemporaneous and authoritative sources before prescribing any medication. Psychosocial interventions should only be used in appropriate contexts under the supervision of (or by) properly trained and registered practitioners.

A list of abbreviations follows, but this contains only abbreviations which are used more commonly. On the whole, abbreviations used within single chapters (and defined therein) have not usually been included in the list.

Philippa Lilford

Julian C Hughes

Abbreviations

ACh	Acetylcholine
ACP	advance care planning
AD	Alzheimer's disease
ALS	amyotrophic lateral sclerosis
BPSD	behavioural and psychological symptoms of dementia
CADASIL	cerebral autosomal dominant arteriopathy with subcortical infarcts and leukoencephalopathy
CBT	cognitive behavioural therapy
ChEIs	cholinesterase inhibitors
CJD	Creutzfeldt–Jakob disease
CNS	central nervous system
CPR	cardiopulmonary resuscitation
CRPD	convention on the rights of persons with disabilities (also UNCRPD)
CSF	cerebrospinal fluid
CT	computerized tomography
CVD	cerebrovascular disease
DLB	dementia with Lewy bodies
DNA	deoxyribonucleic acid
DoLS	deprivation of liberty safeguards
DSM-IV	*The Diagnostic and Statistical Manual of Mental Disorders* (4th edition)
DSM-5	*The Diagnostic and Statistical Manual of Mental Disorders* (5th edition)
ECG	electrocardiogram
ECHR	European Convention on Human Rights (also known as the Convention for the Protection of Human Rights and Fundamental Freedoms)
ECT	electroconvulsive therapy
EEG	electroencephalogram
EMG	electromyography
FDG	fluorodeoxyglucose
FTD	frontotemporal dementia (or degeneration)
GAD	generalized anxiety disorder
GMC	General Medical Council
GP	general practitioner
HIV	human immunodeficiency virus
HMPAO	hexamethylpropyleneamine oxime
ICDs	impulse control disorders
ICD-10	*International Classification of Diseases* (10th edition)
ICU	intensive care unit
IQ	intelligence quotient
MCA	mental capacity act
MCI	mild cognitive impairment
MHA	Mental Health Act 1983

MMSE	mini-mental state examination
MND	motor neurone disease
MRC	Medical Research Council
MRI	magnetic resonance imaging
MS	multiple sclerosis
NHS	National Health Service
NICE	National Institute of Health and Care Excellence
NIHR	National Institute for Health Research
NIMH	National Institute of Mental Health
NINDS–AIREN	National Institute of Neurological Disorders and Stroke and Association Internationale pour la Recherche et l'Enseignement en Neurosciences
NMDA	N-methyl-D-aspartate
NPSA	National Patient Safety Agency
NSAID	non-steroidal anti-inflammatory drug
ONS	Office for National Statistics
PD	Parkinson's disease
PDD	Parkinson's disease dementia
PEG	Percutaneous endoscopic gastrostomy
PET	positron emission tomography
PiB	Pittsburgh Compound B
PTSD	post-traumatic stress disorder
RCT	randomized controlled trial
RR	relative risk
SNRI	serotonin norepinephrine uptake inhibitors
SPECT	single-photon emission computed tomography
SSRI	selective serotonin reuptake inhibitor
SVD	small vessel disease
TCA	tricyclic antidepressant
TIA	transient ischaemic attack
TMS	transcranial magnetic stimulation
TSH	thyroid-stimulating hormone
TSO	The Stationery Office
UK	United Kingdom
USA	United States of America
VaD	vascular dementia
WHO	World Health Organization

Introductory Comments

Julian C Hughes

My first connection with the Royal College of Psychiatrists was when, whilst still a general practice (GP) trainee, I became an inceptor. Inceptorships are now a thing of the past. It's what you could become before you had membership. Now you would be an 'associate member'. But I like the notion of being an inceptor. It's an old-fashioned word. The *Shorter Oxford English Dictionary* says an inceptor is a person 'who incepts or is about to incept at a university'; and to 'incept' means to 'undertake, begin, enter upon', but its use is rare. Still, beginnings are usually exciting and I like the idea of entering upon one's career.

Anyway, I remember being excited to receive my first envelope of journals. One of them was a book review journal. I have to say I've not seen such a publication since. It reviewed a whole range of books. And when I read it, from cover to cover, I remember thinking, 'This is definitely the speciality for me'. It seemed to contain everything I was interested in. I wish I could recall exactly what the subjects were. But I do remember its breadth. It must have reviewed books to do with the brain and with mental illness; there was bound to be stuff on psychotherapy, psychology, and the social determinants of disease. In addition, and this I do remember, there were articles which made reference to subjects such as history, music, and philosophy. Maybe there was some poetry. In any event, it convinced me that here was a subject – psychiatry – which would inspire, engage, and motivate me, as well as bring me pleasure, all within a field of practice that was so obviously worthwhile.

A few years later, now as a trainee in psychiatry, I was pondering on which branch of psychiatry I should pursue. I was in the Royal Air Force (RAF) at the time and, to help me prepare for the membership examination, I was seconded from the RAF to work in old age psychiatry in the National Health Service (NHS). I was fortunate to find a placement in Oxford working with Dr Jane Pearce. The post was arranged by Dr Catherine Oppenheimer. It also involved a little cover of some wards overseen by Dr (later Professor) Robin Jacoby. During my time in Oxford, amongst many other luminaries, I also met Dr (later Professor) Bill Fulford – the doyenne worldwide of philosophy of psychiatry – and Dr (later Professor) Tony Hope – one of the leading ethicists in the world, but also an old age psychiatrist, who later chaired the working group of the Nuffield Council on Bioethics that produced its report *Dementia: Ethical Issues*.

Apart from name-dropping, the reason for mentioning these former colleagues is to reflect both on my good fortune and on the breadth and depth of old age psychiatry. From my first day working with Jane I knew this was the sub-specialty I should pursue. Jane was an inspiring consultant and teacher. Her deep commitment to her patients was obvious, as was her industry and thoughtfulness. I already knew Catherine as someone who wrote about ethical issues in old age psychiatry. She was very helpful to me in finding an avenue to undertake some research. My initial meetings with Robin, for whom I would later be a senior registrar, were either in connection with his long-stay wards, or at the neuroradiology meetings where we would review the brain scans of our patients with the team pursuing the Oxford Project to Investigate Memory and Ageing (OPTIMA). Robin has remained an inspiration for me, mostly because he was – hook, line, and sinker – a brilliant doctor, as well as a brilliant academic, but also because he was another clinician devoted to the care of his patients. Later, with Bill as my supervisor and mentor, which was an immense privilege and pleasure, I undertook doctoral research bringing together my interests in philosophy and dementia. I also conducted a pilot project on ethical issues for family carers of people with dementia under the supervision of Tony, who, apart from being a thinker of the first order is also, as became obvious almost immediately, one of the friendliest people and a man of great integrity.

So, apart from the wonderful characters, who none the less increased what was a delightful experience, I found myself working in an area which required a high degree of clinical expertise and commitment to people with mental illnesses, often in a very vulnerable state, but which also brought to bear sophisticated technology and understanding to aid clinical acumen, drawing on scientific knowledge from a raft of areas, which at the same time required an ethically, psychologically, and socially nuanced approach to care. Old age psychiatry practised what it preached: it truly was a biopsychosocial endeavour. I was still to learn of Kitwood and person-centred dementia care. Later I developed an interest in palliative care, where I heard talk of a biopsychosocial *and spiritual* attitude towards patients and recognized the relevance of this approach to people with dementia. It all induced an excitement concerning the possibilities offered by the profound privilege of working in old age psychiatry.

All of which is relevant to this book. It's been a great pleasure to read the chapters as they have arrived from their authors. The chapters (and the authors) have reaffirmed my feeling that old age psychiatry is a wonderful area in which to work. There is the scientific knowledge we have about the different types of dementia and the wide range of manifestations of mental disorder, which occur as a result of physical as well as 'functional' illnesses. There is the need for careful assessment and thought about where and how assessments and investigations are carried out and the impact they can have on people's lives. Improvements in technology increase our understanding, but raise issues of an ethical nature. The management of mental illness in old age requires a thoughtful and wide-ranging approach, from the deeply biological to the profoundly spiritual, where the person him or herself must always be centre-stage. And all of this must be done in the context of a sure understanding of the relevant laws, which themselves are based on philosophical roots that reflect our deep human concerns.

We hope this book will stimulate its readers just as we have been stimulated and excited by its content. It is but a brief glimpse at the subject matter of old age psychiatry. But we hope one that will enthuse you in the way that I was enthused when I entered upon the field. For those who are longer in the tooth, we hope that the book will remind you of the richness of our discipline.

I shall resist the narcissistic tendency to tell you about the rest of my career, which is of no importance. It does mean that I shall not tell you of all the other wonderful colleagues and friends with whom I've had the pleasure to work and to whom I remain grateful. A number of them are authors in this book. Nevertheless, rather than looking back, I shall end by looking forwards.

It has been a great pleasure recently to observe, whilst working in an old age psychiatry liaison post, many newly qualified doctors. One or two of them have subsequently decided to pursue careers in psychiatry. Even if they have not, it has been a delight to see their professionalism, their nascent expertise, and their care for their patients. We often hear it said that the NHS is on its knees. Perhaps it is.[1] But at the coalface I have not sensed that *the profession* is on its knees. Things could be better assuredly, but there are bright, enthusiastic, and dedicated doctors (as well as other health and social care professionals) out there working hard. Let's hope that some of them will see their way into old age psychiatry.

All of which allows me to segue to Pip Lilford, the co-editor of this book. Pip is far from being newly qualified. But at the time of writing she remains just a couple of rungs below consultant level. Nevertheless, she epitomizes all of what I have just said about younger professionals in this field. She has been a delight to work with on this project. Her intelligence, hard work, knowledge, and common sense have helped to shape the book and bring it to fruition, all achieved whilst she was working hard clinically, passing exams, undertaking a Masters in Law and Ethics, securing Wellcome Trust clinical primer funding, and marrying into the bargain! Doctors like Pip (but lest I'm later berated I should include my daughter, Emma, and daughter-in-law, Anna) suggest that the future is bright.

---

[1] This was written some time before we knew anything about COVID-19. Re-reading it now, in the midst of the coronavirus pandemic, when the NHS has so far withstood its rigours, it is clear that the NHS was not on its knees except insofar as it was simply under-resourced. We've all bemoaned the under-funding by successive governments for years. Perhaps things will be different in the future! But the pandemic has certainly confirmed that in terms of staff and expertise there never was a problem. The same can be said of social care and of social care workers too.

Epidemiology and Mental Health in Old Age

Philippa Lilford and Julian C Hughes

Introduction

Epidemiology is the study of disease and its determinants in populations. Epidemiological studies investigate what the patterns of diseases are and why they develop in particular populations.[1] Epidemiology is important in improving our understanding of what causes disease. Similarly, understanding epidemiology and how to interpret observational data is crucial to avoid inaccurate causal inferences. Unfortunately, critically evaluating all of the data on mental health problems in old age was outside the scope of this chapter, but we try to highlight some important limitations and gaps in the literature. There are exciting developments in epidemiology which will guide our knowledge about the determinants of psychiatric disease. For example, genome-wide association studies (GWAS) are increasing our understanding of genetic associations with psychiatric diseases. In Alzheimer's disease (AD), epidemiology has revealed genetic susceptibilities and identified modifiable environmental risk factors, as well as leading to improved diagnostic criteria through the use of biomarkers (see Chapter 10). It has been estimated that modifying risk factors could 'delay or prevent a third of dementia cases',[2] which has enormous implications for the information that clinicians give to their patients, as well as for public health policies.

Definitions

Descriptive epidemiology describes the spread of diseases and their severity in populations. In descriptive epidemiology the disease pattern is established with regard to time, place and person (see Box 1.1). Thus, for example, we might consider the population affected, the characteristics of the disease and how it changes over time. Analytical epidemiology seeks to explain *why* people get the disease.

In analytical epidemiology, the association between the exposure and the outcome is studied to try to establish whether certain exposures are risk factors for the development of disease.

Observational studies allow associations to be derived from observing populations, rather than from performing experiments. This means it is harder to establish whether associations are causal. One of the most significant difficulties in interpreting observational data is determining whether the exposure (A) caused the outcome (B). Without experimental conditions, it is difficult to reach this conclusion since B may have caused A (reverse causation), or C may have caused A and/or B (confounding factors).

Basic measurements in epidemiology include prevalence and incidence rates (see Box 1.2).

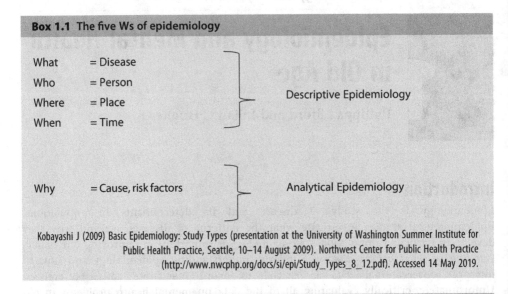

Box 1.1 The five Ws of epidemiology

What	= Disease	
Who	= Person	
Where	= Place	Descriptive Epidemiology
When	= Time	

| Why | = Cause, risk factors | Analytical Epidemiology |

Kobayashi J (2009) Basic Epidemiology: Study Types (presentation at the University of Washington Summer Institute for Public Health Practice, Seattle, 10–14 August 2009). Northwest Center for Public Health Practice (http://www.nwcphp.org/docs/si/epi/Study_Types_8_12.pdf). Accessed 14 May 2019.

Box 1.2 Definitions: 1

Prevalence rates 'define the proportion of people in a population who are affected by a disease at one particular time'.

   Incidence rates 'express the rate of occurrence of new cases of a disease and may be defined as the frequency of some event related to a disease (e.g. onset of symptoms, hospital admission) related to the size of the population and a specified time period'.

(pages 47–48)

Barker DJP, Rose G (1976) Epidemiology in Medical Practice (2nd edn). Churchill Livingstone

The gold standard experimental design to try to establish causality is a randomized controlled trial; however, this is not always practical or ethical. You cannot randomize people to a treatment thought to increase the risk of disease. Therefore, careful observational studies with appreciation of their limitations are an important source for understanding diseases and their determinants.

Observational Study Designs

There are different types of observational studies which we shall briefly discuss here. The main study designs are descriptive studies of population prevalence, cross-sectional surveys, case–control studies and cohort studies.

Descriptive Studies

Prevalence is the proportion of a population who have a specific disease. The point prevalence is the prevalence of the disease measured at a particular time point. The period prevalence is the prevalence during a time interval. The prevalence of dementia increases significantly with age; therefore, prevalence for this condition is often expressed for age brackets. Prevalence of dementia according to five-year age groups can be reviewed in Table 1.1. Roughly, the prevalence of dementia doubles every five years after 65 years of age.[3]

Table 1.1 The prevalence of dementia according to five-year age groups

Age	Population prevalence (%) of late-onset dementia
60–64	0.9
65–69	1.7
70–74	3.0
75–79	6.0
80–84	11.1
85–89	18.3
90–94	29.9
95+	41.1

Jorm AF, Korten AE, Henderson AS. The prevalence of dementia: A quantitative integration of the literature. Acta Psychiatr Scand. 1987; 76(5): 465–479. DOI: 10.1111/j.1600-0447.1987.tb02906.x

The prevalence is roughly the same as the incidence multiplied by the disease duration; diseases with short durations, therefore, have similar prevalence and incidence rates. For dementia, a chronic condition, the prevalence is far greater than the incidence. Incidence is not always a useful way to describe mental illnesses. Most mental illnesses, for example, schizophrenia and bipolar affective disorder, have relapsing and remitting courses which can be hard to capture in a single incidence study. In any case, both prevalence and incidence figures depend on the definition of a case and its operational criteria.[4]

Cross-Sectional Surveys

A cross-sectional survey is a type of observational study that measures relevant data on a sample population at a specific time point.[1] In a cross-sectional study a sample population is chosen and then a survey is conducted to determine whether the population has the disease or the risk factor of interest. Cross-sectional surveys are quick and cheap to perform. However, they may be prone to selection bias if those responding to the survey are not representative of the general public. They are an inefficient method of determining prevalence of rare diseases and it is hard to establish cause and effect. The sample population that is surveyed must be considered carefully because certain diseases will be over-represented in certain populations. For example, the prevalence of late-onset schizophrenia is higher in inpatient settings and nursing homes than in the community.[5]

Case–Control Studies

Case–control studies are more useful than cross-sectional surveys in studying rare diseases. Rather than studying a whole representative population, cases are chosen as individuals who have the disease of interest. Controls are then chosen as individuals who are disease-free. The risk factors between the cases and controls are then examined to determine whether a particular

Box 1.3 Definitions: 2

	Disease	No disease
Exposure	a	b
No exposure	c	d

Derived from Woodward M. Epidemiology. Chapman and Hall/CRC, 2013. DOI: 10.1201/b16343

Relative risk (RR) is the ratio of the probability of developing the disease in the exposure group, compared to the non-exposure group

$$RR = (a/(a+b))/(c/(c+d))$$

The **odds ratio** is the ratio of the odds of the disease in the exposure group compared to the odds of the disease in the control group

$$OR = (a/b)/(c/d) = ad/bc$$

risk factor is associated with developing the disease. In this way an odds ratio (OR) can be calculated. An OR determines the odds of the outcome developing in the exposure group, as compared with the odds of the outcome developing in the control group (see Box 1.3).

In old age psychiatry, case–control studies have been most commonly used to investigate risk factors for the development of dementia. There are disadvantages to this type of study, for example, they are prone to biases. Individuals in the case group may have been more extensively investigated or they may be more likely to recall exposures to risk factors than those in the control group. In addition, reverse causality can be problematic. For example, depression has been identified as a risk factor for dementia; contrariwise, perhaps dementia causes depression; or there may be a common pathophysiological pathway (e.g. cerebro-vascular disease or inflammation) to cause both.[6,7] Given these limitations, cohort studies where participants are followed up over time may be used to help ascertain causality.

Cohort Studies

Cohort studies are a form of longitudinal study where individuals are chosen based on whether they have had exposure to a risk factor of interest, and then followed up to ascertain whether they develop the disease.[1] The ratio of the probability of developing the outcome in the exposure group compared to the non-exposure group is expressed as the RR (see Box 1.3). RR = 1 suggests no difference in risk between the two groups; RR >1 suggests an increased risk in the exposed group, whereas RR <1 suggests a reduced risk in the exposed group.

Cohort studies are more helpful in determining causality than other types of observational study. The individuals chosen are disease free to begin with, which makes it more likely that the exposure caused the outcome. However, cohort studies are costly because they require a large number of individuals and long follow-up periods.[1]

Epidemiology of Dementia

Dementia is a syndrome caused by a range of diseases that cause progressive cognitive decline, severe enough to affect functioning.[8] There are many different causes of dementia. In this chapter, we shall only discuss the epidemiology of the three leading causes of dementia: Alzheimer's disease, vascular dementia and dementia with Lewy bodies (DLB). Although there are some forms of dementia that affect younger people (see Chapter 3), dementia is in general a disease of older people, with age being the biggest risk factor. Consequently, with an ageing global population, the prevalence of dementia worldwide has been increasing. However, a review of world literature found stable or decreasing incidence and prevalence for dementia in high-income countries.[9] In the United Kingdom, for instance, two consecutive Cognitive Function and Ageing Studies (CFAS I and CFAS II) showed that over the course of two decades there was a 23% reduction in the prevalence of dementia in three areas of England (Cambridgeshire, Newcastle and Nottingham): on the basis of the data from CFAS I, the researchers would have expected 8.3% (884,000 people) to have dementia, whereas the figure was 6.5% (670,000 people), representing a decrease of 1.8%.[10] An important limitation to consider in light of these findings is the difference in response rates between the two studies. CFAS I had a response rate of 80%, compared to 56% in CFAS II, which makes interpretation of the findings difficult.

However, the CFAS results have been replicated in other countries[9] and they provide a rich source of further information. For example, first, when combined with neuropathological findings, the CFAS raise fundamental questions about the basis of cognitive impairment. Wharton et al. have shown: a high prevalence of mixed Alzheimer's and vascular pathology; a significant population of people who die with dementia, but whose brains show less of the pathology associated with dementia; and a group with a lot of pathology, but little dementia.[11] This reflects the earlier findings of the Nun Study,[12] which focused on nuns in the Order of Notre Dame in the United States of America (USA). Second, the studies have been used to show that people living with dementia are now relying much more on unpaid care than are people with other long-term conditions.[13] Third, there has been much speculation around the reasons for the decrease in the prevalence of dementia in higher-income countries. They probably reflect changes in lifestyle. For instance, there is evidence that reduced salt intake has led to decreases in blood pressure, which may have contributed to decreases in mortality from stroke and ischaemic heart disease.[14] Such changes would presumably have an impact on dementia pathology too. Meanwhile, the CFAS have shown that higher educational attainment, a more complex mid-life occupation and late-life social engagement are all associated with preserved cognitive function in later life.[15]

There is a lack of epidemiological data from low- and middle-income countries, but it is likely that, with their populations ageing, the prevalence of dementia is increasing. There are an estimated 47 million people living with dementia worldwide with estimates that this will rise to 48.1 million people by 2020 and to 90.3 million by 2040.[16] For some years, the 10/66 Dementia Research Group has looked at ageing in low- and middle-income countries.[17] In the regions covered by the 10/66 investigators, the prevalence of dementia has been estimated to be between 5.6% and 11.7% in those aged 65 and over.[18] Their research shows great variation in prevalence rates, especially in comparison with European studies.[4]

Alzheimer's Disease

The leading cause of dementia is AD. Alois Alzheimer first described the pathological hallmarks of AD-plaques and neurofibrillary tangles-in 1907, but even then there were vascular components too.[19] There is an overlap between the risk factors for AD and other forms of dementia, and these are laid out in Table 1.2. Identifying these risk factors has led to recommendations to delay

Table 1.2 Risk factors for dementia and AD

Risk factor	Explanation
Age and sex	The largest risk factor for the development of dementia and AD is advancing age. Women of all ages have higher prevalence and incidence of dementia than men.
Education and intellectual stimulation	There is an association between lower education levels and higher incidence of dementia and AD. The cognitive reserve hypothesis is a possible explanation for this finding.[74] This theory suggests that education and intellectual stimulation extend neural reserve; therefore, the brain can withstand more insults before developing clinical symptoms of dementia. The 'use it or lose it' theory has also been used to explain the finding that lower levels of cognitive stimulation in early and middle life are associated with a higher prevalence of AD.[75]
Psychosocial factors	Longitudinal studies have shown that increased social engagement is associated with lower rates of cognitive decline and grand-parenting (up to a certain duration) is also associated with a reduced incidence of dementia.[76] As discussed earlier, depression has been identified as a possible risk factor for developing dementia.[7]
Genetic susceptibility	Compared to the general population, first-degree relatives of people with AD have a higher risk of developing the condition. The genetic basis for AD is best understood for the development of young-onset AD where mutations in three genes have been identified as the main genetic cause of young-onset AD: the amyloid precursor protein (APP), *presenilin 1* and *presenilin 2*. In late-onset AD it is more complicated with fewer direct downstream genetic effects and more complex interplay between genetic predisposition and environmental risk factors. The most widely recognized implicated gene in the causal pathway is the apolipoprotein E (APOE) ε4 allele, although there have been other susceptibility genes which have been implicated through GWAS.[77]
Vascular risk factors	Smoking, high cholesterol, high blood pressure and diabetes mellitus have all been associated with an increased risk of AD. [78]

and prevent the development of dementia. These include active treatment of hypertension and diabetes, alongside smoking cessation advice and management of hearing loss.[2]

Vascular Dementia

Vascular dementia is a form of dementia which is caused by diminished cerebral blood flow (see Chapter 2). It often presents as cognitive impairment following a stroke, although it can present as cognitive impairment with established cerebrovascular disease and no history of stroke.[20]

The classification of dementia is debated – how helpful are such classifications? – and we know that often we are not describing discrete entities.[21] Generally, people presenting with cognitive impairment in their 60s and 70s are more likely to have a single aetiology underlying their dementia. Older people, however, as we have already seen, are more likely to have mixed pictures.[11]

Vascular dementia is the second most common cause of dementia after AD. Some degree of cerebrovascular disease is seen in 80% of dementias.[20] Summing up a variety of studies, Kalaria suggested that 'the worldwide frequency of [vascular dementia] in autopsy-verified cases is determined to be 10–15%, being marginally less than when clinical criteria alone are used'.[22] Again, the prevalence of vascular dementia rises with age: among people 65 years and over the prevalence is 1.6%, but it rises from 0.1% in females and 0.5% in males between 65 and 69 years to 5.8% in females and 3.6% in males who are 90 years or above.[23]

Lewy Body Dementia

Dementia with Lewy bodies is the most common cause of dementia after AD and vascular dementia. Lewy bodies are neuronal inclusion bodies and the location in the brain where they aggregate determines the clinical syndrome that predominates. Lewy bodies largely located in the basal ganglia lead to Parkinson's disease. Cerebral Lewy bodies are associated with DLB, although they are not specific to it and are also found at autopsy in patients with AD.[24] Like other dementias, the prevalence of DLB increases with age. The average age at presentation is 75 years.[25] Lewy body pathology is identified more commonly than Lewy body disease is diagnosed clinically. In one systematic review where dementia classification was in accordance with the criteria of the fourth edition of the *Diagnostic and Statistical Manual of Mental Disorders* (DSM-IV) and DLB subtype was diagnosed using the original (1996) or revised (2005) International Consensus Criteria, DLB accounted for 4.2% of all diagnosed dementias in the community, a figure that rose to 7.5% in secondary care.[26] The incidence of DLB was 3.8% of new dementia cases.[26] The exact prevalence of DLB is debated. Elsewhere it has been estimated to be 10–22% of the dementias in people 65 years or over, suggesting that 1% of this population have DLB.[4] But the diagnostic rate depends on the diagnostic criteria used.[26] Men have a higher prevalence of DLB than women, with one study showing a male-to-female preponderance in the ratio of 4:1.[27] Possible reasons for this male preponderance include environmental risk factors and male sex hormones. Alternatively, women may be more likely to develop Alzheimer's pathology and, therefore, have their cognitive decline attributed to AD.[28]

Behavioural and Psychological Symptoms of Dementia

Behavioural and psychological symptoms of dementia (BPSD) include irritability, apathy, psychotic symptoms, agitation, 'wandering' (although it must be acknowledged that this term is unhelpful given that it covers a variety of behaviours, many of which are not purposeless as might be suggested by 'wandering'), disinhibition, aggression (which, like 'wandering', might from a different viewpoint represent a perfectly reasonable response to a frustrating situation), restlessness, depression, sleep and appetite changes. A systematic review of longitudinal studies of BPSD, the majority from the USA, Canada and Europe, showed a high prevalence of apathy, depression, agitation and 'wandering', and a low prevalence of anxiety and hallucinations.[29] Affective symptoms such as apathy and depression tend to persist rather than occur episodically. Included studies used a variety of assessment measures. For example, studies that used the informant-based Behavioural Pathology in Alzheimer's Disease Rating Scale (BEHAVE-AD) to measure BPSD demonstrated a higher prevalence than studies using the Neuropsychiatric Inventory (NPI).[29]

Comorbid Disease

Of course, dementia tends not to come alone. Older people are prone to a variety of comorbid physical diseases. In the Newcastle 85+ cohort study, people aged 85 years or older had on average five diseases, the most prevalent being hypertension (57.5%) and osteoarthritis (51.8%), with moderate to severe cognitive impairment featuring in 11.7%.[30] Data from CFAS I and CFAS II, mentioned earlier, demonstrated that in the 10 years between the two studies the prevalence of diabetes and visual impairment in diabetes increased, which provides evidence that can be correlated with other possible comorbidities.[13] But it is also possible that more than one mental illness might be present at one time. This is a complicated area because of difficulties ensuring that the same diagnostic criteria have been applied across studies and because of the possibility that one condition leads to or is part of the other. In one systematic review and meta-analysis of comorbid mental illnesses in people with dementia compared with their healthy peers, the mean prevalence of depression ranged from 20% in AD, to 37% in frontotemporal degeneration and to 13% in healthy controls.[31] When all the different types of dementia were combined, the prevalence of depression increased to 25%, whereas in the controls it was 13%. In the same study, the prevalence of anxiety in all types of dementia was 14%, but this was not statistically different from the rate in the healthy controls (3%), albeit the anxiety analyses were thought to be underpowered (i.e. the sample sizes were not sufficient to show statistical differences). The authors of the review also considered the literature on post-traumatic stress disorder (PTSD) and dementia. They did not find enough (only two studies) to perform a meaningful statistical analysis, but the overall prevalence of PTSD in dementia was 4.4%.[31]

Dementia and Dying

In a study in the north of England looking at people who had been diagnosed with early-onset dementia (called 'pre-senile dementia' in the paper, which referred to people between the ages of 45 and 64 years identified from records between 1985 and 1989) who had died by the end of 1998, 19.3% died at home, 24.5% in nursing or residential homes and 56.3% in hospital.[32] In people aged over 65 years, dementia is one of the leading causes of death, and for those who have died from another cause with dementia as a contributory factor, stroke, Parkinson's disease and ischaemic heart disease are the most common causes.[33]

Indeed, cognitive impairment is strongly associated with an increased mortality; a UK population study gives a median survival time from diagnosis of dementia to death as 4.1 years.[34] A large cohort study of nursing-home residents in the USA revealed that, compared with residents with terminal cancer, residents with advanced dementia received more active and non-palliative interventions, less advanced care planning and palliative symptoms were not as well controlled.[35] Similar patterns are seen in the UK. For example, in a study in London between 2012 and 2014, of 85 people living with advanced dementia in nursing homes or their own homes, pain (11% at rest, 61% on movement) and significant agitation (54%) were common and persistent.[36] Aspiration, dyspnoea, septicaemia and pneumonia were more frequent in those who had died by the end of the study (mortality at 9 months was 37%). The researchers found that 76% had 'do not resuscitate' orders, 30% had an advance care plan, 40% had a documented preferred place of death and 40% had a lasting power of attorney.[36]

The Epidemiology of Functional Illnesses and Suicide in the Elderly

Depression

Depression is one of the most common mental health conditions to affect older people, although it is not a normal part of ageing. Depression in older people is associated with impaired functioning,[37] increased use of healthcare services[38] and an increase in mortality.[39] Given that depression is a readily treatable disorder, this is a potential target for a significant improvement in morbidity and mortality in older people.[38] Older people suffer bereavements and social role transitions such as retirement or loss of independent living. Despite this, major depression is not common in older people, with a review of the literature finding a prevalence of 1–5% (most studies report prevalence figures closer to 1%) in large studies in the USA of community-dwelling older adults.[40] These studies tended to use DSM-IV criteria to define major depressive disorder. Minor depression, however, is common. The prevalence of depression was 8.7% (95% confidence interval (CI): 7.3–10.2) in those living in the community in England and Wales,[41] and it was as high as 27.1% in a large UK-based cohort study of those living in institutions.[42] The definition of minor depression varies between studies. In some it refers to clinically significant depression that does not meet criteria for major depressive disorder. In others, however, it denotes subclinical depressive symptoms. Which of these definitions is adopted will have a significant effect on prevalence and highlights the importance of the diagnostic criteria adopted by any particular study. Similarly, studies that use depression symptom checklists rather than diagnostic criteria can overestimate rates of depression in older people because positive responses can relate to physical symptoms or bereavement rather than depression.[40] Data from 47 studies of older adults in acute hospitals show that the prevalence of depression is 29%.[43]

Bipolar Affective Disorder

Similar to the prevalence of unipolar depression in older people, the prevalence of bipolar affective disorder varies according to the setting in which it is being studied. In the USA, the prevalence of bipolar disorder in the community is 0.1%,[44] but is higher in nursing homes – between 3%[45] and 10%.[44] A more recent study, albeit less rigorous in its definition of bipolar affective disorder, found a prevalence of 0.5% in those over 65 years in the community in the USA.[46] Bipolar disorder usually starts in younger adults, with a mean age at onset between 20 and 30 years.[47] It has been estimated that 90% of individuals with bipolar disorder would have developed their illness before the age of 50,[48] which is supported by an Australian study which found that only 8% of patients with bipolar disorder presented for the first time to mental health services once they were over the age of 65 years.[49] Interestingly, whereas the prevalence for bipolar disorder among men and women is similar in younger adults, in older people a systematic review found a preponderance of women: 69% of individuals presenting with bipolar disorder over the age of 65 were reported to be women.[50] A critical review of epidemiological studies of bipolar disorder in older people found that the majority of the studies included used convenience sampling of psychiatric inpatients who were mostly in a manic phase of their illness.[47] We know less about those living in the community between episodes or during depressive periods. In addition, a range of different diagnostic

---

Box 1.4 Definitions: 3

In 1911, Eugen Bleuler was the first to publish the observation that a small number of people with schizophrenia seemed to develop the disease in their middle to old age. There has typically been confusion concerning nomenclature in this field and the tendency is for psychosis in old age to be thought of as organic. The International Late-Onset Schizophrenia Group has established accepted terminology for these conditions to try to improve diagnosis of functional psychosis in older people, the consensus being that schizophrenia developing between the ages of 40 and 60 is named late-onset schizophrenia, and after the age of 60 it is very-late-onset schizophrenia.[73]

---

classifications was used, including DSM-III, DSM-IV and the *International Classification of Diseases* (ICD) revisions eight to ten.[47]

Late-Onset Schizophrenia

Late-onset schizophrenia refers to schizophrenia which develops after the age of 40 while very-late-onset schizophrenia is the term used for those developing symptoms after 60 years. Individuals with late-onset schizophrenia are more likely to suffer from sensory impairment,[51] particularly hearing loss.[52]

The prevalence of late-onset schizophrenia is higher in individuals with a positive family history of schizophrenia, although this association is not as strong as in those with early-onset schizophrenia.[52] Similarly to bipolar disorder in older people, there is a female preponderance for late-onset schizophrenia. The incidence for late-onset schizophrenia has been found to be 12.6 per 100,000 population.[5] A systematic review of literature published between 1960 and 2016 found that the pooled incidence of very-late-onset schizophrenia (in this study defined as those over 65) was 7.5 per 100,000 person-years at risk, with an increased risk in women (OR = 1.6, 95% CI 1.0–2.5).[53] Included studies used a range of different diagnostic classifications (ICD revisions 8–10, DSM-III and DSM-IV), and organic causes were excluded. One review reported that 23.5% of patients with schizophrenia had symptom onset after the age of 40 years.[52]

Delirium

Delirium is the most common psychiatric condition among general hospital inpatients (see Chapter 18). The prevalence on medical wards is 20–30% in the UK, and this rises to nearly 50% of patients who have surgery.[54] In the community, understandably, the prevalence is lower, at 1–2%. Individuals who develop delirium have more comorbidities and greater polypharmacy.[55] One limitation with epidemiological data on delirium is that a diagnosis of delirium relies on a retrospective account of premorbid functioning and this can often be subject to recall bias. This can make it difficult to distinguish between delirium and pre-existing dementia. In addition, studies often exclude participants who have delirium on top of pre-existing cognitive impairment, which leaves a paucity of information on the clinical presentation of delirium in those with dementia.[56] A large population-based cohort study in Finland showed that delirium was strongly associated with a future risk of developing dementia (OR = 8.7, 95% CI 2.1–35).[57] The study relied on retrospective recall of episodes

Table 1.3 Prevalence of neurotic disorders

Diagnosis	One-month prevalence (%)
Phobic disorder	4.8
Panic disorder	0.1
Obsessive-compulsive disorder	0.8
Generalized anxiety disorder	1.9

Regier DA, Boyd JH, Burke JD et al. One-month prevalence of mental disorders in the United States. *Arch Gen Psychiatry*. 1988;45(11)"977. DOI:10.1001/archpsych.1988.01800350011002

of delirium, and it should be noted that hyperactive delirium is more likely to be remembered than hypoactive delirium.

Anxiety-Related Disorders

The prevalence of new presentations of anxiety-related illnesses reduces with age. This may in part reflect a reduction in care-seeking behaviour by older people, or a reduced rate of detection by clinicians or it might be that older people with anxiety are inappropriately referred to medical or surgical services for treatment of somatization.[58] Table 1.3 summarizes the 1-month prevalence of different anxiety-related disorders in people over the age of 65 from the US Epidemiologic Catchment Area (ECA) study.[59] The ECA sampled community residents and those in institutions and used personal interviews in line with the Diagnostic Interview Schedule. Diagnoses were made according to DSM-III. There are few epidemiological studies looking at the prevalence of anxiety-related conditions in older people and the ECA study remains one of the most widely used sources for determining how common anxiety disorders are in older people living in the community. A more recent study, the MentDis_ICF65+, is a cross-sectional multicentre survey based on a selection of European countries. Diagnoses were made with an adapted version of the Composite International Diagnostic Interview (CIDI), the CIDI65+. According to this study the overall 12-month prevalence of anxiety disorders was higher than in previous epidemiological studies, with a 12-month prevalence of 3.8% for panic disorder, 4.9% for agoraphobia, 1.4% for PTSD and 9.2% for any simple phobia.[60]

Eating Disorders

Although young women are most at risk of developing eating disorders, eating disorders do affect men and women of all ages. There are very few incidence studies of eating disorders among older people. Prevalence is estimated at 3–4% in women and 1–2% in men over the age of 40.[61] In women, childhood sexual abuse has been associated with binge-eating disorders. In men, excessive exercise is associated with binge-eating disorders, which often masks symptoms and makes diagnosis more difficult.[61]

Personality Disorders

There are numerous methodological concerns and a poverty of information regarding the epidemiology of personality disorders in old age. One common criticism is that the diagnostic criteria for personality disorders are focused on diagnosis for younger people and may not be valid in an older age group where biological and psychological factors of ageing will affect the behaviour necessary for a diagnosis. [62] The prevalence varies in different meta-analyses, but is reported to be between 2.8% and 13% of older people living in the general population and between 5% and 33% of patients in psychiatric outpatient settings.[63] The idea that personality disorders 'burn out' in later life may not hold true. A cross-sectional study in The Netherlands showed that the prevalence of personality disorders is similar in old age; however, the prevalence of specific personality disorders changes.[64] This study used the self-report Questionnaire of Personality Traits, which is based on DSM-III and ICD-10. Older people were found to display more schizoid and anankastic personality traits and fewer emotionally unstable and paranoid personality traits.[64]

Substance Misuse

Substance misuse among older people is a growing area of concern. Harmful drinking is falling in most age groups in most countries, yet in 'baby boomers' (people born between 1946 and 1964) harmful drinking has been increasing.[65] Alcohol is the most common substance misused, but drug misuse, mainly of prescription drugs, is also increasing in older people (see Chapters 6 and 7).[65] Prevalence studies of alcohol misuse in older people are likely to give an underestimate owing to (a) reluctance of older people to disclose this information, (b) less suspicion from clinicians and (c) fewer well-validated screening tools for this age group.[66] The prevalence of alcohol misuse in individuals over the age of 65 in the USA as diagnosed by DSM-IV is 1.2%, and is estimated at 0.24% for alcohol dependence.[67] If this is extended to individuals over the age of 50, the prevalence of alcohol use disorders is 2.98%.[67] Older people take more prescribed and over-the-counter medications and, although often taken appropriately, these medications are prone to misuse. One review found that psychotropic medications are commonly prescribed to older adults worldwide, particularly benzodiazepines, antipsychotics and antidepressants, namely selective serotonin reuptake inhibitors.[65] Polypharmacy is frequent in older people and adverse drug reactions are much more likely when four or more drugs are prescribed.[68] The prevalence of illicit drug dependence decreases with age, although rates do vary according to the cohort, with baby boomers using more illicit drugs than previous generations.[65] In the USA, the prevalence of illicit drug dependence in older people is less than 1%, compared with 17% in 18- to 29-year-olds.[69]

Suicide

Suicide rates vary according to country, and in the UK suicide has been decreasing among older people since the 1950s.[70] Recent figures from the Office for National Statistics (ONS) show that suicide rates increase with age up to the highest rates amongst 45- to 49-year-olds.[71] The rates then decrease until the age of 80, when they begin to rise again (Figure 1.1); suicide rates in the very old have stayed relatively static over time. Reduction in suicide rates among older people in the UK has been associated with a reduction in access to lethal means and a rise in gross domestic product (GDP).[70]

As the baby boomer generation move into old age, however, the general fall in suicides in the UK could change. This cohort is associated with higher rates of suicide than other generations and has higher rates of substance misuse than other age groups,[65] which may predispose to suicide.

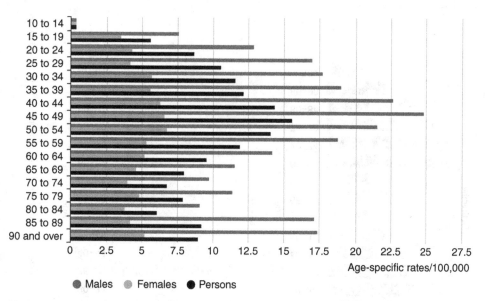

Figure 1.1 Age-specific suicide rates by sex and five-year age groups, UK, registered in 2017
Office for national statistics. Suicides in the UK: 2017 registrations. *ONS*. 2017.

Conclusion: Mental Illness and Mental Health in Old Age

The epidemiological evidence shows a high burden of mental illness in the population of older people. Mental illness in older people can often present differently (e.g. anxiety-related disorders may present as physical illnesses), or go undiagnosed. Identifying and treating mental illness is one aspect of improving the lives of older people, but another aspect is optimizing mental health in general and improving quality of life. Quality of life in old age in the UK has improved over time. There are fewer older people living in poverty; household incomes and the physical health of older people have improved. The ONS has found that life satisfaction actually rises after age 59, peaks in those aged 70–74 and begins to fall in those over 75 years; however, in people aged over 90 years there are higher levels of life satisfaction than people in their middle age (see Figure 1.2).[70] People over 90, however, did show falling levels of feeling worthwhile and falling levels of happiness. Poor health, loneliness and isolation may all contribute to this and are important targets of polices aiming to improve the overall mental health of older people.[72]

In this brief overview, therefore, we have shown that older people have significant psychiatric morbidity, may present differently from younger people, but present opportunities for both curative and palliative care. Epidemiology and public health research generally help to focus our attention on what matters and on what might be done to alleviate morbidity and associated mortality. The well-being of older people remains a worthwhile and attainable goal.

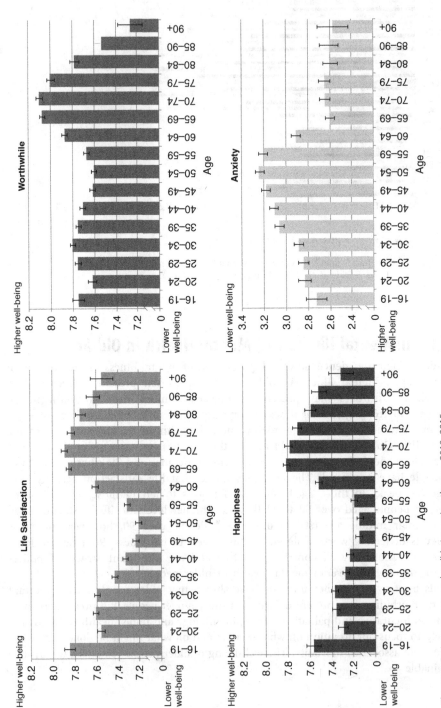

Figure 1.2 Average personal well-being ratings by age, 2012–2015 Measuring National Well-being – Office for National Statistics. www.ons.gov.uk/peoplepopulationandcommunity/wellbeing/articles/measuringnationalwellbeing/qualityoflifein theuk2018. Accessed October 21, 2019.

Acknowledegements

We should like to thank the reviewers of the original article in *BJPsych Advances*, as well as the reviewers of this book for their input. Their very helpful comments have definitely improved this chapter and saved us from error. Any persisting faults remain our responsibility.

For information, the original paper on which this chapter is based was:

Lilford P, Hughes JC. Epidemiology and mental health in old age. *Adv Psychiatr Treat* 2020; **26** (2):92–103. DOI: 10.1192/bja.2019.5

References

1. Woodward M. *Epidemiology.* Chapman and Hall/CRC, 2013. DOI:10.1201/b16343

2. Livingston G, Sommerlad A, Orgeta V et al. Dementia prevention, intervention, and care. *Lancet.* 2017;**390**(10113):2673–2734. DOI:10.1016/S0140-6736(17)31363-6

3. Jorm AF, Korten AE, Henderson AS. The prevalence of dementia: a quantitative integration of the literature. *Acta Psychiatr Scand.* 1987;**76**(5):465–479. DOI:10.1111/j.1600-0447.1987.tb02906.x

4. Minett T, Stephan B, Brayne C. Epidemiology of old age psychiatry: an overview of concepts and main studies. In Oxford Textbook of Old Age Psychiatry (2nd edn) (eds Dening T, Thomas A): 57–85. Oxford University Press, 2013

5. Castle DJ, Murray RM. *The Epidemiology of Late-Onset Schizophrenia.* Vol 19; 1993. https://academic.oup.com/schizophrenia bulletin/article-abstract/19/4/691/1888798. Accessed 13 February 2019.

6. Jorm AF. History of depression as a risk factor for dementia: an updated review. *Aust New Zeal J Psychiatry.* 2001;**35**(6):776–781. DOI:10.1046/j.1440-1614.2001.00967.x

7. Singh-Manoux A, Dugravot A, Fournier A et al. Trajectories of depressive symptoms before diagnosis of dementia. *JAMA Psychiatry.* 2017;**74**(7):712. DOI:10.1001/jamapsychiatry.2017.0660

8. Sosa-Ortiz AL, Acosta-Castillo I, Prince MJ. Epidemiology of dementias and Alzheimer's disease. *Arch Med Res.* 2012;**43**(8):600–608. DOI:10.1016/j.arcmed.2012.11.003

9. Yu-Tzu Wu A, Beiser AS, B Breteler MM et al. The changing prevalence and incidence of dementia over time-current evidence. *Nat Rev Neurol.* 2017;**13**(6):327. DOI:10.1038/nrneurol.2017.63

10. Matthews FE, Arthur A, Barnes LE et al. A two-decade comparison of prevalence of dementia in individuals aged 65 years and older from three geographical areas of England: results of the Cognitive Function and Ageing Study I and II. *Lancet (London, England).* 2013;**382**(9902):1405–1412. DOI:10.1016/S0140-6736(13)61570-6

11. Wharton SB, Brayne C, Savva GM et al. Epidemiological neuropathology: the MRC cognitive function and aging study experience. *J Alzheimer's Dis.* 2011;**25** (2):359–372. DOI:10.3233/JAD-2011-091402

12. Snowdon DA, Nun Study. Healthy aging and dementia: findings from the Nun Study. *Ann Intern Med.* 2003;**139**(5 Pt 2):450–454. DOI:10.7326/0003-4819-139-5_part_2-200309021-00014

13. Bennett HQ, Norton S, Bunn F et al. The impact of dementia on service use by individuals with a comorbid health condition: a comparison of two cross-sectional analyses conducted approximately 10 years apart. *BMC Med.* 2018;**16**(1):114. DOI:10.1186/s12916-018-1105-8

14. He FJ, Pombo-Rodrigues S, MacGregor GA. Salt reduction in England from 2003 to 2011: its relationship to blood pressure, stroke and ischaemic heart disease mortality. *BMJ Open.* 2014;**4**(4):e004549. DOI:10.1136/bmjopen-2013-004549

15. Marioni RE, Valenzuela MJ, van den Hout A, Brayne C, Matthews FE, MRC cognitive function and ageing study. Active cognitive lifestyle is associated with positive cognitive health transitions and

compression of morbidity from age sixty-five. Fielding R, ed. *PLoS One*. 2012; 7(12):e50940. DOI:10.1371/journal. pone.0050940

16. Prince M, Bryce R, Albanese E et al. The global prevalence of dementia: a systematic review and metaanalysis. *Alzheimer's Dement*. 2013;9(1):63–75.e2. DOI:10.1016/ j.jalz.2012.11.007

17. Prince M, Ferri CP, Acosta D et al. The protocols for the 10/66 dementia research group population-based research programme. *BMC Public Health*. 2007;7 (1):165. DOI:10.1186/1471-2458-7-165

18. Rodriguez JJL, Ferri CP, Acosta D et al. Prevalence of dementia in Latin America, India, and China: a population-based cross-sectional survey. *Lancet*. 2008;372 (9637):464–474. DOI:10.1016/S0140-6736(08)61002-8

19. Stelzma RA, Norman Schnitzlein H, Murllagh FR. *An English Translation of Alzheimer's 1907 Paper, 'Ijber Eine Eigenartige Erlranliung Der Hirnrinde'*; Vol 8; 1995. http://citeseerx.ist.psu.edu/view doc/download?doi=10.1.1.664.1065&rep=r ep1&type=pdf. Accessed 6 February 2019.

20. Smith EE. Clinical presentations and epidemiology of vascular dementia. *Clin Sci (Lond)*. 2017;131(11):1059–1068. DOI:10.1042/CS20160607

21. Hughes JC. *Thinking Through Dementia*. Oxford University Press, 2011. DOI:10.1093/ med/9780199570669.001.0001

22. Kalaria RN. The neuropathology of vascular dementia. In *Dementia* (eds Ames D, O'Brien JT, Burns A): 643–59. 5th ed. CRC Press, 2017.

23. Lobo A, Launer LJ, Fratiglioni L et al. Prevalence of dementia and major subtypes in Europe: a collaborative study of population-based cohorts. Neurologic Diseases in the Elderly Research Group. *Neurology*. 2000;54(11 Suppl. 5):S4–S9. www.ncbi.nlm.nih.gov/pubmed/10854354. Accessed 6 February 2019.

24. Hamilton RL. Lewy bodies in Alzheimer's disease: a neuropathological review of 145 cases using alpha-synuclein immunohistochemistry. *Brain Pathol*.

2000;10(3):378–384. www .ncbi.nlm.nih.gov/pubmed/10885656. Accessed 21 October 2019.

25. Barber R, Panikkar A, McKeith IG. Dementia with Lewy bodies: diagnosis and management. *Int J Geriatr Psychiatry*. 2001; 16 (Suppl. 1):S12–8. www .ncbi.nlm.nih.gov/pubmed/11748785. Accessed 6 February 2019.

26. Vann Jones SA, O'Brien JT. The prevalence and incidence of dementia with Lewy bodies: a systematic review of population and clinical studies. *Psychol Med*. 2014; 44 (04):673–683. DOI:10.1017/ S0033291713000494

27. Savica R, Grossardt BR, Bower JH et al. Incidence of dementia with Lewy bodies and Parkinson disease dementia. *JAMA Neurol*. 2013; 70(11): 1396. DOI:10.1001/ jamaneurol.2013.3579

28. Nelson PT, Schmitt FA, Jicha GA et al. Association between male gender and cortical Lewy body pathology in large autopsy series. *J Neurol*. 2010;257(11):1875–1881. DOI:10.1007/s00415-010-5630-4

29. van der Linde RM, Dening T, Stephan BCM et al. Longitudinal course of behavioural and psychological symptoms of dementia: systematic review. *Br J Psychiatry*. 2016; 209(5): 366–377. DOI:10.1192/bjp.bp.114.148403

30. Collerton J, Davies K, Jagger C et al. Health and disease in 85 year olds: baseline findings from the Newcastle 85+ cohort study. *BMJ*. 2009; 339: b4904. DOI:10.1136/bmj.b4904

31. Kuring JK, Mathias JL, Ward L. Prevalence of depression, anxiety and PTSD in people with dementia: a systematic review and meta-analysis. *Neuropsychol Rev*. 2018; 28(4): 393–416. DOI:10.1007/s11065-018-9396-2

32. Kay DWK, Forster DP, Newens AJ. Long-term survival, place of death, and death certification in clinically diagnosed pre-senile dementia in northern England. *Br J Psychiatry*. 2000;177(2):156–162. DOI:10.1192/bjp.177.2.156

33. Data Analysis Report: Dying with Dementia. National Dementia Intelligence. https://assets.publishing.service.gov.uk/go

vernment/uploads/system/uploads/attachment_data/file/733065/Dying_with_dementia_data_analysis_report.pdf. Accessed 21 October 2019.

34. Xie J, Brayne C, Matthews FE, Medical research council cognitive function and ageing study collaborators. Survival times in people with dementia: analysis from population based cohort study with 14 year follow-up. *BMJ.* 2008;**336**(7638):258–262. DOI:10.1136/bmj.39433.616678.25

35. Mitchell SL, Kiely DK, Hamel MB. Dying with advanced dementia in the nursing home. *Arch Intern Med.* 2004; **164**(3): 321. DOI:10.1001/archinte.164.3.321

36. Sampson EL, Candy B, Davis S et al. Living and dying with advanced dementia: a prospective cohort study of symptoms, service use and care at the end of life. *Palliat Med.* 2018; **32**(3): 668–681. DOI:10.1177/0269216317726443

37. Ormel J, VonKorff M, Ustun TB et al. Common mental disorders and disability across cultures. Results from the WHO Collaborative Study on Psychological Problems in General Health Care. *JAMA.* 1994; **272**(22): 1741–1748. www.ncbi.nlm.nih.gov/pubmed/7966922. Accessed 8 February 2019.

38. Beekman AT, Copeland JR, Prince MJ. Review of community prevalence of depression in later life. *Br J Psychiatry.* 1999;**174**:307–311. www.ncbi.nlm.nih.gov/pubmed/10533549. Accessed 8 February 2019.

39. Djernes JK, Gulmann NC, Foldager L, Olesen F, Munk-Jørgensen P. 13 year follow up of morbidity, mortality and use of health services among elderly depressed patients and general elderly populations. *Aust New Zeal J Psychiatry.* 2011;**45** (8):654–662. DOI:10.3109/00048674.2011.589368

40. Fiske A, Wetherell JL, Gatz M. Depression in older adults. *Annu Rev Clin Psychol.* 2009; **5**(1): 363–389. DOI:10.1146/annurev.clinpsy.032408.153621

41. McDougall FA, Kvaal K, Matthews FE et al. Prevalence of depression in older people in England and Wales: the MRC CFA study.

Psychol Med. 2007; **37**(12): 1787–1795. DOI:10.1017/S0033291707000372

42. McDougall FA, Matthews FE, Kvaal K, Dewey ME, Brayne C. Prevalence and symptomatology of depression in older people living in institutions in England and Wales. *Age Ageing.* 2007; **36**(5): 562–568. DOI:10.1093/ageing/afm111

43. Royal College of Psychiatrists (RCPsych). Improving the Outcome for Older People Admitted to the General Hospital: Guidelines for the Development of Liaison Mental Health Services for Older People. 2005. www.rcpsych.ac.uk/docs/default-source/members/faculties/liaison-psychiatry/cr183liaisonpsych-every-acute-hospital.pdf?sfvrsn=26c57d4_2. Accessed 21 October 2019.

44. Koenig HG, Blazer DG. Epidemiology of geriatric affective disorders. *Clin Geriatr Med.* 1992;**8**(2):235–251. DOI:10.1016/S0749-0690(18)30476-2

45. Tariot PN, Podgorski CA, Blazina L, Leibovici A. Mental disorders in the nursing home: another perspective. *Am J Psychiatry.* 1993; **150**(7): 1063–1069. DOI:10.1176/ajp.150.7.1063

46. Hirschfeld RMA, Calabrese JR, Weissman MM et al. Screening for bipolar disorder in the community. *J Clin Psychiatry.* 2003;**64**(1):53–59. DOI:10.4088/jcp.v64n0111

47. Rowland TA, Marwaha S. Epidemiology and risk factors for bipolar disorder. *Ther Adv Psychopharmacol.* 2018;**8** (9):251–269. DOI:10.1177/2045125318769235

48. Oostervink F, Boomsma MM, Nolen WA. Bipolar disorder in the elderly; different effects of age and of age of onset. *J Affect Disord.* 2009; **116**(3): 176–183. DOI:10.1016/j.jad.2008.11.012

49. Almeida OP, Fenner S. Bipolar disorder: similarities and differences between patients with illness onset before and after 65 years of age. *Int Psychogeriatrics.* 2002; **14**(3): 311–322. www.ncbi.nlm.nih.gov/pubmed/12475092. Accessed 11 February 2019.

50. Depp CA JD. *Bipolar Disorder in Older Adults: A Critical Review*; 2004. https://onlinelibrary.wiley.com/doi/pdf/10.1111/j.1399-5618.2004.00139.x. Accessed 11 February 2019.

51. Pearlson G, Rabins P. The late-onset psychoses: possible risk factors. *Psychiatr Clin North Am.* 1988; **11**(1): 15–32. DOI:10.1016/S0193-953X(18)30514-8

52. Harris J, Jeste D. Late onset schizophrenia: an overview. *Schizophr Bull.* 1988;**14**(1). https://watermark.silverchair.com/14-1-39.pdf?token=AQECAHi208BE49Ooan9kkhW_Ercy7Dm3ZL_9Cf3qfKAc485ysgAAAmQwggJgBgkqhkiG9w0BBwagggJRMIICTQIBADCCAkYGCSqGSIb3DQEHATAeBglghkgBZQMEAS4wEQQMvceOJVaLG0qgF17IAgEQgIICF5zX95t5l1-5fbYYWAFNEcw1miHR3xVYimna1ALr3KE4Q4P. Accessed 13 February 2019.

53. Stafford J, Howard R, Kirkbride JB. The incidence of very late-onset psychotic disorders: a systematic review and meta-analysis, 1960–2016. *Psychol Med.* 2018; **48**(11): 1775–1786. DOI:10.1017/S0033291717003452

54. Overview | Delirium: prevention, diagnosis and management | Guidance | NICE. www.nice.org.uk/guidance/cg103. Accessed 21 October 2019.

55. Folstein MF, Bassett SS, Romanoski AJ, Nestadt G. The epidemiology of delirium in the community: the Eastern Baltimore Mental Health Survey. *Int Psychogeriatrics.* 1991; **3**(2): 169–176. www.ncbi.nlm.nih.gov/pubmed/1811771. Accessed 13 February 2019.

56. Davis DHJ, Kreisel SH, Muniz Terrera G et al. The epidemiology of delirium: challenges and opportunities for population studies. *Am J Geriatr Psychiatry.* 2013; **21**(12): 1173–1189. DOI:10.1016/j.jagp.2013.04.007

57. Davis DHJ, Muniz Terrera G, Keage H et al. Delirium is a strong risk factor for dementia in the oldest-old: a population-based cohort study. *Brain.* 2012;**135**(9):2809–2816. DOI:10.1093/brain/aws190

58. Blazer D, George L HD. The epidemiology of anxiety disorders: an age comparison. – PsycNET. https://psycnet.apa.org/record/1991-97050-002. Published 1991. Accessed 13 February 2019.

59. Regier DA, Boyd JH, Burke JD et al. One-month prevalence of mental disorders in the United States. *Arch Gen Psychiatry.* 1988;**45**(11):977. DOI:10.1001/archpsyc.1988.01800350011002

60. Andreas S, Schulz H, Volkert J et al. Prevalence of mental disorders in elderly people: the European MentDis_ICF65+ study. *Br J Psychiatry.* 2017; **210**(2): 125–131. DOI:10.1192/bjp.bp.115.180463

61. Mangweth-Matzek B, Hoek HW. Epidemiology and treatment of eating disorders in men and women of middle and older age. *Curr Opin Psychiatry.* 2017;**30**(6):446–451. DOI:10.1097/YCO.0000000000000356

62. van Alphen SPJ, Engelen GJJA, Kuin Y, Derksen JJL. The relevance of a geriatric sub-classification of personality disorders in the DSM-V. *Int J Geriatr Psychiatry.* 2006; **21**(3): 205–209. DOI:10.1002/gps.1451

63. van Alphen SPJ (Bas), Derksen JJL (Jan), Sadavoy J (Joel), Rosowsky E (Erlene). Features and challenges of personality disorders in late life. *Aging Ment Health.* 2012; **16**(7): 805–810. DOI:10.1080/13607863.2012.667781

64. Engels GI, Duijsens IJ, Haringsma R, van Putten CM. Personality disorders in the elderly compared to four younger age groups: a cross-sectional study of community residents and mental health patients. *J Pers Disord.* 2003; **17**(5): 447–459. www.ncbi.nlm.nih.gov/pubmed/14632377. Accessed 13 February 2019.

65. Rao R, Roche A. Substance misuse in older people. *BMJ.* 2017; **358**: j3885. DOI:10.1136/BMJ.J3885

66. Khan N, Davis P, Wilkinson T, Sellman JD GP. Drinking patterns among older people in the community: hidden from medical attention? | Request PDF. *New Zeal Med J.* 2002; **115**(1148): 72–75. www

.researchgate.net/publication/11450449_D rinking_patterns_among_older_people_i n_the_community_Hidden_from_medica l_attention. Accessed 21 October 2019.

67. Kuerbis A, Sacco P, Blazer DG, Moore AA. Substance abuse among older adults. *Clin Geriatr Med.* 2014;**30**(3):629–654. DOI:10.1016/j.cger.2014.04.008

68. Cadieux RJ. Drug interactions in the elderly. *Postgrad Med.* 1989;**86**(8):179–186. DOI:10.1080/00325481.1989.11704506

69. Hinkin CH, Castellon SA, Dickson-Fuhrman E, Daum G, Jaffe J, Jarvik L. Screening for drug and alcohol abuse among older adults using a modified version of the CAGE. *Am J Addict.* 2001; **10** (4): 319–326. www.ncbi.nlm.nih.gov/pub med/11783746. Accessed 21 October 2019.

70. Gunnell D, Middleton N, Whitley E, Dorling D, Frankel S. Why are suicide rates rising in young men but falling in the elderly? A time-series analysis of trends in England and Wales 1950–1998. *Soc Sci Med.* 2003;**57**(4):595–611. www .ncbi.nlm.nih.gov/pubmed/12821009. Accessed 20 February 2019.

71. Office for National Statistics. Suicides in the UK: 2017 registrations. *ONS.* 2017.

72. Measuring National Well-being – Office for National Statistics. www.ons.gov.uk/people populationandcommunity/wellbeing/arti cles/measuringnationalwellbeing/qualityofli feintheuk2018. Accessed 21 October 2019.

73. Howard R, Rabins PV, Seeman MV, Jeste V. *Late-Onset Schizophrenia and Very-Late-Onset Schizophrenia-Like Psychosis: An International Consensus and the International Late-Onset Schizophrenia Group.* Vol 157; 2000. https://ajp .psychiatryonline.org/doi/pdfplus/10.1176 /appi.ajp.157.2.172. Accessed 19 February 2019.

74. Katzman R. Education and the prevalence of dementia and Alzheimer's disease. *Neurology.* 1993;43: 13–20.

75. Staff R, Hogan M, Williams D, et al. Intellectual engagement and cognitive ability in later life (the 'use it or lose it' conjecture): longitudinal, prospective study. *BMJ.* 2018;363: k4925.

76. Burn K, Szoeke C. Is grandparenting a form of social engagement that benefits cognition in ageing? *Maturitas.* 2015;80: 122–5.

77. Daw EW, Payami H, Nemes EJ, et al. The number of trait loci in late onset Alzheimer disease. *American Journal of Human Genetics.* 2000;66: 196–204.

78. Breteler MM. Vascular risk factors for Alzheimer's disease: an epidemiological perspective. *Neurobiology of Aging.* 2000;21: 153–60.

Chapter 2

Vascular Dementia

Hugh Series and Margaret Esiri

Introduction

Over the course of the last hundred years our understanding of dementia has undergone considerable change. For much of that time 'senility' was seen as an almost inevitable concomitant of ageing and was usually attributed to atherosclerosis. In the post-war period, a concept of multi-infarct dementia emerged,[1] but at the same time Alzheimer's disease (AD) came to be seen not as a rare young-onset disorder but as the cause of most cases of dementia. Indeed, the concept of dementia itself was built around the impairments seen in AD, notably the impairment of memory. With greater understanding of dementia, particularly its pathological basis, it came to be realized that many different kinds of pathology can produce a dementia syndrome and that multiple types of pathology are the rule rather than the exception. This chapter aims to review our current understanding of how cerebrovascular disease contributes to cognitive impairment in order to assist those involved in the assessment and management of people with cognitive impairments to understand the strengths and limitations of our current concepts, and to inform diagnosis and management. We try to reach pragmatic conclusions, not to provide a comprehensive account of a complex area of research.

Vascular cognitive impairment (VCI) is a term that includes the full range of cognitive impairments which occur in people with cerebrovascular disease, ranging from mild cognitive impairment (MCI) to vascular dementia (VaD).[2] This is perhaps slightly confusing as the term 'mild cognitive impairment' refers to a condition which, unlike VCI, falls short of dementia in its severity.

The pathology of VaD and VCI is not well defined at the present time. There are several reasons why this is so: the clinical definitions of VaD and VCI are not well delineated and there are several different clinical schemes for assessing and diagnosing it; the clinico-pathological correlation is not very good and varies from one series of cases to another, in part based on the source of cases, e.g. whether in the context of post-stroke cognitive performance or memory clinics; and cerebrovascular pathology itself is highly heterogeneous with a lack of clear agreement about how to characterize it and how different components relate to cognitive problems. Some skewing of views has stemmed from the attempts, when arriving at definitions, to distinguish clearly between AD and VaD/VCI despite many cases of dementia, as is increasingly recognized, showing both AD pathology and vascular disease in the same brain. (This is shown schematically in Figure 2.1, which emphasizes how difficult it can be to find 'pure' cases of vascular pathology, especially when some pathology remains symptomatically silent.) Indeed, in a recent autopsy study of dementia nine different combinations of pathology were found and in more than 74% of cases there were two or more forms of neuropathology.[3] An indication of the prevalence of vascular disease as

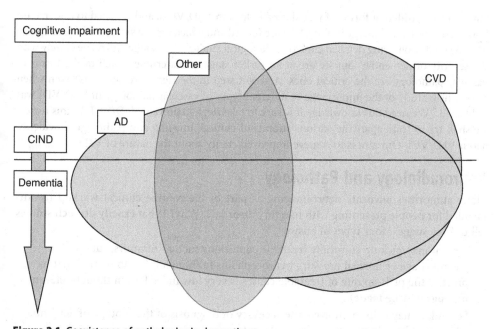

Figure 2.1 Coexistence of pathologies in dementia.
Schematic diagram to show the extensive coexistence of different types of pathology in many individuals and the corresponding low frequency of pure forms of pathology. The degree of cognitive impairment increases from top to bottom of the diagram, and the horizontal line represents the point at which impairments are sufficiently great to be classified as dementia. CIND – cognitive impairment no dementia; AD – Alzheimer's disease (presence of pathology, not necessarily with dementia syndrome); CVD – cerebrovascular disease (pathology, not necessarily with dementia syndrome). 'Other' includes many forms of pathology which can give rise to cognitive impairment, such as Lewy bodies

a cause of cognitive impairment or dementia is provided by the extensive study of Power *et al.*, who found, in a study of 1,362 autopsies on elderly subjects, 44% of whom had dementia, that vascular pathology accounted for 32% of the association between age and dementia while amyloid/tau pathology accounted for 24%, TDP-43 pathology and hippocampal sclerosis for 43% and Lewy body disease for 1%.[4] However, differing prevalences of types of neuropathology are apparent, depending on the source of cases, as exemplified by another study of 132 autopsy cases of dementia, in which 84 cases had mixed pathology and Lewy body pathology figured prominently (with differing amounts of AD pathology), but vascular disease with AD was the commonest form of mixed pathology.[5] Another level of complexity in linking vascular pathology to dementia arises from the very important added contribution to the debate that has come from neuroimaging studies over the last 20–30 years. The ease with which vascular lesions can be seen on imaging may lead to the overdiagnosis of vascular disease as the cause of dementia or cognitive impairment in some cases. At least this is the suggestion from a clinico-pathological study in which 42 autopsied subjects had the clinical diagnosis of the cause of their dementia compared with the autopsy findings. Thirty-eight per cent of these cases were given a clinical diagnosis of VaD, but at autopsy only 19% of the cases were so diagnosed.[6]

It could be said that in some respects our understanding of the pathological basis of VaD/VCI now is at the same stage as our understanding of the pathological basis of AD in the early 1980s. In both conditions there are complex, distinct components to the pathology (plaques and tangles in AD, different forms of vascular pathology in VaD/VCI), and we need to understand how these types of pathology in VaD/VCI are related and which are the key contributors. In AD we now know, following detailed clinico-pathological studies, that tangles correlate closely with the severity of dementia;[7] but we are at an earlier stage of discerning which of the forms of vascular pathology are the critical ones. A recent step in the right direction was taken when a consensus study of the importance of different types of vascular pathology in VaD/VDI was published.[8] We need this knowledge if we are to take steps to prevent VaD/VCI. In this review we shall try to tease apart the various strands of clinical, imaging and pathological evidence about VaD/VCI. Our aim is to achieve improved clarity about the nature of VaD.

Neuroradiology and Pathology

Many authorities advocate neuroimaging as part of the routine clinical workup recommended for people presenting with memory disorders. Why? What exactly do such studies tell us? We suggest four types of answer.

- First, it may pick up surgically treatable conditions such as tumours, subdural haemorrhage or normal pressure hydrocephalus (although it has to be said that in practice the pick-up rate of treatable causes is very low indeed, even though relevant findings may be made).
- Second, it may help to improve the accuracy of diagnosis of the subtype of dementia, which may have implications for treatment.
- Third, it can be helpful for those affected and their families to see for themselves that the problems they struggle with have a real physical cause and to feel that everything possible is being done to identify and treat the problem. The ability to use the picture archiving and communication system (PACS) to show images to patients in the clinic can be a source of information and explanation, and a valuable aid to discussing diagnosis. For some people with limited insight into their condition, it can help them to understand that there is a problem for which assistance might be beneficial.
- Finally, neuroimaging has a growing role in research, and there is reason to hope that it can assist in early diagnosis and disease monitoring. As new treatments are developed which may be effective in the early stages of disease, it will become increasingly important to identify disease early. In the case of CVD, early identification of brain changes, perhaps even before clinical signs of dementia, may mean that there is stronger motivation to manage risk factors energetically at a relatively early stage. Neuroradiology has reached a level of development where some authors have argued that neuroradiology rather than pathology should be considered the gold standard against which new diagnostic criteria should be judged.[9]

Space does not allow a full treatment of the wide variety of new imaging techniques now available (but see Chapter 13).[10] We will focus in this section on computerized tomography (CT) and magnetic resonance imaging (MRI) and on the pathology that these imaging techniques show.

Forms of Pathology which May Contribute to VaD/VCI

Major Stroke

Large vessel disease includes single and multiple infarcts that can be readily seen by CT or MRI. They can be in the territory of main arteries or in the watershed zones between the main arterial territories. Vascular dementia can be caused by multiple or single strategic infarcts (i.e. infarcts in locations critical for cognitive function such as thalamus, anterior thalamic radiation or angular gyrus), and the NINDS–AIREN criteria (devised by the National Institute of Neurological Disorders and Stroke and Association Internationale pour la Recherche et l'Enseignement en Neurosciences) specify in which brain regions infarcts should be for diagnosis of VaD. For large vessel infarcts to be sufficient for diagnosis of VaD they should be multiple, bilateral or in the dominant hemisphere. Studies of patients after they have suffered an ischaemic stroke show that progressive dementia is significantly more common than in an age- and sex-matched control population. Thus, in a study of 251 patients aged over 60 years, dementia was found in 26% of patients 3 months after they had suffered a stroke compared with 3.2% in a control sample.[11] In a meta-analysis of dementia after stroke, dementia was present in 10% of patients before the stroke developed and in a further 10% there was evidence of dementia developing after one stroke, while this rose to more than 30% in those who had suffered more than one stroke.[12] In a more recent study, post-stroke dementia was particularly likely after a severe stroke.[13] This evidence points to the significant contribution that major ischaemic stroke can make to dementia. A deficiency in most of the stroke literature is that post-mortem studies have not been performed so that the relative contributions of AD pathology, perhaps 'unmasked' by vascular disease, and the vascular disease itself were not assessed.

Lacunar Stroke

Lacunes are small subcortical infarcts from 3 to 20 mm in size, usually round or oval. They may be clinically silent but may be accompanied by the history of a transient ischaemic attack (TIA) or stroke. Lacunar infarcts in the thalamus can cause prominent cognitive problems. At least two lacunes are required for a diagnosis of VaD. There is good evidence that lacunar infarcts can form a substrate for VaD. They are often multiple and bilateral and are associated with disease affecting the small arteries and arterioles subserving the deep grey matter and white matter (see Figure 2.2).

Microinfarcts

These are ischaemic lesions that are too small to be seen with the naked eye and are detected when microscopic histology is carried out. They can occur in the subcortical tissue but are most frequently found in the cortex, where it is estimated they can occur in their hundreds. They are difficult to detect in vivo. They can result from a number of different disease processes in vessel walls, e.g. vasculitis, but most are probably caused by cerebral amyloid angiopathy (CAA) or subcortical small vessel disease (see the following section) or by embolic occlusion of small arteries by microemboli.

Diffuse Subcortical Small Vessel Disease

Diffuse subcortical small vessel disease (SVD) is damage to the small subcortical vessels that supply the deep grey matter and white matter. The vessels affected are small arteries and arterioles that branch from proximal parts of the major cerebral arteries to supply the basal ganglia and thalamus, and penetrating arterioles from the pial surface that reach through the cerebral cortex to supply the white matter. In SVD the perivascular Virchow–Robin spaces around these vessels are frequently widened, and the vessel wall is thickened by fibrosis and the lumen narrowed. Smooth muscle cells in the walls of small arteries and arterioles are replaced

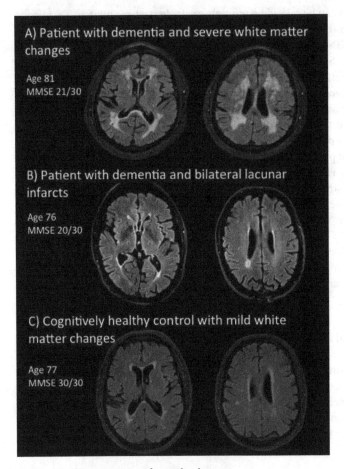

A) Patient with dementia and severe white matter changes

Age 81
MMSE 21/30

B) Patient with dementia and bilateral lacunar infarcts

Age 76
MMSE 20/30

C) Cognitively healthy control with mild white matter changes

Age 77
MMSE 30/30

Figure 2.2 MRI appearance of vascular damage.
Examples of two patients with dementia and diffuse white matter changes (a) and bilateral lacunar infarcts (b), and of a cognitively healthy control with mild white matter changes (c). MMSE – mini-mental state examination. Images were acquired with a FLAIR sequence in 3T MRI scanner

by collagen. The tissue supplied by these small vessels may suffer from lacunar infarction or hypoperfusion of blood that renders it ischaemically damaged but not dead. The myelin in regions affected by diffuse SVD is reduced and microglia and macrophages infiltrate the tissue. In a study of brains from elderly subjects in whom pathology of AD and other neurodegenerative dementing conditions was absent, it was only those cases with the most severe extent of SVD that had dementia, and in those cases the severity of dementia within a short time of death was less than in AD.[14] Neuroimaging changes of SVD are very commonly seen in scans of older people, and it is likely that this pathology accounts for the largest proportion of VaD.[15, 16] Erkinjuntti et al. have proposed specific radiological criteria for subcortical ischaemic VaD.[17]

A number of types of small vessel disease are seen on imaging (see Figure 2.2). White matter hyperintensities (WMH) appear bright on T2-weighted and FLAIR MRI images (FLAIR images use a technique called 'fluid attenuation inversion recovery'). When seen in CT, they appear dark and are referred to as hypodense areas or leukoaraiosis. They become more common with increasing age and are associated with cognitive impairment. As they are so commonly seen, the NINDS–AIREN criteria set an arbitrary cut-off that 25% of the total white matter should be affected for a diagnosis of VaD. White matter hyperintensities can be seen around the lateral ventricles, often starting at the poles, and in subcortical areas, although these two types of distribution are thought to have different aetiologies. They are often rated either by eye or using an automated process as mild (punctiform), moderate (beginning confluent) or severe (confluent).[18] An unusual but informative form of subcortical small vessel disease occurs in the rare inherited condition of cerebral autosomal-dominant arteriopathy with subcortical infarcts and leukoencephalopathy (CADASIL), in which a mutation in the *Notch3* gene results in deposition of granular material in the walls of small arteries and arterioles, narrowing of vessel lumens and destruction of smooth muscle cells in their walls. Cerebral autosomal-dominant arteriopathy with subcortical infarcts and leukoencephalopathy is discussed further in Chapter 4.

Cerebral Amyloid (Congophilic) Angiopathy

Cerebral amyloid (congophilic) angiopathy refers to the deposition of abnormal protein in the form of twisted beta-pleated sheets in the walls of small arteries and arterioles where it eventually replaces the smooth muscle. It principally affects the leptomeningeal and cortical vessels. In most cases the protein is the amyloid beta protein that also forms the characteristic parenchymal amyloid plaques of AD. Cerebral amyloid angiopathy occurs to a variable extent in almost all cases of AD, but it also occurs in about a third of elderly subjects who do not meet criteria for pathological AD, and in these cases it can be shown to contribute to VaD or VCI. Criteria for clinical diagnosis of CAA have been developed.[19, 20] With imaging, a key feature of CAA is microbleeds, which are small dots best seen in T2*-weighted images. They represent leakage of haemosiderin from damaged small blood vessels and, though present at low level in community populations, are much more common in stroke and VaD populations.

Mixed or Multiple Forms of Vascular Pathology

As indicated earlier, it is commonly the case that in an elderly brain there may be more than one of these forms of vascular pathology and it can be difficult to define the exact component of mixed pathology that contributes most to VaD or VCI. In the unselected community-based population of elderly subjects that contributed to the Medical Research Council (MRC) Cognitive Function and Ageing Study (CFAS) it was only in cases that had more than one form of vascular pathology that vascular disease contributed to dementia,[21] but it is noteworthy that in almost all cases one form of vascular pathology was SVD. Thus, there is good reason to believe that SVD, including lacunes that it gives rise to, is a particularly important contributor to VaD/VCI.

What Is the Mechanism by Which Vascular Pathology Causes VaD/VCI?

Given the importance of SVD in VaD and VCI it is reasonable to suggest that cognitive dysfunction results at least in part from interruption of axonal connections between one part of the cerebral cortex and another and between the cerebral cortex and deep grey matter. Small vessel disease affects particularly the frontal lobe white matter and the closely related basal ganglia, so it is not surprising that the cognitive dysfunction commonly seen in

VaD involves executive activity, which is known to be a function of the frontal lobe (see the following section). It is interesting that in CADASIL the cognitive dysfunction closely resembles that seen in elderly sporadic cases of VaD/VCI.[22] Cerebral amyloid angiopathy may also affect white matter function because this is the final destination for the blood flowing in the cortical arterioles affected by this condition. In macroinfarction, lacunes and microinfarction it is loss of neurons that is thought to be important, and there is evidence that after a stroke dementia is more likely if the stroke was a large one, therefore destroying more neurons.

Diagnostic Criteria

At least eight different sets of diagnostic criteria for VaD have been published, including the Hachinski Ischaemic Scale, the *DSM-5* and its predecessors, the *ICD 10* and its predecessors, and criteria from the State of California Alzheimer's Disease Diagnostic and Treatment Centers (ADDTC) and from the NINDS–AIREN.[23] In order to determine how effective these criteria are at identifying patients with VaD in life, Wiederkehr *et al.* conducted a literature search to identify studies which compared lifetime diagnoses using one or other of these criteria against post-mortem pathological diagnoses.[23] Only six studies of this kind were identified. Sensitivities across the studies ranged from 20% to 100%, mostly in the range 20–60%, while specificities ranged from 13% to 100%, mostly in the range 60–90%. The NINDS–AIREN criteria tended to have the highest specificity, though lower sensitivity. Sensitivities were usually lower than specificities. One problem with the use of sensitivity and specificity is that they are affected by the prevalence of the disorder. In order to avoid this problem, likelihood ratios (LR) may be calculated. LR+ is the odds in favour of the disease being present given a positive test result, and LR– is the odds against this. Based on standard criteria, Widerkehr *et al.* found that, taking an LR+>10 and LR–<0.1 as the threshold of acceptability for a diagnostic test, only the NINDS–AIREN criteria reached this threshold, with ADDTC coming close in one study.[23]

Two studies comparing the published criteria against clinical judgement found the *DSM-IV* criteria were most sensitive, while the NINDS–AIREN were the most specific.[24, 25] Another comparative study found that all of seven sets of criteria agreed in only 8 out of 124 cases of dementia.[26]

Thus, even in research centres it is difficult to achieve accurate diagnoses in life. Among the factors that contribute to the difficulty are issues in the diagnosis of the dementia syndrome – that it may not be appropriate to base this on definitions of dementia derived largely from AD, the heterogeneity of pathology in cerebrovascular disease and the lack of agreement on pathological criteria for diagnosis. More research is needed to determine which of the many pathological cerebrovascular processes contribute to VCI and in what way.

Most diagnostic criteria specify that there must be a dementia syndrome and then set out criteria to classify it as cerebrovascular in origin. However, as AD is the predominant form of dementia, this can dominate the clinical concept of the dementia syndrome, e.g. by emphasizing the memory aspect. Studies comparing cognitive changes in AD with those in VaD have found that for similar levels of cognitive deficit VaD patients were more likely to have relatively better-preserved verbal episodic memory and poorer frontal-executive functioning.[27, 28] That there should be differences is not surprising in view of the different pathologies and the tendency of Alzheimer's pathology to start in hippocampal areas involved in processing memories. However, not all studies have confirmed that VCI does affect executive functioning in such a distinct way.[29] *DSM-5* draws attention to deficits prominent in complex attention (including processing speed) and frontal executive function.

There is widespread awareness that current criteria and definitions are an inadequate basis for the research that is necessary to resolve some of these complex issues, and so an expert group has proposed a set of harmonization standards for the collection of research data in this area.[30] These do not constitute new diagnostic criteria but may inform their development.

Epidemiology

The difficulties referred to above in agreeing clinical criteria for diagnosis and the variability of sources of cases mean that epidemiological studies also lack agreement. In population-based studies estimates of the prevalence of VaD in Europe and North America vary between 1.2% and 4.2% in individuals over the age of 65 years.[31] In Japan they are higher.[32, 33] The prevalence and incidence of VaD increases with age over the age of 65 years. Thus, in a major European study incidence rose from 0.7 per 1,000 person years at 65–69 years to 8.1 per 1,000 person years at 90+ years.[34] However, this is much less steep a rise with age than for AD and pathological studies on selected populations suggest that the frequency of pure VaD is actually considerably lower than these epidemiological studies indicate.

Risk factors for VaD include hypertension (though the risk is less than for stroke and AD – it was only a risk factor for females in a Canadian study),[35] orthostatic hypotension, cardiac disease, diabetes, smoking, obesity, major surgery, elevated blood homocysteine level and hyperlipidaemia.

Clinical Assessment

The goals of clinical assessment in VCI include not only diagnosis, but also identification of specific therapeutics targets in each particular patient. Box 2.1 provides details of the content of clinical assessment, which may need to be adapted to the presentation of the particular patient. It is clear that many patients have more than one pathological process present, and cerebrovascular disease is common, so clinicians should have a low threshold for considering that CVD may be present and contributing to the presentation, even if another pathological process such as AD has also been identified.[36] The VaD harmonization standards group has set out a range of items which should be considered in assessing subjects for research studies, and these are also helpful, though perhaps rather inclusive, in clinical settings.[30] Wilcock and colleagues present an old but useful account of clinical assessment procedures,[37] and for a very helpful account of cognitive assessments see Hodges.[38]

Treatment

Treatment of Cognitive Changes

Two randomised controlled trials have examined the efficacy of donepezil in VaD and found only modest efficacy.[43, 44, 45] A trial of galantamine in patients with mixed AD with CVD found small benefit only,[46] although benefit was seen in the subgroup with probable VaD.

Box 2.1 Clinical assessment

History: Time and mode of onset of cognitive impairment, relation to stroke, TIA, myocardial infarction. Full health history, diabetes, hypertension, hyperlipidaemia. Alcohol, drugs, smoking. Family history of cardiovascular or neurological disease.

Collateral history: Confirm extent of functional loss (required to diagnose dementia syndrome).

Physical examination: Focal neurological signs, asymmetries of power, tone, reflexes and sensation, tremor, balance, and gait abnormalities. Cardiovascular system, signs of relevant systemic disease such as diabetes mellitus. Other associated degenerative disorders such as Parkinson's disease. Extrapyramidal signs could be a feature of CVD, but also of Parkinson's disease, progressive supranuclear palsy, other dementias, or neurological disorders such as multiple sclerosis. 'Classic' physical signs associated with VaD include dysarthria, pseudo-bulbar palsy, gait abnormalities, and emotional lability, but it is doubtful how far they positively support a diagnosis of VaD.

Psychiatric disorders: Depression may impact on the diagnostic assessment and require treatment in its own right. Psychosis, whether chronic or acute, can produce cognitive impairment.

Investigations: Blood screen, including vitamin B12 and folate. Growing evidence that homocysteine is a risk factor for dementia, and may prove to be a useful treatment target.[39, 40] NICE does not recommend routine screening for syphilis or HIV unless the history is suggestive.[41] Chest X-ray and an electrocardiogram (ECG) should be considered if relevant, but electroencephalogram (EEG) should be reserved for those who have seizures or in whom Creutzfeld–Jacob disease (CJD) or fronto-temporal dementia (FTD) is possible. Cerebrospinal fluid (CSF) analysis is not widely used in UK clinical practice, and not recommended by NICE, but is more common in Scandinavia. Neuroimaging is recommended. While CT is widely available and helpful, MRI provides more information, though is more expensive and may be less well tolerated. Many other types of imaging, notably single-photon emission computed tomography (SPECT) or positron emission tomography (PET) to investigate regional blood flow, are useful.

Neuropsychological testing: To establish breadth and depth of cognitive impairments. Sometimes the diagnosis will be apparent with only very limited testing such as the Mini-Mental State Examination (MMSE), but in CVD there may well be significant breadth of impairment requiring more extensive testing; and the MMSE is rather insensitive to impairment of executive functioning. The harmonisation group recommended the use of a five-minute screening test based on subscales of the Montreal Cognitive Assessment (the MOCA, available free of charge at www.mocatest.org) as a quick and useful instrument which can be used by telephone if necessary.[30] Screening tests for depression may be useful, such as the Cornell scale for depression in dementia.[42]

Two studies have examined the effects of oral rivastigmine in VaD: one found no significant difference,[47] while the other found a modest but statistically significant advantage in cognitive response at 24 weeks.[48] Two randomised controlled studies have tested the effects of memantine in VaD and both found only modest efficacy.[49, 50] Neither memantine nor any of the cholinesterase inhibitors is licensed in VaD, and the National Institute of Health and Care Excellence (NICE) does not recommend their use for this indication.[51] A variety of other types of agent has been tested: calcium channel blockers (e.g. nimodipine) nootropics (e.g. piracetam, citicoline), xanthenes (e.g. pentoxifylline), vasodilators, ergot derivatives, antithrombotics (e.g. aspirin, gingko), and others. Most have not been shown to have any effect and none has more than modest effects.[52, 53] A Cochrane review of cognitive training and cognitive rehabilitation for people with mild AD or VaD failed to demonstrate a benefit.[54]

Symptomatic Treatment

Depression is common and requires treatment, whether or not there is any aetiological relation to cognitive impairment. There is an emerging concept of vascular depression,[55] and, while attempts to treat it are appropriate, treatment may be less successful than in other types of depression.[56] Depression is a risk factor for dementia. Psychosis may also be present and may require treatment in its own right, although clinicians need to be mindful of the evidence that antipsychotic medication may increase cerebrovascular mortality in people with dementia and note the advice to avoid use of antipsychotics if possible.[57]

As in any form of dementia, appropriate support and information for both patients and carers are essential, and arguably contribute more to well-being than currently available drug treatments.

Control of Vascular Risk Factors

There is no shortage of potential targets for management of VCI risk factors, but perhaps surprisingly the evidence that managing these effectively reduces rates of onset or progression is limited. A Cochrane review failed to find convincing evidence that lowering blood pressure prevents the development of dementia or cognitive impairment in hypertensive patients without prior CVD,[58] although the Syst-Eur and PROGRESS studies showed small but significant reductions in dementia from treating hypertension.[59, 60] Several studies have failed to show a benefit of statins on VaD, which Bowler suggests may be because subcortical VCI is the commonest form of VCI and hypertension is its strongest treatable risk factor, while cholesterol has little association with small vessel disease.[61] Nevertheless, most clinicians would consider that it is appropriate to treat vascular risk factors in any case.

Summary and Conclusion

Vascular dementia is a form of dementia associated with a group of diverse pathologies affecting the cerebrovascular circulation. It is commonly associated with other dementia pathologies, particularly AD, and rather rarely on its own. There is a spectrum of severity of CVD ranging from people who have pathology but no cognitive impairment, through those with mild cognitive impairment to those with a dementia syndrome. Where present, CVD can magnify the impact of other pathologies such as AD. Current criteria for diagnosing vascular dementia are inadequate. Neuroimaging can be very helpful in defining the extent of pathology. Assessment needs to take into account a wide range of issues. Specific evidence-based treatments are limited, but attention should be given to managing risk factors and associated psychiatric problems such as depression.

In conclusion, the points we would wish to emphasize are as follows:

- vascular dementia is not a single entity, but any form of dementia arising from a wide variety of impairments in the cerebrovascular circulation;
- not everyone with evidence of cerebrovascular disease has a cognitive impairment;

- the term 'vascular cognitive impairment' includes vascular dementia, but also mild cognitive impairment of vascular origin;
- even in research centres, the ability to diagnose vascular dementia in life as indicated by post-mortem pathology later is limited;
- pure vascular dementia is rare: it is most commonly associated with AD;
- treatment of vascular risk factors is appropriate, though the evidence base is small; and
- cholinesterase inhibitors have only small benefit in vascular dementia and are not licensed in VaD.

Acknowledgement

We are extremely grateful to Dr Giovanna Zamboni for providing the MRI images.

For information, the original paper on which this chapter is based was:
Series H, Esiri M. Vascular dementia: a pragmatic review. *Adv Psychiatr Treat* 2012; **18**: 372–80.

References

1. Hachinski VC, Lassen NA, Marshall J. Multi-infarct dementia: a cause of mental deterioration in the elderly. *Lancet* 1974; **304**: 207–9.

2. Erkinjuntti T, Gauthier S. Diagnosing vascular cognitive impairment and dementia: concepts and controversies. In *Vascular Cognitive Impairment in Clinical Practice* (eds Wahlund LO, Erkinjuntti T, Gauthier S): 3–10. Cambridge University Press, 2009.

3. Boyle PA, Yu L, Wilson RS et al. Person-specific contribution of neuropathologies to cognitive loss in old age. *Ann Neurol* 2018; **83**: 74–83.

4. Power MC, Mormino E, Soldan A et al. Combined neuropathological pathways account for age-related risk of dementia *Ann Neurol* 2018; **84**: 10–22.

5. De Reuck J, Maurage C-A, Deremacourt V et al. Aging and cerebrovascular lesions in pure and in mixed neurodegenerative and vascular dementia brains: a neuropathological study. *Folia Neuropathol* 2018; **56**: 81–87.

6. Niemantsverdriet E, Feyen BFE, Le Bastard N et al. Overdiagnosing vascular dementia using structural brain imaging in dementia work-up. *J Alz Dis* 2015; **45**: 1039–43.

7. Nagy ZS, Esiri MM, Jobst KA et al. Relative roles of plaques and tangles in the dementia of Alzheimer's disease: correlations using

three sets of neuropathological criteria. *Dement Geriat Cogn Dis* 1995; **6**: 21–31.

8. Skrobot OA, Attems J, Esiri M et al. Vascular cognitive impairment neuropathology guidelines (VCING): the contribution of cerebrovascular pathology to cognitive impairment *Brain* 2016; **139**: 2957–69.

9. Moorhouse P, Rockwood K. Vascular cognitive impairment: current concepts and clinical developments. *Lancet Neurology* 2008; **7**: 246–55.

10. Barkhof F, Fox NC, Bastos-Leite AJ, Scheltens P. *Neuroimaging in Dementia.* Springer, 2011.

11. Tatemichi TK, Desmond DW, Mayeux R et al. Dementia after stroke. *Neurology* 1992; **42**: 1185.

12. Pendlebury ST, Rothwell PM. Prevalence, incidence, and factors associated with pre-stroke and post-stroke dementia: a systematic review and meta-analysis. *Lancet Neurology* 2009; **8**: 1006–18.

13. Pendlebury ST, Rothwell PM for the Oxford Vascular Study.Incidence and prevalence of dementia associated with transient ischaemic attack and stroke: analysis of the population-based Oxford Vascular Study. *Lancet Neurology* 2019; **18**:248–58.

14. Smallwood A, Oulhaj A, Joachim C et al. (2012) Cerebral subcortical small vessel

disease and its relation to cognition in elderly subjects: a pathological study in the Oxford Project to Investigate Memory and Ageing (OPTIMA) cohort. *Neuropathol Appl Neurobiol* 2012; **38**: 337–43.

15. Dichgans M and Leys D. Vascular cognitive impairment. *Circ Res* 2017; **120**: 573–91.

16. van der Flier W, Staekenborg SS, Barkhof F et al. Structural neuroimaging: CT and MRI. In *Vascular Cognitive Impairment in Clinical Practice* (eds Wahlund L, Erkinjuntti T, Gauthier S): 58–69. Cambridge University Press, 2009.

17. Erkinjuntti T, Inzitari D, Pantoni L et al. Research criteria for subcortical vascular dementia in clinical trials. *J Neural Transm. Supple* 2000; **59**: 23–30.

18. Scheltens P, Erkinjuntti T, Leys D et al. White matter changes on CT and MRI: an overview of visual rating scales. *Eur Neurol* 2000; **39**: 80–9.

19. Linn J, Halpin A, Demacrel P et al. Prevalence of superficial siderosis in patients with cerebral congophilic angiopathy. *Neurology* 2010; **74**: 1346–50.

20. Charimidou A, Gang Q, Werring DJ. Sporadic cerebral amyloid angiopathy revisited: recent insights into pathophysiology and clinical spectrum. *J Neurol, Neurosurg Psychiatry* 2012; **83**: 124–37.

21. Ince G, Neuropathology Group of the Medical Research Council Cognitive Function and Ageing Study–MRC CFAS. Pathological correlates of late-onset dementia in a multicentre, community-based population in England and Wales. *Lancet* 2001; **357**: 169–175.

22. Charlton RA, Morris RG, Nitkunan A, Markus HS. The cognitive profiles of CADASIL and sporadic small vessel disease. *Neurology* 2006; **66**: 1523.

23. Wiederkehr S, Simard M, Fortin C et al. Validity of the clinical diagnostic criteria for vascular dementia: a critical review. Part II. *J Neuropsychiatry Clin Neurosci* 2008; **20**: 162–77.

24. Fischer P, Jellinger K, Gatterer G et al. Prospective neuropathological validation

25. of Hachinski's Ischaemic Score in dementias. *J Neurol, Neurosurg Psychiatry* 1991; **54**: 580.

25. Rockwood K, Davis H, MacKnight C et al. The Consortium to Investigate Vascular Impairment of Cognition: methods and first findings. *Can J Neurol Sci* 2003; **30**: 237–43.

26. Verhey FRJ, Lodder J, Rozendaal N et al. Comparison of seven sets of criteria used for the diagnosis of vascular dementia. *Neuroepidemiology* 1996; **15**: 166–72.

27. O'Brien JT, Erkinjuntti T, Reisberg B et al. Vascular cognitive impairment. *Lancet Neurology* 2003; **2**: 89–98.

28. Sachdev PS, Looi JCL. Neuropsychological differentiation of Alzheimer's Disease and vascular dementia. In *Vascular Cognitive Impairment: Preventable Dementia* (eds Bowler JV, Hachinski V): 152–176. Oxford University Press, 2003.

29. Price CC, Jefferson AL, Merino JG et al. Subcortical vascular dementia. *Neurology* 2005; **65**: 376–82.

30. Hachinski V, Iadecola C, Petersen RC et al. National institute of neurological disorders and stroke-Canadian stroke network vascular cognitive impairment harmonization standards. *Stroke* 2006; **37**: 2220–41.

31. Hebert R, Brayne C. Epidemiology of vascular dementia. *Neuroepidemiology* 1995; **14**: 240–57.

32. Ueda K, Kawano H, Hasuo Y et al. Prevalence and etiology of dementia in a Japanese community. *Stroke* 1992; **23**: 798.

33. Ikeda M, Hokoishi K, Maki N et al. Increased prevalence of vascular dementia in Japan. *Neurology* 2001; **57**: 839.

34. Fratiglioni L, Launer LJ, Andersen K et al. Incidence of dementia and major subtypes in Europe: a collaborative study of population-based cohorts. *Neurology* 2000; **54**: S10–5.

35. Hebert R, Lindsay J, Verreault R et al. Vascular dementia: incidence and risk factors in the Canadian study of health and aging. *Stroke* 2000; **31**: 1487.

36. Lopez OL, Wolk DA. Clinical evaluation: a systematic but user-friendly approach. In *Vascular Cognitive Impairment in Clinical Practice* (eds Wahlund L, Erkinjuntti T, Gauthier S): 32–45. Cambridge University Press, 2009.

37. Wilcock GK, Bucks RS, Rockwood K. *Diagnosis and Management of Dementia: A Manual for Memory Disorders Teams.* Oxford University Press, 1999.

38. Hodges JR. *Cognitive Assessment for Clinicians.* 3rd edn. Oxford University Press, 2018.

39. Smith AD, Smith SM, de Jager CA et al. Homocysteine-lowering by B vitamins slows the rate of accelerated brain atrophy in mild cognitive impairment: a randomized controlled trial. *PloS One* 2010; 5: e12244.

40. Wald DS, Kasturiratne A, Simmonds M. Serum homocysteine and dementia: meta-analysis of eight cohort studies including 8669 participants. *Alz Dement* 2011; 7: 412–17.

41. NICE. Dementia: supporting people with dementia and their carers in health and social care. Clinical Guideline 42 (amended March 2011). National Institute for Health and Clinical Excellence.

42. Alexopoulos GS, Abrams RC, Young RC et al. Cornell scale for depression in dementia. *Biol Psychiat* 1988; 23: 271–84.

43. Black S, Román GC, Geldmacher DS et al. Efficacy and tolerability of donepezil in vascular dementia: positive results of a 24-week, multicenter, international, randomized, placebo-controlled clinical trial. *Stroke* 2003; 34: 2323–32.

44. Wilkinson D, Doody R, Helme R et al. Donepezil 308 Study Group. Donepezil in vascular dementia: a randomized, placebo-controlled study. *Neurology* 2003; 61: 479–86.

45. Wilkinson DG, Doody RS, Black SE et al. Donepezil in vascular dementia: combined analysis of two large-scale clinical trials. *Dement Geriatr Cogn Disord* 2005; 20: 338–44.

46. Erkinjuntti T, Kurz A, Gauthier S et al. Efficacy of galantamine in probable vascular dementia and Alzheimer's disease combined with cerebrovascular disease: a randomised trial. *Lancet* 2002; 359: 1283–90.

47. Mok V, Wong A, Ho S et al. Rivastigmine in Chinese patients with subcortical vascular dementia. *Neuropsychiatr Dis Treat* 2007; 3(6): 943–8.

48. Ballard C, Sauter M, Scheltens P et al. Efficacy, safety and tolerability of rivastigmine capsules in patients with probable vascular dementia: the VantagE study. *Curr Med Res Opin* 2008; 24 (9):2561–74.

49. Orgogozo J, Rigaud A, Stoffler A et al. Efficacy and safety of memantine in patients with mild to moderate vascular dementia: a randomized, placebo-controlled trial (MMM 300). *Stroke* 2002; 33: 1834–9.

50. Wilcock G, Möbius HJ, Stöffler A. A double-blind, placebo-controlled multicentre study of memantine in mild to moderate vascular dementia (MMM500). *Int Clin Psychopharmacol* 2002; 17: 297–305.

51. NICE. Alzheimer's disease – donepezil, galantamine, rivastigmine and memantine. Technology Appraisal 217. National Institute for Health and Clinical Excellence, 2011.

52. Erkinjuntti T, Román G, Gauthier S et al. Emerging therapies for vascular dementia and vascular cognitive impairment. *Stroke* 2004; 35: 1010.

53. Román G. Therapeutic strategies for vascular dementia. In *Dementia* (eds Burns A, O'Brien J, Ames, D): 574–600. Hodder Arnold, 2005.

54. Bahar-Fuchs A, Clare L, Woods B. Cognitive training and cognitive rehabilitation for mild to moderate Alzheimer's disease and vascular dementia. *Cochrane Database of Systematic Reviews* 2013, Issue 6. Art. No.: CD003260.

55. Alexopoulos GS, Meyers BS, Young RC et al. 'Vascular depression' hypothesis. *Arch Gen Psychiat* 1997; 54: 915–22.

56. Sheline YI, Pieper CF, Barch DM et al. Support for the vascular depression

hypothesis in late-life depression: results of a 2-site, prospective, antidepressant treatment trial. *Arch Gen Psychiat* 2010; **67**: 277–85.

57. Banerjee, S. *The Use of Antipsychotic Medication for People with Dementia: Time for Action.* Department of Health, London, 2009.

58. McGuinness B, Todd S, Passmore P et al. Blood pressure lowering in patients without prior cerebrovascular disease for prevention of cognitive impairment and dementia. *Cochrane Database.* John Wiley & Sons, 2009.

59. Forette F, Seux ML, Staessen JA et al. The prevention of dementia with antihypertensive treatment: new evidence from the Systolic Hypertension in Europe (Syst-Eur) study. *Arch Int Med* 2002; **162**: 2046–52.

60. Tzourio C, Anderson C, PROGRESS Collaborative Group et al. Effects of blood pressure lowering with perindopril and indapamide therapy on dementia and cognitive decline in patients with cerebrovascular disease. *Arch Int Med* 2003; **163**: 1069–75.

61. Bowler JV. Modern concept of vascular cognitive impairment. *Br Med Bull* 2007; **83**: 291–305.

Young-Onset Dementias

Kate Jefferies and Niruj Agrawal

Introduction

Dementia is stereotypically associated with older people. However, it can affect people in their forties and fifties, or even younger. Currently, even among healthcare professionals, there is a lack of awareness and a dearth of appropriate services for such patients. Despite the attention given to this condition by National Institute for Health and Care Excellence (NICE) guidelines, provision of specialist young-onset dementia services in the United Kingdom (UK) remains patchy. Carers and patients often find themselves being passed 'from pillar to post' between psychiatry and neurology, and also between adult, old age and liaison psychiatry. The responsibility for identifying available and appropriate help is often left with carers. This leads to unnecessary delays, causes undue distress to patients and places an added burden on carers. The aim of this chapter is to review how things are in the field of young-onset dementia and provide an overview of this important topic.

Young-onset dementias are a fascinating group of disorders that present challenges in diagnosis, management and service provision. It has become accepted practice that 'young-onset' refers to dementias that occur before the age of 65 years.

ICD–11 defines dementia as follows:

Dementia is an acquired brain syndrome characterized by a decline from a previous level of cognitive functioning with impairment in two or more cognitive domains (such as memory, executive functions, attention, language, social cognition and judgment, psychomotor speed, visuoperceptual or visuospatial abilities). The cognitive impairment is not entirely attributable to normal aging and significantly interferes with independence in the person's performance of activities of daily living. Based on available evidence, the cognitive impairment is attributed or assumed to be attributable to a neurological or medical condition that affects the brain, trauma, nutritional deficiency, chronic use of specific substances or medications, or exposure to heavy metals or other toxins.[1]

The diagnosis of dementia involves a decline in cognitive functions sufficient to impair activities of daily living. It should also be remembered that dementias, particularly in younger people, often present with symptoms other than memory decline as the predominant feature.

Differences between Young-Onset Dementias and Dementias in Later Life

Young-onset dementia is less common than dementia in later life. The differential diagnosis is broader and younger people are more likely to have a rarer form of dementia, as explored in Chapter 4. Both the diagnosis and the symptoms of the condition can have a devastating impact on patients, carers and their families. Younger people are likely to have different needs and commitments to older people. They are more likely to be in work at the time of diagnosis, have dependent family or children, and have heavy financial commitments (e.g. a mortgage). They are also likely to be physically fit and active, and aware of their problems. As a consequence, they are prone to feel distressed and frustrated. Yet access to information and support can be difficult and limited. Spouses of patients with young-onset dementia have many concerns, especially worries about financial and health matters, a feeling of lack of support and social isolation.[2]

Prevalence of Young-Onset Dementia

In 1998, an estimated 18,500 people had young-onset dementia in the UK.[3] The disorder was more common in men than in women: in people between 30 and 64 years of age there were 78.2 cases per 100,000 men and 56.4 cases per 100,000 women. Prevalence increased sharply with age, with two-thirds of patients aged 55 and over (see Figure 3.1). About a decade later, Knapp & Prince reported a comparable prevalence, with young-onset dementias accounting for 2.2% of all people with dementia in the UK.[4] They calculated that there are at least 15,034 people with young-onset dementia. In 2013, this estimate had risen again, to suggest there were 42,325 people with young-onset dementia in the UK.[5] However, this estimate is based on the number of referrals to services, and the true figure may be up to three times higher.

Diagnosis of Young-Onset Dementia

Distribution of Diagnoses

The distribution of diagnoses of dementia differs dramatically between older and younger patients. Alzheimer's disease (AD) is the most common cause of dementia in both groups,

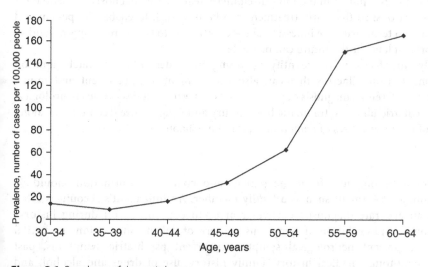

Figure 3.1 Prevalence of dementia by age
Data derived from Harvey R. *Young Onset Dementia: Epidemiology, Clinical Symptoms, Family Burden, Support and Outcome.* Dementia Research Group, 1998.

Box 3.1 Differential diagnosis of young-onset dementia

1. Delirium
2. Amnesic syndromes:
   Korsakoff's syndrome
   anoxic brain damage
   herpes simplex encephalitis
3. Mild cognitive impairment
4. Pseudodementia:
   depressive
   dissociative
5. Traumatic brain injury
6. Neurological illness (e.g. normal-pressure hydrocephalus, stroke, encephalitis, vasculitis, multiple sclerosis)
7. General medical conditions (e.g. endocrine, B12 deficiency, systemic lupus erythematosus, sarcoidosis)
8. Drugs (e.g. alcohol, benzodiazepines)

accounting for almost two-thirds of cases in older people, but only a third of cases in younger people. Frontotemporal dementia (FTD) occurs much more commonly in younger than in older populations. Rarer causes of dementia also occur with greater frequency in the younger population (see Chapter 4).

Clinical Approach to Assessment

Assessment requires input from the multidisciplinary team. Early diagnosis is essential for a number of reasons: so that early treatment can be provided; to enable the person and family to come to terms with the illness; to allow early access to the correct support; and so that appropriate plans for the future can be made.

Clinically, the focus is on identifying young-onset dementia accurately and on differentiating it from illnesses that can also cause cognitive impairment and mimic dementia. The differential diagnosis of young-onset dementia includes various neurological illnesses, psychiatric illnesses, traumatic brain injury and drug misuse (see Box 3.1), along with some of the rarer causes of dementia explored in Chapter 4.

History

History should be obtained from the patient and collateral information should be gathered from an informant such as a family member. An informant's account is often the key to an accurate diagnosis. Particular areas to concentrate on during history-taking are onset and evolution of symptoms, pattern of deficits, fluctuations in mental state, past or present neurological symptoms, current psychiatric symptoms, past psychiatric symptoms, medical history, family history, use of drugs and alcohol, and risk assessment.

Cognitive Testing

Detailed neuropsychological testing is an important component of the diagnostic process. It can reveal the precise nature and location of the cognitive deficits. Neuropsychological testing can also help in teasing out whether there has been any progression of dementia. Using a series of psychological tests, the neuropsychologist establishes the cognitive abilities of the person and compares them with the person's estimated best levels and with those for an average person of the same age. Neuropsychological assessment can also identify where a person's abilities are preserved so that they can be maximized.

Basic bedside testing is also helpful in confirming the nature, degree and location of deficits. The Mini-Mental State Examination (MMSE)[6] has been a widely used screening test for cognitive impairment (but see Chapter 11). It is short, easy to use, has high interrater reliability and is useful for monitoring illness progression. However, it is insensitive to frontal lobe disorders, does not detect focal cognitive deficits and is strongly influenced by previous intelligence quotient (IQ) and education. The Addenbrooke's Cognitive Examination was developed as a more comprehensive screening instrument that also tested frontal lobe functioning.[7] It contains a 100-point test battery that assesses six cognitive domains and takes about 15 to 20 minutes to complete. It included the MMSE, but since 2001 the MMSE has not been available without payment of a fee. A subsequent edition of the test, the ACE-III, developed in 2012, does not include the MMSE.[8]

Bedside tests of frontal lobe functioning, which will often be useful in suspected young-onset dementia, are described in Table 3.1.

Physical Examination

Physical examination is important both in reaching the diagnosis of the subtype of dementia and in identifying any treatable comorbidity. The physical examination is often normal in the early stages of dementia, but the presence of certain symptoms and signs will arouse suspicion of a primary neurological disorder. These include sudden onset of symptoms, focal neurological findings early in the illness, visual hallucinations, incontinence, ataxia and early seizures.

In AD, patients are typically physically well with no neurological signs in the early stages. Later, there may be akinesia and rigidity. In FTD, neurological signs are also usually absent in the early stages. In later stages of the disorder there may be evidence of primitive reflexes, and with further disease progression there may be akinesia and rigidity. Spontaneous features of parkinsonism are one of the core features of dementia with Lewy bodies (DLB). Huntington's disease is evidenced by the presence of chorea and other pyramidal symptoms. In Creutzfeldt–Jacob disease, myoclonus and other extrapyramidal symptoms are often present.

Further Investigations

When arranging for further investigations the priorities are to identify treatable causes of dementia and to guide accurate diagnosis.

We would suggest conducting the following investigations routinely: full blood count; erythrocyte sedimentation rate; C-reactive protein; renal, liver and thyroid function;

Table 3.1 Bedside tests of frontal lobe function

Test	Example	Findings indicative of impairment
Verbal fluency	'Name as many words as you can beginning with the letter T, any words except names of people or places'	Fewer than 13 words a minute
Similarities	'In what way are a banana and an orange alike?'	Inability to identify the similarity
Cognitive estimates	'How tall is the tallest man?' 'How fast can a horse gallop?'	Estimates will be inaccurate and often wildly wrong
Proverb interpretation	'What do you understand by the saying "too many cooks spoil the broth"?'	Concrete (literal) not figurative responses
Luria hand sequence	Fist–edge–palm (the patient is asked to tap the table with a fist, open palm and side of open hand, and to repeat the sequence as quickly as possible)	Inability to follow the sequence; perseveration
Conflicting instructions	'Tap twice when I tap once, and tap once when I tap twice'	Copying the tapping pattern of examiner rather than doing opposite despite clear instruction
Go/No-Go test	'Tap once when I tap once. Do not tap when I tap twice'	Tapping twice when the examiner taps twice

vitamin B_{12} and folate levels; bone profile; lipid profile; glucose; and structural neuroimaging by CT or MRI. Syphilis serology should be tested if there is a history of multiple unprotected sexual contacts and electrocardiogram (ECG) or chest X-ray should be carried out as determined by the clinical presentation, for example a history suggesting treatable comorbidities such as atrial fibrillation.

Structural neuroimaging should be carried out to exclude other pathologies and to help establish the subtype of dementia. MRI is preferable, as CT may not show focal atrophy well (but see Chapter 13 for further discussion of neuroimaging options). Functional imaging may be helpful in the detection of focal brain dysfunction. Hexamethylpropyleneamine oxime (HMPAO) single-photon emission computed tomography scan (SPECT) could help to differentiate the subtype of dementia. Dopaminergic iodine-123-radiolabelled SPECT (DaTscan) can be used to confirm suspected DLB.

In atypical presentations, particularly when dementia is rapidly progressive with features of encephalopathy or focal neurological signs, patients should be referred for neurological opinion; lumbar puncture may be required. Additional investigations such as human immunodeficiency virus (HIV) testing and CD4 count may be considered, depending on the clinical presentation.

Causes of Young-Onset Dementia

The clinical presentations of the following diseases generally do not differ between older and younger populations.

Alzheimer's Disease

AD accounts for almost a third of young-onset dementia cases. The typical presentation of AD includes progressive episodic (day-to-day) memory loss and visuospatial and perceptual deficits, but well-preserved language and social functioning. The posterior cortical variant of the disease, with prominent impairment of parietal lobe functions, is more common in younger people.

AD is more common in women than men. Prevalence increases with increasing age. The average duration of illness is eight years. Alzheimer's disease mostly occurs as a sporadic disorder, even in the younger population. However, inherited forms are more likely in the younger population.

Inheritance is autosomal dominant. There are many reported genetic mutations, but there are three genes that are most commonly affected: the *presenilin 1* gene on chromosome 14, β-amyloid precursor protein on chromosome 21 and the *presenilin 2* gene on chromosome 1.[9]

Vascular Dementia

Vascular dementia (VaD) is the second most common cause of dementia in younger people. Diagnosis is based on the clinical picture, identification of risk factors and brain imaging. The clinical presentation is variable and depends on the site and extent of the lesions (for further discussion see Chapter 2).

VaD has several syndromes:

* multiple cortical infarcts leading to a stepwise deterioration of cognitive functions;
* small vessel disease leading to a more insidious decline of cognitive functioning;
* strategic infarcts – small cryptic strokes that cause cognitive impairment;
* CADASIL (see also Chapter 4).

Frontotemporal Dementia

Frontotemporal dementias occur more frequently in the younger population. Men are more often affected than women. Frontotemporal lobar degeneration, which underpins the different types of FTD, is a heterogeneous group of disorders with an overall prevalence of 81 per 100,000 in the 45- to 64-year-old age group, which is when the condition usually starts.[10] The average duration of illness is eight years. There is a positive family history in up to 50% of patients.

There is an association between FTD and motor neurone disease. The rate of dementia in motor neurone disease is much higher than expected, and indeed a significant minority of patients with FTD develop features of the disease and the other way around.[11] Up to 10% of patients with motor neurone disease show features of dementia. The course of the illness for these individuals is usually aggressive.

The hallmark of the behavioural variant of FTD is the early alteration in personality and social conduct, with relative preservation of memory, perception, visuospatial skills and praxis. (See Chapter 13 (Box 13.5) for a typical case history.) Although presentations are variable and subtle, they are often characterized by behavioural disturbance, personality change, reduced motivation, reduced empathy, impaired planning and judgement, and speech and language problems. International consensus criteria for the behavioural form of FTD have been developed.[12]

As the disease progresses, symptoms of frontal lobe dysfunction may also become apparent. These include behavioural rigidity, disinhibition, loss of social skills and graces, fatuousness, emotional lability, impulsivity, executive dysfunction, reduced verbal fluency, hyperorality and motor and verbal perseveration.

Frontotemporal dementia can take a number of forms which are depicted in Figure 3.2.

Behavioural Form

The frontal (or behavioural) variant primarily affects frontal lobes and affected patients typically show symptoms of frontal lobe dysfunction (as shown in Box 3.2) with relative preservation of day-to-day memory.

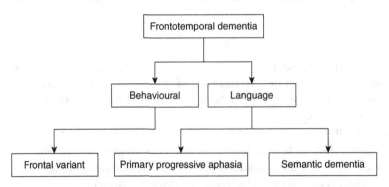

Figure 3.2 Variants of frontotemporal dementia

Box 3.2 Symptoms of frontal lobe dysfunction

- Change in social conduct
- Change in behaviour
- Behaviour inappropriate to the social situation
- Lack of inhibitions
- Impulsivity
- Poor judgement
- Inappropriate sexual behaviour
- Repetitive or compulsive behaviours
- Hyperorality
- Self-neglect
- Lack of insight

Language Forms

Primary Progressive Aphasia

Patients have a progressive decline in their language with a relative absence of other cognitive deficits. Speech is non-fluent and effortful. Speech output becomes increasingly difficult and in the later stages the patient may become mute. Behavioural changes may occur later in the disease. There is predominant atrophy of the left perisylvian region.

Semantic Dementia

Patients have a variety of language difficulties, including naming difficulties, impaired understanding of word meaning and use of substitute words. However, speech is fluent and there is preservation of other cognitive domains. Behavioural difficulties may emerge as the disease progresses. Features of semantic dementia include temporal lobe atrophy (of the left more than the right). The characteristic feature is that atrophy of the anterior temporal lobe is more pronounced than that of the posterior temporal lobe.

Dementia with Lewy Bodies

The core features of DLB include progressive cognitive decline, fluctuating cognition, the presence of parkinsonian symptoms, and visual hallucinations that are typically recurrent, well formed and detailed. Other features that are highly suggestive of DLB include rapid eye movement sleep behaviour disorder, severe antipsychotic sensitivity and low dopamine transporter uptake in the basal ganglia demonstrated by SPECT or positron emission tomography imaging. The full (fourth) set of consensus criteria for DLB can be found in Box 13.4 in Chapter 13.[13]

A positive history of severe antipsychotic sensitivity suggests a diagnosis of DLB, which should be diagnosed when dementia occurs before or concurrently with parkinsonism. Dementia that occurs in the context of well-established Parkinson's disease is best described as Parkinson's disease dementia (PDD).

People with DLB are extremely sensitive to the side effects of typical and atypical antipsychotics. Approximately 50% of patients with this type of dementia will have an adverse reaction to the administration of antipsychotics.

Alcohol-Related Dementia

Heavy, prolonged alcohol use can cause damage to the limbic structures and the frontal lobes, leading to memory and executive impairments. Autobiographical memory is frequently affected and confabulation can occur. The memory loss is often static, although may improve following a period of abstinence. Imaging may be non-specific or it may show generalized cortical atrophy with a frontal preponderance. (For more information on alcohol-related dementia, see Chapter 6.)

Huntington's and Rarer Causes of Young-Onset Dementia

Rarer causes of young-onset dementia, including prion disease and other infectious diseases, are discussed in Chapter 4. Huntington's disease, with a prevalence rate (in the United States (USA) at least) of around five to seven per 100,000, is also an important cause of young-onset dementia and is discussed briefly here.[14]

Huntington's Disease

The characteristic triad of clinical features in Huntington's disease are motor disorder (primarily choreiform involuntary movements), cognitive disorder (with evidence of sub-cortical slowing, apathy, as well as memory problems) and emotional or psychiatric disorders (e.g. depression, irritability, anxiety, with obsessional-compulsive features, and even evidence of schizophrenia). However, there is variation between patients in the time of onset, specific symptoms and the progression of illness. Huntington's disease is an autosomal dominant disorder with complete penetrance caused by expansion of the CAG (cytoscine–adenine–guanine) trinucleotide repeat on the short arm of chromosome 4. Onset is generally in middle life and the typical duration of illness is 15–20 years. Diagnostic and predictive testing is available.

Neuroimaging shows bilateral atrophy of the head of the caudate nucleus and atrophy of the putamen and globus pallidus. Single-photon emission computed tomography scans show cerebral hypoperfusion in the basal ganglia even before atrophy is evident on MRI scan.

Management of Young-Onset Dementia

Accurate diagnosis of young-onset dementia based on comprehensive multidisciplinary assessment and full investigation forms the basis for management. It is important to identify treatable causes of dementia and accurately diagnose underlying neurological or psychiatric conditions. Longer-term support is vital to help manage the cognitive, neuropsychiatric and behavioural symptoms that often accompany these disorders.

Management should encompass pharmacological and non-pharmacological strategies. Non-pharmacological management strategies such as psychoeducation; cognitive strategies such as mental exercise, physical therapy and dietary treatment; and drug therapies may be beneficial in reducing the impact or slowing down the progression of the disease. Medications may be needed for delusions, hallucinations and serious distress or danger from behaviour disturbance or symptoms of depression. Support packages should include appropriate day, respite and intensive home care if required. Support for families and carers is also required, especially in cases where there may be dependants such as children.

Pharmacological Interventions

Pharmacological management strategies include anti-dementia drugs and other psychotropic drugs. It is important to treat any comorbid medical or psychiatric illnesses. The underlying degenerative disorder should also be treated if appropriate. In addition, vascular risk factors should be addressed.

Anti-dementia drugs that are currently licensed in the UK for patients of any age are donepezil, rivastigmine, galantamine and memantine. The available evidence base confirms that the cholinesterase inhibitors (ChEIs) are effective across the spectrum of AD (mild, moderate and severe disease) and they also lead to improvements in non-cognitive symptoms.[15] Results of trials in other types of dementia (VaD, DLB and Parkinson's disease dementia) have been variably positive. NICE has produced guidelines on the use of the anti-dementia agents.[16] In brief, they are recommended in AD and can be offered or considered under certain circumstances in DLB and PDD.[16] Cholinesterase inhibitors should be prescribed with caution to patients with sick sinus syndrome or other supraventricular conduction abnormalities, to those who are susceptible to peptic ulcers and to those with asthma or chronic obstructive pulmonary disease.

Memantine, licensed in the UK for use in moderate to severe AD, is an *N*-methyl-D-asparate (NMDA) receptor antagonist, which may reduce glutamate-mediated neuronal excitotoxicity.

Antipsychotic Agents

Symptoms that may respond to antipsychotic medication include physical aggression and psychotic symptoms. They should be used for the shortest time possible, at the lowest dose possible, and only after non-pharmacological (psychosocial) approaches (see Chapter 16) have failed and the behavioural symptoms are severe enough to tip the risk–benefit ratio in favour of their use, albeit cautiously.

Antidepressants

Depression occurs frequently in young-onset dementias (see also Chapter 18). Symptoms of mood disturbance should always be asked about. Selective serotonin reuptake inhibitors are used as the first-line treatment because of their favourable side-effect profile and because an antidepressant with strong anticholinergic effects may worsen cognition.

Psychological and Non-Pharmacological Interventions

Symptoms that may respond to non-pharmacological interventions include mild depressive symptoms, wandering and repetitive questioning. The ideal environment for someone with dementia is one that is constant, familiar and non-stressful. Other therapies that have been shown to help to varying degrees in the management of behavioural and psychological symptoms in dementia include aromatherapy, music therapy, recreation, bright light therapy, behaviour therapy, reality orientation, reminiscence therapy and art therapy (see also Chapter 16).[17]

Services for People with Young-Onset Dementia

The ongoing support and care of people with young-onset dementia is complex and requires input from a multidisciplinary team. Patients and their families also benefit from the support offered by voluntary organizations. In particular, *YoungDementia UK* is a dedicated national charity for younger people with dementia and their families.[18] An example of innovative service provision is the charity YPWD: *Younger People with Dementia (Berkshire)* (see www.ypwd.info). However, there are few specific statutory services in the UK and there is limited awareness and understanding of people who develop dementia at an early age, thus making it difficult to access support. In the absence of specific services, some years ago 38 referral pathways and four separate gateways to specialist investigation and care were identified in the city of Leeds in the UK.[19] An earlier UK study had reported 11 different referral pathways in one area.[20] Patients can be referred to two to five different consultants sequentially, leading to significant delays in diagnosis.[19] This is clearly unsatisfactory service provision and causes high rates of patient and carer dissatisfaction.

Younger people with dementia have different needs to older people with the disease. General dementia services are often inappropriate for use by younger people and may not be able to meet their needs. Age can often be a barrier to accessing services, so in some parts of the UK younger people may not be eligible to receive care from general dementia services. We believe the best solution is the development of regional specialist young-onset dementia services in every area and for services to be flexible; some people over the age of 65 may be better suited to services for younger people, whereas some people under the age of 65 may be better catered for by the general dementia services.

National Recommendations

There are recommendations that ratify the need for specialist services for people with young-onset dementia in the UK. The National Institute for Health and Clinical Excellence & Social Care Institute for Excellence joint guidelines published in 2007 stated that specialist multi-disciplinary services allied to existing dementia services should be developed for the assessment, diagnosis and care of younger people with dementia.[21] The current NICE Guideline, published in 2018, makes little specific reference to the needs of people with young-onset dementia. It says that care providers 'should provide additional face-to-face training and mentoring to staff' about 'the specific needs of younger people living with dementia' (section 1.13.2).[22] A recent Royal College of Psychiatrists' report states that there should be a named local clinical lead for early-onset dementia and the service should ensure patients have a named key worker.[23] Patients should have access to a full multidisciplinary team and the specialist team should work with other agencies to enhance the quality and range of services.

To address the needs of these patients and their carers adequately, there must be cooperation and collaboration across all the relevant statutory and voluntary services. Carers regularly report that they would like to see better coordination of services and to receive welfare advice, support and respite care. However, it is often unclear how services should be accessed, with subsequent delays in diagnosis, treatment and provision of appropriate support.

Acknowledgement

For information, the original paper on which this chapter is based was:

Jefferies K, Agrawal N. Early-onset dementia. *Adv Psychiatr Treat* 2009; **15**: 380–388.

References

1. World Health Organization. *International Classification of Diseases 11th Revision.* WHO, 2019. Last accessed on 18 October 2019 via: https://icd.who.int/ct11/icd11_mms/en/release

2. Kaiser S, Panegyres PK. The psychosocial impact of young onset dementia on spouses. *Am J Alzheimers Dis Other Demen* 2006; **21**: 398–402.

3. Harvey R. *Young Onset Dementia: Epidemiology, Clinical Symptoms, Family Burden, Support and Outcome.* Dementia Research Group, 1998.

4. Knapp M, Prince M. *Dementia UK: The Full Report.* Alzheimer's Society, 2007. Last accessed on 18 October 2019 via: www.alzheimers.org.uk/sites/default/files/2018-10/Dementia_UK_Full_Report_2007.pdf?fileID=2

5. Prince M, Knapp M, Guerchet M et al. *Dementia UK: Update. Second edition.* Alzheimer's Society, 2014. Last accessed on 18 October 2019 via: www.alzheimers.org.uk/sites/default/files/migrate/downloads/dementia_uk_update.pdf

6. Folstein MF, Folstein SE, McHugh PR. 'Mini-mental state': a practical method for grading the cognitive state of patients for the clinician. *J Psychiatry Res* 1975; **12**: 189–198.

7. Mathuranath PS, Nestor PJ, Berrios GE, Rakowicz W, Hodges JR. A brief cognitive test battery to differentiate Alzheimer's disease and frontotemporal dementia. *Neurology* 2000; **55**: 1613–1620.

8. Hodges JR, Larner AJ. *Cognitive Screening Instruments: A Practical Approach.* Second Edition. Springer; 2017.

9. Schott JM, Fox NC, Rossor MN. Genetics of the dementias. *J Neurol Neurosurg Psychiatry* 2002; **73**(suppl II): ii27–31.

10. Ratnavalli E, Brayne C, Dawson K, Hodges JR. (2002) The prevalence of frontotemporal dementia. *Neurology* 2002; **58**: 1615–1621.

11. Nestor P. Frontotemporal dementia. In *Dementia (Fifth Edition)* (eds. D Ames, J O'Brien, A Burns): 749–758. CRC Press, Taylor & Francis Group, 2017.

12. Rascovsky K, Hodges JR, Knopman D et al. Sensitivity of revised diagnostic criteria for the behavioural variant of frontotemporal dementia. *Brain* 2011; **134**: 2456–2477. DOI:10.1093/brain/awr179

13. McKeith IG, Boeve BF, Dickson DW et al. Diagnosis and management of dementia with Lewy bodies: fourth consensus report of the DLB Consortium. *Neurology* 2017; **89**: 88–100. DOI:10.1212/WNL.0000000 000004058

14. Chua P, Loi S, Chiu E. Huntingon's disease. In *Dementia (Fifth Edition)* (eds. D Ames, J O'Brien, A Burns): 868–884. CRC Press, Taylor & Francis Group, 2017.

15. Kurz A, Lautenschlager NT. Established treatments for Alzheimer's disease. In *Dementia (Fifth Edition)* (eds. D Ames, J O'Brien, A Burns): 539–553. CRC Press, Taylor & Francis Group, 2017.

16. National Institute for Health and Care Excellence (NICE). *Dementia: Assessment, Management and Support for People Living with Dementia and Their Carers.* NICE Guideline 97. NICE, 2018. Last accessed on 3 October 2019 via: www.nice.org.uk/gui dance/ng97/resources/dementia-assessment-management-and-support-for-people-living-with-dementia-and-their-carers-pdf-1837760199109

17. Scales K, Zimmerman S, Miller SJ. Evidence-based nonpharmacological practices to address behavioral and psychological symptoms of dementia. *Gerontologist* 2018; **58**(Suppl. 1):S88–S102.

18. www.youngdementiauk.org/about-us [Last accessed on 18 October 2019.]

19. Williams T, Dearden AM, Cameron IH. From pillar to post: a study of younger people with dementia. *Psychiatr Bull* 2001; **25**: 384–387.

20. Fuhrmann R. *Early-Onset Dementia in Brighton, Hove and Lewes Area: Prevalence and Service Needs.* Alzheimer's Society (Brighton branch), 1997.

21. National Institute for Health and Clinical Excellence, Social Care Institute for Excellence (NICE-SCIE). *Dementia: Supporting People with Dementia and their Carers in Health and Social Care.* British Psychological Society and Gaskill, 2007.

22. National Institute for Health and Care Excellence (NICE). *Dementia: Assessment, Management and Support for People Living with Dementia and Their Carers.* NICE Guideline 97. NICE, 2018. Last accessed on 3 October 2019 via: www.nice.org.uk/gui dance/ng97/resources/dementia-assessment-management-and-support-for-people-living-with-dementia-and-their-carers-pdf-1837760199109

23. Royal College of Psychiatrists. *Young-Onset Dementia in Mental Health Services CR217.* Royal College of Psychiatrists, 2018. Last accessed on 18 October 2019 via: www.rcpsych.ac.uk/improving-care/cam paigning-for-better-mental-health-policy/college-reports/2018-college-reports/cr217

Rare and Unusual Dementias

Susham Gupta, Olivia Fiertag, Thanakumar Thanulingam,
Bryan Strange, and James Warner

Introduction

Over 95% of cases of dementia are attributable to Alzheimer's disease (AD), vascular dementia (VaD), dementia with Lewy bodies (DLB), and frontotemporal dementia (FTD), as well as mixed Alzheimer's and VaD, and so on. In this chapter we consider some of the rare and unusual causes that account for the remaining 5%. Categorizing them according to aetiological group (degenerative, vascular, and infectious causes, including human prion diseases), we discuss the presentation of these forms and reasons for variations in estimated prevalence rates in the general population. We shall then go on to describe toxic, iatrogenic, nutritional, traumatic, metabolic, neoplastic, and autoimmune causes of dementia. Disorders are graded according to their prevalence, to give an idea of the likelihood of their presentation. Guidance is given on the investigation of uncommon cognitive impairment and dementia. We have tried to avoid repeating information available in Chapter 3 on the causes of young-onset dementias, but inevitably there is some overlap of material.

Dementia is a common and growing problem worldwide. Much is known about its more frequent causes, such as AD, and vascular, Lewy body and FTD, but its numerous rarer forms are less well understood. Reported prevalence rates of these rare forms vary, perhaps owing to inadequate epidemiological studies, regional variations (especially in those with genetic and familial basis), and differences in detection levels and accuracy of diagnosis. However, a European Union project on rarer forms of dementia estimated a prevalence of 5 cases per 10,000 in the community.[1]

Degenerative Causes of Dementia

Box 4.1 summarizes the spectrum of the degenerative causes of dementia.

Familial Alzheimer's Disease

Familial AD is the most common single cause of young-onset dementia, with an estimated 3,000 cases in the UK.[2] It has been discussed in Chapter 3.

Pure Hippocampal Sclerosis (Ageing Subtype)

This rare cause of dementia may mimic AD.[3] It is characterized by severe neuronal loss and gliosis of the hippocampus in the absence of changes present in other common dementias (pure hippocampal sclerosis is very rare). Onset is usually in the very old (over-80s). The rate of progression, clinical signs, and symptoms are similar to those of AD, with prominent

> **Box 4.1** Degenerative causes of dementia
>
> - Familial Alzheimer's disease
> - Pure hippocampal sclerosis
> - Frontotemporal lobar degeneration
> - Primary progressive (non-fluent) aphasia
> - Semantic dementia
> - Progressive supranuclear palsy (Steele–Richardson–Olszewsky syndrome)
> - Corticobasal degeneration
> - Multiple system atrophy (Shy–Drager syndrome)
> - Amyotrophic lateral sclerosis/motor neurone disease (Lou Gehrig's disease)
> - Huntington's disease
> - Spinocerebellar and Friedreich's ataxias
> - Polycystic lipomembranous osteodysplasia with sclerosing leukoencephalopathy (Nasu–Hakola disease)

short-term memory loss. However, behavioural disturbance and subtle neuropsychological deficits also suggest similarities with FTD.[4] The cause is unknown, and association with vascular risk factors is inconclusive. Post-mortem examination is required for definitive diagnosis and there is no known treatment.

Frontotemporal Lobar Degeneration

Frontotemporal dementias are important causes of young-onset dementia and are discussed in Chapter 3.

Corticobasal Degeneration

Corticobasal degeneration affects between 2 and 6 people per 100,000.[1] It is a degeneration of the frontoparietal cortical basal ganglia structures and other subcortical nuclei owing to tauopathy. Corticobasal degeneration is similar to that of progressive supranuclear palsy but with higher putaminal involvement and some vermian atrophy of the cerebellum. It is a sporadic progressive disorder with diverse presentations, including dystonia, myoclonus, rigidity that does not respond to L-dopa, cortical sensory loss (alien hand), apraxia, dysphagia, and aphasia. Frontal executive impairment is common; calculation and visuo-spatial skills are also commonly impaired, but semantic memory is spared and episodic memory loss is less prominent than it is in AD.[5] Electroencephalogram (EEG) changes may be indicative and scans show asymmetrical frontoparietal and midbrain atrophy with third ventricular enlargement greater than that seen in Parkinson's disease.[6]

Multiple System Atrophy (Shy–Drager Syndrome)

Multiple system atrophy is probably more common than was previously thought; estimates have put the prevalence at 16.4 per 100,000 population.[7] It is a neurodegenerative disorder with tauopathy. There is usually cerebellar (olivopontine) and striatonigral degeneration. There is progressive autonomic system failure, with orthostatic hypotension causing light-headedness, constipation, urinary incontinence, inability to sweat, and impotence. Other features include severe dysarthria, falls, myoclonic jerks, disruption of the rapid eye movement phase of sleep, and visual problems. Parkinsonism may be present. Blood pressure monitoring and ophthalmology examination should be included. There are abnormal plasma and urinary levels of noradrenaline and its breakdown products. Magnetic resonance imaging (MRI) helps to distinguish it from progressive supranuclear palsy, as there is higher putaminal involvement, and vermian cerebellar atrophy differs from that of Parkinson's disease.[6] Non-specific treatments such as raising the head-end of the bed, increased dietary salt and fluid intake, and tube-feeding are useful. Alpha-adrenergic, salt-retaining steroids (with close monitoring), and L-dopa may be tried.

Amyotrophic Lateral Sclerosis/Motor Neurone Disease

Amyotrophic lateral sclerosis (ALS), also known as motor neurone disease (MND), has a prevalence of 5–7 per 100,000,[8] has multifactorial causation involving over-activity of the immune system. There is familial clustering, with dominant traits of variable penetrance and expressivity, and, rarely, recessive traits. Average age at presentation is mid-50s, but it can present in young adults. Life expectancy is about 3 years from diagnosis. Clinically, both upper and lower neuron signs are present, progressing to spasticity. Clinical signs include diminished fine motor coordination, bulbar signs, dysarthria, dysphagia, abnormal jaw jerk, and parkinsonism. There is an association between MND and FTD; and in MND patients without dementia there may be subtle frontal executive problems. Electromyography and nerve conduction studies are used to confirm denervation of at least three limbs; MRI may show hyperintensities in corticospinal tracts. Riluzole, a glutamate antagonist, has been shown to have a small effect on improving function and life expectancy, although this remains modest.[9]

Huntington's Disease

Huntington's disease has been discussed in Chapter 3.

Ataxias (Spinocerebellar Ataxias, Friedreich's Ataxia)

Ataxias are an hereditary group of disorders with a worldwide prevalence of 0.3–3 per 100,000 with regional variations. Friedreich's ataxia is the most common.[10] These disorders are inherited as autosomal dominant (spinocerebellar ataxia types 1, 2, and 3; olivopontocerebellar atrophy; Charcot–Marie–Tooth disease), recessive (Friedreich's ataxia, ataxia due to vitamin E deficiency), or, rarely, cross-linked.[11] There is degeneration of the cerebellum, brainstem, and spinal cord. Early symptoms include unsteady and clumsy motion, and fine incoordination. Progression is associated with pyramidal and extrapyramidal signs, peripheral neuropathy, slow saccadic eye movement (especially in spinocerebellar ataxia type 2), nystagmus, ophthalmoplegia, and optic atrophy. Dementia can be progressive and is mild to moderate in some subtypes (e.g. spinocerebellar ataxia type 2). Executive dysfunction and verbal memory deficits occur in others. Magnetic resonance imaging shows cerebellar atrophy; molecular genetic testing identifies the variant. Management includes genetic counselling, speech therapy, and physical rehabilitation. Ataxia with vitamin E deficiency requires lifelong vitamin E treatment. Benzodiazepines and propranolol may reduce tremor.

Polycystic Lipomembranous Osteodysplasia with Sclerosing Leukoencephalopathy (Nasu–Hakola Disease)

This is a very rare disorder of presenile dementia with bone cysts of global distribution. It results from mutations in genes *DAP12* and *TREM2*, which are needed for dendritic maturation. There is localized destruction of adipose tissue, cystic bone lesions, osteoporosis causing spontaneous fractures, and loss of brain white matter owing to progressive sclerosing leukoencephalopathy.[12] Clinically, pain occurs in the bony extremities by the third decade, followed by multiple fractures. By the fourth decade, neuropsychiatric symptoms develop, including profound progressive dementia, generalized seizures, and hypofrontality. Neurological examination shows upper motor neurone signs progressing to dyspraxia and dysphasia (similar to AD). Radiography of joints and EEG are useful. Brain scans show cortical atrophy and calcification of the basal ganglia. There is no known treatment.

Vascular Causes of Dementia

The vascular causes of dementia have been discussed in Chapter 2. It is worth noting that diffuse subcortical small vessel disease, which is common enough, includes what has previously been called Binswanger's disease, which presents with subcortical dementia ('cortical disconnection syndrome') where psychomotor slowness is the most characteristic feature, along with short-term memory impairment, and significant frontal executive and behavioural problems. Physical problems include parkinsonian features, urinary incontinence, and pseudobulbar palsy. Investigations should include electrocardiogram, blood pressure, blood glucose, and lipid monitoring. Treatment is with selective serotonin reuptake inhibitors for depression and anxiety, and atypical antipsychotics (with caution and only if necessary) for behavioural problems. Management of hypertension, diabetes, and arrhythmias may slow disease progression.

Also discussed in Chapter 2 was cerebral amyloid angiopathy, where cognitive impairment is common and may precede intracerebral haemorrhage. The progress of dementia varies but can be rapid. Raised intracranial pressure should be excluded. There is no specific treatment, but treating cardiovascular risk factors and evacuation of haematomata are indicated if required.

Cerebral autosomal dominant arteriopathy with subcortical infarcts and leukoencephalopathy (CADASIL) was also mentioned in Chapter 2, but is discussed further here.

CADASIL

With a prevalence of less than 1 per 100,000, cerebral CADASIL is a non-atherosclerotic, non-amyloid cerebral vasculopathy. Silent lacunar infarcts and white matter changes begin by the third decade, about 10 years before neurocognitive signs become apparent. Predominant multiple small deep ischaemic subcortical infarcts lead to VaD. There is mutation of the *NOTCH3* gene on chromosome 19. Clinical features include migraine with aura, recurrent transient ischaemic attacks, and subcortical dementia with late-stage urinary incontinence and supranuclear palsy.[13] Dementia is global and progressive, with executive dysfunction but with relative preservation of episodic memory. Mean age at onset is the mid-40s. Magnetic resonance imaging shows large areas of leukoencephalopathy with multiple subcortical lacunar infarcts (see imaging for young-onset dementia in Chapter 13). There is no specific treatment. Antiplatelet drugs and statins are used to prevent progression, but they are unlikely to be effective as this is mainly a disease of the arterial media.

Human Prion Diseases

The variety of human prion diseases is shown in Box 4.2.

Sporadic Creutzfeldt–Jakob Disease

Sporadic Creutzfeldt–Jakob disease (CJD) is the most common form of human prion disease. The worldwide average prevalence of CJD is around 0.1 cases per 100,000 persons; 85% of cases are of the sporadic type.[14,15] This is a poorly understood neurodegenerative disease in which accumulation of prion protein affects the grey matter, with neuronal loss, gliosis, and characteristic spongiform change. Although generally non-hereditary, in a minority of cases the disease is transmitted as an autosomal dominant form owing to mutation of the prion protein gene (*PRNP*) on chromosome 20. Most cases occur after the fifth decade. A prodromal period with fatigue, headaches, weight loss, and depression is often present. The classic symptom triad comprises rapidly progressing global dementia, myoclonus, and ataxia, along with progressive pyramidal, extra-pyramidal, and cerebellar dysfunctions with gait, visual (leading to blindness), and speech problems. Typically, 1–2 Hz triphasic periodic sharp-wave changes in EEG are present and cerebrospinal fluid (CSF) proteins are raised. Magnetic resonance imaging shows basal ganglia hyperintensities (characteristically in the putamen and caudate). Treatment is symptomatic. Sodium valproate and clonazepam may reduce the severity of movement disorders.

Iatrogenic CJD

A small fraction of all prion diseases result from inadvertent transmission of CJD between humans, mostly via medical procedures (e.g. contact with surgical instruments, corneal grafts). Spongiform changes and symptoms are similar to those of sporadic CJD, usually with rapid progression. The history of illness is vital for diagnosis. Investigations and treatment are as for sporadic CJD.

Box 4.2 Human prion diseases that cause dementia

- Creutzfeldt–Jakob disease
  - Sporadic
  - Iatrogenic
  - Variant
  - Familial
- Fatal familial insomnia
- Gerstmann–Straussler–Scheinker disease

Variant Creutzfeldt–Jakob Disease (Bovine Spongiform Encephalopathy)

Since being identified in 1996, as of 2013, 174 cases have been diagnosed in the UK.[16] In its *Annual Epidemiological Report for 2016*, the European Centre for Disease Prevention and Control reported as follows: 'For 2016, Italy and the UK each reported a single case of variant CJD. The overall mortality rate remains below 0.01 per 1 million population in this long post-epidemic tail.'[17] Variant CJD is caused by transmission of prion protein variants via food originating from cattle. It is distinct from the other types of CJD in its pathology. Individuals with the disease have diffuse vacuolation, with florid plaques that have a dense core and a halo of spongiform change. Early psychiatric symptoms include depression, personality changes, irritability, aggression, along with neurological deficits such as ataxia, chorea, myoclonus, dysaesthesias, and dementia.[18] Variant CJD occurs in young adults. Survival time after onset of disease is a year or so longer than in sporadic CJD. The pulvinar sign on MRI scan and positive tonsil biopsies for prion protein (negative in sporadic CJD) are helpful indicators. Electroencephalogram is often normal. Treatment is the same as for sporadic CJD.

Familial Creutzfeldt–Jakob Disease (Human Spongiform Encephalopathy)

Familial CJD accounts for 10–15% of CJD cases. It is unusually frequent in some ethnic groups (e.g. Libyan Jews). It has autosomal dominant inheritance due to *PRNP* mutations. Its pathological processes, symptoms, investigations, and treatments are similar to those for sporadic CJD, but age at onset is earlier (40–50 years, but as early as 20 for certain *PRNP* mutations).[15] Genetic testing may identify carriers and early/late-onset varieties, so genetic counselling is important.

Fatal Familial Insomnia

Fatal familial insomnia is extremely rare. It results from a polymorphism at codon 129 of the prion gene on chromosome 20. There is gliosis and neuronal loss mainly in the thalamus, inferior olives, and to a lesser extent in the cerebellum.[19] It is most common in the fourth decade (range 20–70 years). The illness results in progressive insomnia, along with movement disorders such as myoclonus, dysautonomia, inattention, confusion, psychosis (complex hallucination), and dementia (severe memory impairment with relatively preserved intellectual functioning). Death usually occurs within 12 months of onset. Genetic screening and counselling are available and treatment is supportive.

Gerstmann–Straussler–Scheinker Disease

This extremely rare disease results from heterogeneous mutations of a prion gene, associated with multicentric cerebellar amyloid plaque depositions and symptoms of olivopontocerebellar degeneration. There are typical (but fewer) spongiform changes, gliosis, and neuronal loss. Neurofibrillary tangles may be present. Onset is in the third and fourth decades. Clinical presentation varies, with initial signs of cerebellar dysfunction (e.g. clumsiness, ataxia, and dysmetria) progressing to rigidity, hypo-reflexia, and dementia. Extrapyramidal signs, gaze palsies, pseudobulbar palsies, and cortical blindness may occur.[2]

Death occurs 3–8 years after onset. Electroencephalogram may show characteristic changes and MRI may demonstrate mild cerebral and cerebellar atrophy. Post-mortem examination is confirmatory.

Infectious Causes of Dementia

There is a variety of infective agents that can cause or contribute to dementia, as summarized in Box 4.3.

Lyme Disease

The infective agent of Lyme disease is the spirochaete *Borrelia burgdorferi*, transmitted in tick bites. The disease occurs sporadically in parts of North America, Europe, and Asia, but true prevalence is unknown. Lyme disease typically causes a red rash (erythema migrans) which sometimes has a central clearing, is not itchy, and becomes visible 1–4 weeks after the tick bite. Lyme disease should be considered in patients presenting with subsequent fever, fatigue, muscle/joint pains, cognitive impairment, neurological symptoms (such as facial palsy), cardiac problems (e.g. heart block), or uveitis.[20] Lyme disease can be difficult to recognize as it causes many symptoms across multiple systems. Testing for Lyme disease should only occur if there is clinical suspicion, and should not be based on a tick bite alone. Treatment is with antibiotics, the choice of which depends on the symptoms.[20]

Neurosyphilis

Syphilis infection rates are low in Western Europe. Although no longer very prevalent, untreated neurosyphilis is an important cause of dementia, which can present more than a decade after initial infection.[21] Human immunodeficiency virus (HIV)-related neurosyphilis tends to have a poorer outcome. The infective agent is the spirochaete *Treponema pallidum*. There is diffuse meningovascular inflammation and parenchymal involvement, often associated with brain infarcts and focal neurological deficits. Later stages cause tabes dorsalis, a degeneration of the ascending fibres of the dorsal root ganglia affecting the posterior columns of the spinal cord. Clinical presentation varies, from asymptomatic neurosyphilis, acute meningitis, subacute or chronic meningovascular syphilis, tabes dorsalis to general paralysis of the insane with frontotemporal symptoms. Neuropsychiatric symptoms include apathy, irritability, elation, grandiosity, depression, personality changes,

---

Box 4.3 Infective causes of dementia

- Lyme disease
- Neurosyphilis
- Cerebral toxocariasis
- Neurocysticerosis
- Viral encephalitis
- HIV-related dementia
- Progressive multifocal leukoencephalopathy
- Subacute sclerosing panencephalitis

and psychosis (rarely), along with neurological signs such as coarse tremor, ataxia, hyper-reflexia, dysarthria, Argyll Robertson pupil, seizures, and late-stage spasticity. An accurate medical and treatment history is vital. Investigations include the Venereal Disease Research Laboratory (VDRL), Rapid Plasma Reagin, *T. pallidum* haemagglutination, and fluorescent treponemal antibody absorption tests; the last two have good reactivity to tertiary syphilis. Treatment is with high doses of intramuscular penicillin (over 10–14 days), doxycycline, or ceftriaxone. Jarisch–Herxheimer reaction may cause initial worsening of symptoms.

Cerebral Toxocariasis

Toxocara canis, the parasitic roundworm of dogs, can infect humans through the widespread dissemination of its ova in the environment. The larvae exhibit a predilection for the host's central nervous system (CNS), migrating to the brain as infection progresses. Clinically, it may mimic dementia, especially in elderly people. Blood and CSF eosinophilia and positive antibody titre are helpful; treatment with antihelmintic agents such as albendazole reverses cognitive impairment.[22]

Neurocysticerosis

The infective agent *Taenia solium* is acquired from eating infected meat. This is exceptional in the West but more common in low- and middle-income countries. Central nervous system presentation is very rare and potentially reversible. This may be clinically silent, but usually manifests with neurological symptoms such as headaches, focal signs, seizures, hemiparesis, psychiatric, and cognitive problems. Anaemia is common and stool examination may identify worms. Computed tomography or MRI demonstrates space-occupying lesions. Serological tests have low sensitivity and specificity. Treatment with antihelmintics (e.g. albendazole), antiepileptics (for controlling seizures), and steroids (for raised intracranial pressure) is useful.

Viral Encephalitis

Encephalitis is inflammation of the brain parenchyma and can be caused by a number of different microorganisms including viruses, and herpes viruses are the most common cause of viral encephalitis. Encephalitis can also be triggered by the immune system after the infection itself has subsided.

The main agents of viral encephalitis are herpes simplex virus types 1 and 2, Epstein–Barr virus, human herpes virus types 6 and 7 in immunocompetent hosts, and cytomegalovirus and varicellazoster virus in immunocompromised patients. The classic presentation of viral encephalitis includes fever, vomiting, headache, neurological signs, and altered consciousness. Presentations can, however, be more subtle and mimic psychiatric conditions or dementia, with behavioural changes and disorientation. All patients who have a fever and altered behaviour or consciousness should have investigations for a CNS infection. Treatment of viral encephalitis is with acyclovir as well as treatment of associated complications.[23]

HIV and Acquired Immune Deficiency Syndrome Dementia Complex

Incident rates of HIV-related dementia have fallen significantly in the West owing to antiretroviral therapy (ART), but the effect of longevity on cognition is still uncertain. Anti-retroviral therapy data show that dementia occurs in 5–15% of untreated patients.[24]

Opportunistic infections such as *Toxoplasma gondii*, cryptococcal meningitis, neurosyphilis, tuberculous meningitis, cytomegalovirus encephalitis, increased vascular risk factors, and tumours (e.g. lymphomas) can also contribute to a dementia syndrome. HIV can cause encephalitis, leukoencephalopathy, cerebral vasculitis, and neuronal damage, often leading to cortical atrophy with greater subcortical dementia associated with basal ganglia pathology. Acquired immune deficiency syndrome dementia complex occurs with a very low CD4 count (<200) and raised viral load. Cognitive impairment is usually global and moderately severe. Common associated symptoms are inattention, psychomotor slowing, dysexecutive syndrome, poor verbal memory (impaired recall but not recognition), psychosis, mood, and personality problems. Reversibility of symptoms has improved with newer ART drugs, which have greater CSF penetrability. Intravenous drug misuse is associated with a poorer prognosis.

Subacute Sclerosing Panencephalitis

Adult-onset subacute sclerosing panencephalitis is a very uncommon and delayed sequel to persistent measles infection. The prevalence is greatly reduced in countries with high vaccination levels. It leads to progressive and usually fatal encephalitis. There is astrogliosis, neuronal loss, and demyelination. Mean age at onset is in the early twenties, and the disease occurs predominantly in men. In adults it can mimic a degenerative dementia and usually presents many years after the initial infection, with death occurring within 1–3 years. Early changes may be subtle, with attention and behaviour problems. Characteristic features include dementia, seizures, myoclonus, visual problems, pyramidal, and extrapyramidal signs.[25] Subacute sclerosing panencephalitis should be suspected in young patients with dementia and myoclonus. Serum measles antibodies may be detected. There is no established therapy and treatment is supportive; antiepileptics may be useful to control seizures and intraventricular α-interferon appears to be effective.[25]

Further Exogenous and Endogenous Rare Causes of Dementia

We shall now describe other rare and unusual causes of dementia, which we categorize as being of 'exogenous' (toxicity, vitamin deficiency, brain damage) or 'endogenous' (endocrine and other organ failure, compromised metabolism, neoplasia, autoimmunity) origin. We shall start with exogenous factors (Box 4.4). As in the rest of this chapter, we have not attempted to describe purely medical matters in relation to the conditions we are discussing, whether to do with diagnosis or treatment, but have focued on the psychiatric issues, in particular those that relate to cognitive impairment and dementia. Specialist texts should be consulted for fuller discussion of these conditions and specialist clinical input would be required to manage them.

Toxicity

Heavy Metals

Lead

Dementia caused by heavy metals poisoning is most commonly caused by chronic exposure to lead. Causes of chronic lead poisoning include exposure in industrial workplaces, drinking water supplied through lead pipes, and accidental ingestion, for example by ingesting paint.[26]

Box 4.4 Exogenous causes of rare dementias

Toxicity

- Heavy metals, e.g. lead, mercury, arsenic, manganese
- Organophosphates and pesticides
- Medications, e.g. steroids, interferon
- Alcohol and recreational drugs

Vitamin Deficiency

- Thiamine
- Folate
- Vitamin B$_{12}$

Head Trauma and Diffuse Brain Damage

- Dementia pugilistica ('punch drunk' syndrome)
- Anoxic brain injury/delayed post-anoxic encephalopathy
- Head injury
- Normal-pressure hydrocephalus
- Chronic subdural haematoma

Inorganic forms of lead (e.g. in paint, as well as ground and surface water) typically affect the central and peripheral nervous systems and the haematopoietic, renal, gastrointestinal, and reproductive systems. The rarer organic forms (such as tetraethyl lead used in petroleum products) affect the CNS. Lead poisoning presents with a combination of gastrointestinal, haematological (lead interferes with haemoglobin synthesis), and neurological symptoms, including fatigue, depression, confusion, peripheral neuropathy, cognitive impairment, encephalopathy, and seizures. A grey or bluish black lead line may be visible at the gingival border.

Diagnosis is based on history (particularly occupational exposure), clinical features, and venous blood levels. A blood lead level >10 µg/dL is considered toxic. Normocytic or microcytic anaemia and non-specific red cell basophilic stippling on peripheral blood smears are common.

Treatment with chelating agents such as edentate calcium disodium, dimercaptosuccinic acid, or dimercaprol reduces the body stores of lead.[27]

Mercury, Arsenic, and Manganese

Dementia caused by chronic mercury poisoning presents in some industrial workers (mercury occurs in certain batteries, paints, and industrial wastes). Symptoms include peripheral neuropathy, ataxia, and fine tremor, progressing to cerebellar (intention) tremor, choreoathetosis, and dementia. Chronic arsenic ingestion causes confusion, memory loss, peripheral neuropathy, 'raindrop pigmentation' of the skin, and transverse white lines on the fingernails (Mae's lines). Treatment for both mercury and arsenic poisoning is chelation therapy.[26]

Manganese toxicity has been suggested as a cause of dementia.[28] In conjunction with genetic predisposition, manganese exposure might play an important role in causing parkinsonian disturbances, possibly enhancing physiological ageing of the brain.[29]

Aluminium

Aluminium toxicity (dialysis dementia syndrome) can occur secondary to dialysis using water containing aluminium. The syndrome has been mostly eliminated by the use of deionized water.

Untreated patients can develop progressive encephalopathy, confusion, memory loss, agitation, lethargy, myoclonic jerks, and stupor. Electroencephalogram shows non-specific generalized changes. Post-mortem studies show high brain aluminium content without neurofibrillary tangles or amyloid plaques.

A causal link between aluminium and AD had been suggested, but a direct relationship has not been found.[30]

Organophosphates and Pesticides

It has been suggested that environmental exposure to organophosphates and other pesticides is associated with various neurodegenerative processes.[31] There is mounting evidence that chronic moderate exposure to pesticides is neurotoxic and increases the risk of Parkinson's disease, ALS, mild cognitive impairment (similar to that described in the Gulf War syndrome), and dementia.[32]

Medications

Lithium

The relationship between lithium and dementia is unclear. Subjective complaints by those taking lithium of mental slowness are not uncommon but a longer-term effect remains controversial. One review found a subtle impairment of psychomotor speed and verbal memory but not of visuospatial ability, attention, or concentration.[33] Other studies have suggested that lithium in bipolar affective disorder has a protective effect against dementia, owing to its inhibition of AD pathogenesis.[34] Acute lithium toxicity can present with cognitive impairment. Investigations in patients on lithium showing cognitive impairment should include measurement of lithium level and routine blood, renal (to exclude chronic renal failure), and thyroid function tests. Adjunctive thyroid hormone may improve cognitive functioning as thyroid levels are restored.

Antipsychotics

There is much debate around the relationship between long-term antipsychotic use and cognitive impairment. Observational studies have revealed that long-term use of antipsychotics is associated with smaller brain volume and increased ventricular spaces. Moreover, reduced brain volume has been associated with reduced cognitive performance.[35] However, these are observational studies, and confounding by illness course and severity may well account for the association.

Anticholinergic Medication and Antidepressants

It has long been known that anticholinergic medication can impair cognitive function, causing confusion and disorientation. But this was considered a temporary phenomenon which would reverse as soon as the medication was stopped. Even so, anticholinergics have caused dilemmas for clinicians and patients for many years, the classic being the use of antimuscarinic medication (such as oxybutynin) for urinary incontinence or an overactive bladder in an older person with mild cognitive problems. Given a requirement for the long-term use of many such medications, the possibility of resulting increased confusion tips the risk–benefit scale in favour of not using the anticholinergics. But this seemingly condemns the patient to the indignities of, for example, urinary incontinence.

In recent years, however, evidence has accumulated that the resulting confusion may not be reversible and that anticholinergics are associated with dementia. In a study from the USA of 3,434 participants aged 65 years and over with no dementia at the start of the study, it was found that higher cumulative anticholinergic use over 10 years was associated with an increased risk of dementia.[36] In a UK study of 40,770 patients aged between 65 and 99 years with a diagnosis of dementia compared to 283,933 controls without dementia, the researchers observed a 'robust association' between some classes of anticholinergic drugs (in particular, antidepressants, urological, and antiparkinsonian drugs) and the incidence of future dementia.[37] A further UK study looked at exposure to anticholinergic drugs 'in 58,769 patients with a diagnosis of dementia and 225,574 controls 55 years or older matched by age, sex, general practice, and calendar time'.[38] They found a significant increase in the risk of dementia in those taking anticholinergic antidepressants, antiparkinsonian drugs, antipsychotics, bladder antimuscarinic drugs, and antiepileptic drugs.[38] These studies, therefore, caution against the prolonged use of anticholinergic drugs in middle age or older people because of the risk of dementia.

Moreover, there is a specific worry about antidepressant medication, which may not solely relate to their anticholinergic properties. In a meta-analysis of observational studies, researchers from Taiwan demonstrated 'that antidepressant use is significantly associated with an increased risk of developing dementia'.[39] The risk was highest for monoamine oxidase inhibitors (relative risk (RR) = 2.791), but was high for tricyclics too (RR=2.131), and was also raised for selective serotonin reuptake inhibitors (RR=1.75).[39] As in the case of any anticholinergic drugs, the message is not to avoid antidepressants altogether, but to use them judiciously.

Interferon

Interferon is used in immunotherapy for treatment of cancer and viral infections and has numerous neuropsychiatric side effects. Neurological effects of interferon alpha are more common in older age groups, in those treated with higher doses, in those with longer treatment duration, and when used in combination with other medications that affect cognition. Patients may exhibit mild to moderate symptoms of frontal subcortical brain dysfunction, including cognitive slowing, apathy, and executive dysfunction. There has been at least one report of a dementia-like syndrome which persisted.[40] Neurotoxicity may be mediated through neuroendocrine, neurotransmitter, or cytokine pathways. Neuroimaging studies show decreased prefrontal metabolism with interferon alpha therapy. Opiate antagonists could be helpful in treating the cognitive impairment.[41]

Steroids

Iatrogenic glucocorticosteroid dementia syndrome is often unrecognized but occurs in about 1 in 250 people treated with steroids and is more common in the elderly.[42] The syndrome may reflect steroid neurotoxicity. Glucocorticosteroids may affect hippocampal volume.[43] Clinically, there is transient impairment of attention, concentration, and memory. Cushingoid features such as facial puffiness and weight gain may be present. Diagnosis requires a history of glucocorticosteroid use and cortisol assay. Symptoms are usually reversible with discontinuation but in rare cases problems may initially worsen or persist.

Alcohol and Recreational Drugs

Alcohol and other recreational drugs can have psychological sequelae and these can include cognitive impairment and dementia. Chapters 6 and 7 discuss these issues.

Vitamin Deficiency

Niacin Deficiency (Pellagra)

Pellagra is mostly found in parts of the world with niacin- or tryptophan-poor diets. In the West, it is most common in alcoholism, Hartnup disease (a congenital defect in tryptophan absorption), and in carcinoid syndrome (increased conversion of hydroxytryptophan to serotonin).

The classic presentation includes dementia, haemorrhage, dermatitis (Casal collar – dermatitis around the neck), and diarrhoea. Myoclonus, ataxia, and seizures may also occur.[26]

The diagnosis is based on detection of low levels of the urinary metabolites 2-methylnicotinamide and 2-pyridone. Treatment is with oral niacin.

Folate Deficiency

Congenital errors of folate transport and metabolism produce developmental delay, cognitive deterioration, motor and gait abnormality, seizures, vascular and demyelinating changes. Deficiency is caused by inadequate intake, increased requirements, malabsorption, and impaired metabolism. Folate and vitamin B_{12} deficiency both lead to impaired methylation and accumulation of homocysteine. In AD, high plasma homocysteine levels are associated with more rapid atrophy of the medial temporal lobes.[44]

Patients may present with peripheral neuropathy, depression, apathy, withdrawal, and mild to moderate dementia. Investigations show megaloblastic anaemia, low serum and CSF folate, and raised homocysteine. Neuropsychological symptoms respond much more slowly to folate replacement than do haematological symptoms.

Vitamin B_{12} Deficiency

Vitamin B_{12} deficiency can be caused by inadequate intake (e.g. in the vegan diet), malabsorption due to defective release of gastric intrinsic factor (gastric achlorhydria, partial gastrectomy), inadequate production of intrinsic factor (pernicious anaemia, total gastrectomy), disorders of the terminal ileum (tropical and non-tropical spruce, intestinal resection), competition for cobalamin (fish tapeworm, 'blind loop' syndrome), drugs (colchicines, neomycin), and Crohn's disease. The mechanism of neurological damage may be related to S-adenosylmethionine deficiency. Damage to cerebral myelinated fibres may also cause dementia. Neurological complications include sensory neuropathy (more common in the upper limbs), myelopathy, optic nerve dysfunction, positive Romberg's test, and altered cognition. Spinal cord involvement may occur. Blood tests may show low vitamin B_{12} level, megaloblastic anaemia, macrocytosis, and target cells, but neurological dysfunction can occur with normal haematological parameters.[26]

Early treatment with parenteral vitamin B_{12} stops progression but rarely reverses advanced damage to the nervous system. In cases of both folate and vitamin B_{12} deficiencies, the latter should be replaced first, to prevent precipitation of subacute combined degeneration of the spinal cord.

Head Trauma and Diffuse Brain Damage

Dementia Pugilistica ('Punch Drunk' Syndrome)

Dementia pugilistica, caused by recurrent head trauma, is most commonly found in boxing, affecting about 20% of professional boxers. Symptoms are progressive and begin late (even many years after retirement). Severity depends on length of career and on the number of head injuries. There is profound loss of pigmented neurons in the substantia nigra, without Lewy bodies.[45] The extent of dementia is variable, with slow progression. The syndrome is characterized by extrapyramidal symptoms, ataxia, intention tremor, cognitive, and personality change, which help to differentiate it from AD. There is progressive social decline. Treatment with drugs for AD or parkinsonism may be useful.

Soccer and Dementia

There has for a long time been speculation and clinical concern that older soccer players have an increased prevalence of dementia, probably in connection with heading heavy leather footballs. A retrospective cohort study from Glasgow has shown that mortality from neurodegenerative disease was 3.45 times higher (but 5.07 times higher for AD) amongst former professional soccer players ($n = 7676$) in comparison with matched controls ($n = 23,028$).[46] The use of lighter footballs might affect the prevalence of dementia amongst soccer players in the future, but large prospective studies would provide more conclusive evidence.

Anoxic Brain Injury/Delayed Post-Anoxic Encephalopathy

Severe cerebral hypoxia is usually caused by carbon monoxide poisoning, cardiac or respiratory arrest, and attempted hanging. Most patients with carbon monoxide poisoning recover well, but 10–30% develop delayed neuropsychiatric sequelae such as cognitive and personality changes, incontinence, dementia, and psychosis.[47] About 10% develop parkinsonism.[48] Memory impairment is probably due to hippocampal changes.[49] Computed tomography and diffusion weighted MRI show low density in the cerebral white matter and lesions in the globus pallidus.

Head Injury

Acute head injury with loss of consciousness can cause anterograde and retrograde amnesia. The relationship between remote head injury and dementia is unclear. One large study found that mild head trauma did not increase the risk of dementia or AD in older people.[50] However, other studies have suggested that previous head trauma is associated with risk of developing AD.[45]

Normal-Pressure Hydrocephalus

Normal-pressure hydrocephalus is seen in 6–10% of all dementia patients.[1] The pathophysiology is unclear but there is a possible cerebrovascular role. The classic triad includes: (a) early gait disturbance characterized by proximal weakness and short, shuffling, broad-based gait; (b) urinary incontinence; and (c) dementia – predominantly subcortical with frontal lobe involvement in later stages, characterized by prominent memory loss and bradyphrenia. Cortical features such as aphasia, agnosia, and apraxia are generally absent. Computed tomography or MRI shows ventricular enlargement, a prominent flow void in the aqueduct and third ventricle (the 'jet sign'), and rounding of the frontal horns. In 50% of cases, EEG shows beta oscillations with bursts of monorhythmic bilateral theta and delta waves. Lumbar puncture to measure CSF pressure is considered the diagnostic gold standard, but it has a high incidence of false negatives. Insertion of a ventriculoperitoneal shunt improves symptoms in 30–40% of patients, but with a relatively high incidence of complications such as strokes or seizures.

Chronic Subdural Haematoma

Chronic subdural haematoma is a common treatable cause of dementia, with an annual population prevalence of between 1.2 and 7.3 per 100,000 and a male to female ratio of 2:1.[51] Older individuals with cerebral atrophy are vulnerable and 25–50% of patients have no identifiable history of head trauma (spontaneous or idiopathic subdural haematoma). It may be that blockages to dural lymphatic drainage play a role in the pathogenesis of cognitive impairment in connection with chronic subdural haematoma.[52] Risk factors for chronic subdural haematoma include chronic alcoholism, epilepsy, arachnoid cyst, coagulopathy, anticoagulation therapy, and cardiovascular disease. Clinical presentation is often insidious, with altered consciousness, focal neurological deficits (subtle changes to hemiparesis), headache, gait and balance abnormalities, and seizures. Brain scans help diagnosis. Treatment is by surgical evacuation. Patients with chronic alcoholism and pneumocephalus have poor outcomes.

We shall now examine various 'endogenous' causes of rare dementias (Box 4.5).

Endocrine and Other Organ Failure

Hypothyroidism or Raised Thyroxine

Hypothyroidism is up to six times more common in women than in men.[53] Its clinical features include: cold, thickened skin; malar flush; coarse, brittle hair; cerebellar signs; slowed reflexes; bradycardia; deafness; and carpal tunnel syndrome. Memory impairment can progress from mild cognitive blunting to severe dementia. Depression, psychosis, apathy, irritability, and fatigue are common. Proximal myopathy, respiratory problems, cardiac failure, cardiac arrhythmia, and coma are serious complications. Other findings include elevated cholesterol and autoantibodies in Hashimoto's thyroiditis. ECG may show cardiomegaly. Treatment is with thyroid replacement (levothyroxine) and may reverse the cognitive impairment.

On the other hand, higher total and free thyroxine levels have been associated with an increased risk of dementia and AD in particular; and higher total thyroxine levels at autopsy have been associated with higher numbers of plaques and tangles (the neuropathological hallmarks of AD) in the brain.[54]

Hyperparathyroidism

Primary hyperparathyroidism is caused by solitary adenomas (80%) or as part of multiple endocrine neoplasia. In people over 60 years of age the incidence of primary hyperparathyroidism may be as high as 0.2%, with a prevalence of 1.0% or greater in this elderly

---

Box 4.5 Endogenous causes of rare dementias

Endocrine and Other Organ Failure
- Hypothyroidism
- Hyperparathyroidism
- Hypoparathyroidism/hypocalcaemia
- Diabetes mellitus
- Renal encephalopathy
- Hepatic encephalopathy

Metabolic and Other Conditions
- Wilson's disease (hepatolenticular degeneration)
- Hemochromatosis
- Metachromatic leukodystrophy
- Adrenoleukodystrophy/ adrenomyeloneuropathy
- Pantothenate kinase-associated neurodegeneration (PKAN), formerly Hallervorden–Spatz syndrome
- Neuroacanthocytosis
- Cerebral lipidoses – adult variant

Neoplasms and Paraneoplastic Disorder
- Including paraneoplastic limbic encephalitis

Inflammatory/Autoimmune Causes
- Autoimmune encephalitis
- Multiple sclerosis
- Neurosarcoidosis
- Vasculitis

---

population.[55] The incidence peaks between the third and fifth decades. Patients present with recurrent renal calculi, peptic ulcers, and extensive bone resorption. Over half of those affected present with neuropsychiatric manifestations such as depression, apathy, and cognitive impairment. Some develop psychosis, stupor, and delirium. A high level of corrected serum calcium with elevated parathyroid hormone supports the diagnosis. A technetium (^{99m}Tc) sestamibi scan can reveal an adenoma. Treatment is either medical or surgical. Some of the severe neuropsychiatric manifestations may be reversed by parathyroidectomy.

Hypoparathyroidism/Hypocalcaemia

Hypoparathyroidism may be idiopathic, hereditary, or acquired. Hypocalcaemia is caused by hypoparathyroidism, chronic renal failure, vitamin D deficiency, and hypomagnesaemia. Clinical manifestations are irritability, anxiety, psychosis, dementia, hallucinations, depression, confusion, and neuromuscular irritability. Treatment involves replacement of vitamin D or calcitriol with oral calcium.

Diabetes Mellitus

In patients with young-onset diabetes and those with poor glycaemic control, the presence of micro- and macrovascular disease may cause early cognitive deficits. Hypertension, dyslipidaemia, and obesity are associated with diabetes and increase the risk of dementia. A meta-analysis of longitudinal studies showed that diabetes was a risk factor for dementia of any type (RR = 1.51), but including AD (RR = 1.46) and VaD (RR = 2.48), as well as mild cognitive impairment (RR = 1.21).[56] The most common impairments are in verbal memory, attention, semantic and language functions, and processing speed, with relatively preserved visuospatial functioning.[57] Cognitive deficits are also observed in older, untreated patients but improve with glycaemic control.

Renal Encephalopathy

Dementia due to renal failure usually has potentially reversible causes. These include uraemic encephalopathy with parathyroid hormone dysfunction, dialysis dementia syndrome, and dialysis-associated encephalopathy. The treatment of renal encephalopathy requires addressing any hypertension, diabetes, lipid problems, acidosis, and hyperkalaemia, in a specialist setting. Dialysis may reverse uraemic encephalopathy, but can be associated with dementia.[58]

Hepatic Encephalopathy

Chronic neuropsychiatric conditions are seen in cirrhosis, portal hypertension, fulminant hepatic failure, and following portosystemic shunt procedures. This potentially reversible condition is caused by accumulation of toxic metabolites such as ammonia, which bypass the liver and alter brain neurotransmitter balance. Acute onset is often precipitated by high dietary protein intake, gastrointestinal haemorrhage, constipation, infection, electrolyte imbalance, shunting procedures, and drugs (such as CNS depressants). Neurological signs include poor attention, restlessness, and lethargy, which progress to delirium, stupor, seizures, and coma. There may be a chronic progressive course with cognitive blunting and confusional states.[1] Physical signs include asterixis, foetor hepaticus, constructional apraxia, and decreased mental ability. Diagnosis is clinical, supported by routine biochemistry. An EEG will show decreased alpha and increased delta waves.

Management consists of restricting protein intake, correcting electrolyte imbalances, and treating the underlying cause. Lactulose (which helps excrete ammonia) and rifaximin (an antibiotic to stop the growth of certain bacteria in the intestinal system) can induce transient improvement. A liver transplant may be needed.

Metabolic and Other Conditions

Wilson's Disease

Wilson's disease has a population prevalence of 3.3/100,000. Cognitive impairment is rare and ranges in severity from mild to moderate.[59] It is an autosomal recessive disorder caused by mutations of the copper-transporting adenosine triphosphatase (ATPase) gene on chromosome 13q. There is abnormal copper deposition in the liver (causing cirrhotic changes), brain (lenticular nuclei), kidneys, and corneas (Kayser–Fleischer rings), caused by impaired biliary copper excretion. Onset usually occurs between 5 and 30 years of age and rarely after middle age. Affect, behaviour, and personality abnormalities are common clinical features. Neurological features include orofacial dystonia, dysarthria, dysphagia, dystonic postures, tremor, and cognitive impairment.

Diagnosis is based on neurological and ophthalmological examination, ceruloplasmin levels, and liver function abnormality and is confirmed by liver biopsy. Brain imaging may indicate enlarged ventricles with cortical and brainstem atrophy in addition to T_2 hyperintensities in the basal ganglia.

Treatment is with the copper-chelating agent penicillamine.

Haemochromatosis

Haemochromatosis is an inherited condition caused by the mutation of the *HFE* gene, which results in high levels of iron. Haemochromatosis typically affects the liver; increasingly, however, it has been observed that it can cause cognitive impairment. It should be suspected in patients presenting with fatigue, arthralgia, impotence, late-onset diabetes, or signs of liver disease.

Metachromatic Leukodystrophy

Metachromatic leukodystrophy is a demyelinating storage disease caused by deficiency of the lysosomal enzyme arylsulfatase A (ARSA). It is an autosomal recessive inherited metabolic disease with late juvenile and adult onset. Clinical presentation includes personality and behavioural changes, gradual loss of motor skills, optic atrophy, seizures, cognitive deficits, and dementia.[60] Non-specific white matter lesions are evident on MRI. Cerebrospinal fluid proteins may be increased and ARSA enzyme activity may be decreased in leukocytes or in cultured skin fibroblasts. Deoxyribonucleic acid mutation analysis can be undertaken. Treatment is symptomatic and supportive.

Adrenoleukodystrophy and Adrenomyeloneuropathy

This disorder affects 1/20,000 males either as cerebral adrenoleukodystrophy in children or as adrenomyeloneuropathy in adults. The neonatal form is autosomal recessive, whereas the adult form is X-linked. The defect lies in the gene *ABCD1*. There is an accumulation of very long-chain saturated fatty acids such as hexacosanoate in lipid-containing tissue in the brain, with characteristic lamellar inclusions in the Schwann cells of the CNS and the adrenal cortex. These lead to non-inflammatory axonopathy involving the spinal cord.

Adrenomyeloneuropathy is the milder form, with onset at 15–30 years of age and a progressive course. It affects the brain, spinal cord, adrenal glands, and testes. Clinical features include spastic paraparesis, ataxia and sensory loss of lower limbs, language difficulties, and adrenal insufficiency. Rarely, focal signs and memory problems may mimic AD. Treatment is symptomatic with adrenal hormone replacement and haematopoietic stem cell transplantation. Psychological support and physiotherapy are helpful.

Pantothenate Kinase-Associated Neurodegeneration, Formerly Hallervorden–Spatz Syndrome

There are about 100 published cases of this condition.[1] Familial occurrences are more common, with autosomal recessive inheritance. There is neuroaxonal dystrophy and iron accumulation in the basal ganglia. Common clinical features include dementia with early personality changes. Extrapyramidal symptoms with motor dysfunctions, gait disorder, hypotonia, rigidity, nystagmus, optic atrophy, abnormal movements, and seizures may occur. Duration of illness can vary widely. A CSF analysis may show increased non-protein-bound iron. Electromyography shows rigidospasticity (fluctuating rigidity) and EEG shows generalized slowing with spikes and sharp waves. Brain scans show generalized cortical atrophy with prominent basal ganglion, brainstem, and cerebellar atrophy. Positron emission tomography shows hypoperfusion of the head of the caudate nucleus, pons, and cerebellum. Levodopa and dopamine agonists may provide symptomatic relief.

Neuroacanthocytosis

This is a group of phenotypically and genetically heterogeneous disorders. Neuroacanthocytosis occurs through autosomal dominant, autosomal recessive, or X-linked inheritance or, in sporadic cases, with recessive mutations in the chorein gene on chromosome 9 or X-linked mutation.[61] There may be choreiform or parkinsonian features, neuropathy, muscle wasting, dementia, and acanthocytosis. Depression, personality changes, and paranoia may occur. Symptoms may progress slowly. At least half of patients develop subcortical dementia with executive and visuospatial difficulties and anomia in later stages. Onset is usually in early middle age. Blood tests show acanthocytes and serum creatinine kinase may be abnormal. Computed tomography often shows caudate or generalized atrophy; T_2-weighted MRI may show abnormal signals from basal ganglia. No specific treatment exists for the primary disease. Antipsychotics or tetrabenazine may be useful for chorea.

Cerebral Lipidoses – Adult Variant

Cerebral lipidoses are a group of lysosomal storage diseases, with X-linked or autosomal recessive transmission. Rare adult forms may cause cognitive impairment. Tay–Sachs disease (also known as hexosaminidase A deficiency) and Sandhoff disease (Jatzkewitz–Pilz syndrome, hexosaminidase A and B deficiency) are caused by mutation in the *HEXA* or *HEXB* genes on chromosome 15. They present with progressive lower limb weakness, cerebellar atrophy, denervation MND, and dementia.

Chronic type I (non-neuropathic) Gaucher disease, which rarely affects adults, can lead to dementia, spastic paraplegia, seizures, behavioural problems, and psychosis. Types C and D, Niemann–Pick disease (sphingomyelin lipidosis, sphingomyelinase deficiency), present with neurological and cognitive impairment owing to accumulation of sphingomyelin. No established treatment is available for improving cognitive impairment, although enzyme replacement (in Gaucher disease) and a low-cholesterol diet (in Niemann–Pick disease) have been tried.

Neoplasms and Paraneoplastic Disorder

Cerebral tumours are a rare cause of dementia. The most prevalent are multiple metastases and temporal gliomas. Clinical features are related to the site of the tumour, its extent, and progress. Paraneoplastic symptoms are caused by immune changes as a result of malignancy rather than as a local effect of the cancer itself.[62] Paraneoplastic symptoms have a subacute progression which may precede the diagnosis of malignancy. Paraneoplastic limbic encephalitis leads to personality changes, irritability, memory loss (anterograde or retrograde), seizures, altered consciousness, and focal deficits. Brainstem involvement causes diplopia, gaze abnormalities, facial numbness, dysarthria, and dysphagia. Cerebellar symptoms include problems with balance, gait, and ataxia. Underlying primary malignancy such as lung, testicular, or breast carcinomas need to be excluded. Routine blood tests may be abnormal. Testing for tumour markers such as carcinoembryonic antigen, cancer antigen 125, and prostate-specific antigen should be considered. The autoantibody involved can give rise to clinical suspicion regarding where the cancer may originate, for example anti-NMDAR (*N*-methyl D-aspartate receptor) antibodies are associated with teratomas of the ovaries. Brain MRI may show temporal lobe abnormalities but is non-specific. Inflammatory cells and negative cytology are apparent on lumbar puncture. Treatment of the underlying cancer will not necessarily lead to improvement of symptoms. Specific immunosuppressive therapies have been tried.[63]

Inflammatory/Autoimmune Causes

Inflammatory and autoimmune disorders affecting the CNS have various aetiologies. Some of the rare heritable causes of cognitive impairment and dementia are listed in Box 4.5.

Autoimmune Limbic Encephalitis

More recently it was discovered that limbic encephalitis is not only a paraneoplastic phenomenon, it has also been associated with autoimmunity without the presence of cancer. Voltage-gated potassium channel (VGKC) and NMDA antibodies are most commonly associated with autoimmune limbic encephalitis. Antibodies target proteins associated with particular ion channels, such as leucine-rich glioma inactivated protein 1 (LGI1) and contactin-associated protein-like 2 receptor (CASPR2), which are both associated with the VGKC. When LGI1 is affected, the clinical picture tends to be one of seizures (particularly faciobrachial), hyponatraemia, and cognitive impairment. When CASPR2 is targeted the symptoms of autonomic disturbance, insomnia, and amnesia predominate.[64] Diagnosis is confirmed by the detection of autoantibodies in the blood and CSF, which is more specific than blood alone. EEGs are often abnormal and there may be temporal T2 high signal on MRI.

Multiple Sclerosis

Over half of people with multiple sclerosis (MS) develop some cognitive impairment, especially in the progressive forms. Multiple sclerosis is a multifocal demyelinating disorder usually characterized by periods of relapse and remission, although it can have a progressive pattern. It is more common in women than in men. Depression is common and the risk of suicide is increased compared to the general population.[65] Psychosis is uncommon in MS and is distinct from schizophrenia as it has a later age at onset, quicker resolution, fewer relapses, better response to treatment, and a better prognosis.[66] Psychosis may be secondary to steroid treatment. Cognitive deficits may precede other symptoms, progress slowly, and can be severe. The main cognitive decline occurs in attention, concentration, verbal fluency, comprehension, naming, executive functioning, and memory. Magnetic resonance imaging reveals brain atrophy and ventricle enlargement. Donepezil therapy for memory and cognitive dysfunction has undergone trials with some positive results.[67]

Neurosarcoidosis

This multisystemic granulomatous disease principally affects the lungs. It can also involve the CNS, causing cranial nerve palsies (e.g. facial palsy), delirium, seizures, and peripheral neuropathy. It can occur at any age, but is most common in young adults. Women and people from certain ethnic groups are most likely to be affected (e.g. African Americans). Around 10% of patients have cognitive, psychotic, and neuropsychiatric complications.[68] Multiple white matter lesions are evident on MRI. A history of sarcoidosis, chest X-ray, and nerve biopsy can confirm the diagnosis.

Systemic and CNS Vasculitis

Vasculitis is a systemic disorder of heterogeneous origin. It commonly involves the vertebral and basilar arteries (posterior circulation) and may lead to cerebellar and cerebral infarction. The cause can be primary, for example giant cell arteritis or Takayasu's arteritis (inflammation of the aorta); secondary, for example rheumatoid disease or infections (hepatitis B, HIV); or the cause can be iatrogenic from drugs such as sulfonamides.

Vasculitis may present with fever, night sweats, and MS-like symptoms with a relapsing–remitting course. Severe headaches are common. Optic neuropathy, mood problems, personality changes, multifocal/focal neurological deficits, or rapidly progressive dementia may occur. Contrast angiography and MRI can be helpful but are non-specific.[69] Immunotherapy achieves a partial response of cognitive and psychiatric features.

Coeliac Disease (Non-Tropical Sprue)

About 10% of people with coeliac disease experience CNS complications, but there are few recorded cases of dementia, mostly in case series.[70, 71] Coeliac disease is an auto-immune disease with genetic preponderance. There may be a higher prevalence of gluten sensitivity in some genetic neurodegenerative disorders. Chronic immune-mediated inflammation, lymphocytic infiltration, or vasculitis of the CNS leads to irreversible neuronal, glial, or axonal damage. Gastrointestinal symptoms include weight loss, steatorrhoea, and diarrhoea (malabsorption syndrome). Neurological complications include migraine, chorea, encephalopathy, cerebellar ataxia, peripheral neuropathy, symptoms similar to those of Guillain–Barré syndrome, epilepsy, and depression. Dementia is of a frontosubcortical type with rapid onset and progression. It may be associated with macrocytic anaemia, leukocytosis, and raised antigliadin/antiganglioside positive antibodies. Hyperintensities on T_2-weighted MRI scans and diffuse slowing on EEG are non-specific findings. Neurological symptoms may be difficult to stabilize but depression may respond to pyridoxine (vitamin B_6) treatment.

Behçet Disease

The aetiology of Behçet disease is unknown. It is a chronic, relapsing, multisystemic inflammatory disorder. Neurological complications include encephalopathy, sterile meningoencephalitis, cranial neuropathies, cortical motor, and sensory deficits. Chronic, progressive involvement of the CNS occurs in 10–20% of patients with Behçet disease, particularly males in whom the disease began at an early age. In the terminal stage of the disease, 3–6% of patients develop dementia.[72] When present, dementia is insidious with slow progression.[73] The classical triad of symptoms includes (a) oral aphthous ulcerations, (b) genital ulcerations, and (c) ocular lesions (uveitis). There can be underlying vasculitis, with arthritis, thrombophlebitis, erythema nodosum, acneiform nodules, and papulopustular lesions. Depression, pseudobulbar palsy (brainstem involvement), and parkinsonism may be present. Cerebral venous sinus thrombosis is a serious complication. Computed tomography shows single- or multiple-density subcortical and brainstem lesions.

The acute phase of neurological involvement responds well to high-dose systemic corticosteroids, which can be supplemented with cytotoxic agents (cyclophosphamide, chlorambucil, and methotrexate). In contrast, chronic progressive CNS disease responds poorly to treatment. In one study, 20% of patients with chronic neurological involvement died within 7 years.[74]

Systemic Lupus Erythematosus

Systemic lupus erythematosus is a multisystemic autoimmune disorder that has direct effects on the CNS. These can be caused by autoantibodies (antiphospholipid, antiribosomal-P protein autoantibodies), cytokines, and the long-term side effects of glucocorticosteroids. The disease is more common in women. Clinical features include fever, malaise, maculopapular rash, photosensitivity, oral ulcers, and non-erosive arthritis. Common complications include pneumonitis, pleurisy, pericarditis, endocarditis, and glomerulonephritis. Between 30% and 70% of patients have neuropsychiatric symptoms such as psychosis, depression, personality changes, anxiety, seizures, chorea, neuropathies, stroke, and cognitive changes. Cognitive effects are usually subtle.[75]

If suspected, encephalopathy should be excluded. Non-specific cerebral atrophy, focal hyperintensities, and widespread vasculopathy may be detected on MRI. Treatment includes corticosteroids with or without immunosuppressive drugs. Lupus-inducing psychotropic drugs such as chlorpromazine, carbamazepine, and lithium should be avoided.

Sjögren Syndrome

This is an autoimmune disorder which targets moisture-producing glands, causing mouth and eye dryness. It is often associated with other autoimmune disorders, such as rheumatoid arthritis, systemic lupus erythematosus, and scleroderma. It occurs more commonly in women. Cognitive impairment can occur but is rare and subtle. General treatments include artificial tears, eye ointment (methylcellulose), steroids, and immunosuppressive drugs.[76]

Conclusion: The Psychiatrist's Role

Often, rare dementias present initially to neurologists, especially in younger patients with physical symptoms. However, psychiatric teams may be involved at various stages of management of the illness. A significant proportion of patients present to psychiatry services with cognitive difficulties or other psychiatric symptoms. Others are referred to psychiatrists after diagnosis for the management of psychological comorbidities, such as mood, psychotic, or behavioural disturbances. With the introduction of young-onset dementia services (see Chapter 3), many patients may now be directly referred to these teams. A better understanding of the epidemiology and presentation of the numerous rarer forms would improve detection and management.

It is important that patients presenting with dementia, particularly at a younger age than usual, receive an appropriate work up. Unless diagnosed early, these individuals are at risk of losing out on treatment that could alleviate, control, or even reverse some of the symptoms. Clues to the underlying cause of a rare dementia may be sparse, although a family history may point to an inherited condition (Box 4.6). A comprehensive clinical examination with appropriate investigations will help diagnosis, and seeking a specialist opinion from a physician or neurologist is highly recommended for atypical presentations.

Although psychiatrists might have theoretical knowledge of rare dementias, they are unlikely to encounter many cases in day-to-day practice. We hope that the overview of causes and estimated prevalence rates (Table 4.1) presented in this chapter will guide

---

Box 4.6 Autosomal inheritance of rare dementias

Autosomal Dominant

- Familial Alzheimer's disease
- Frontotemporal lobar degenerations
- Spinocerebellar atrophy types 1, 2, and 3
- Olivopontocerebellar atrophy and Charcot–Marie–Tooth disease
- Huntington's disease
- Amyotrophic lateral sclerosis[a]
- Motor neurone disease[a]
- CADASIL
- Sporadic Creutzfeldt–Jakob disease
- Familial Creutzfeldt–Jakob disease
- Neuroacanthocytosis
- Di George syndrome

Autosomal Recessive

- PLOSL
- Friedreich ataxia and ataxia with vitamin E deficiency
- Amyotrophic lateral sclerosis[a]
- Motor neurone disease[a]
- Wilson's disease
- Neuroacanthocytosis
- Metachromatic leukodystrophy
- Adrenoleukodystrophy (neonates)
- PKAN (formerly Hallervorden–Spatz syndrome)

X-linked

- Rare ataxias
- Neuroacanthocytosis
- Adrenoleukodystrophy (males only)

> CADASIL, cerebral autosomal dominant arteriopathy with subcortical infarcts and leukoencephalopathy; NBIA1, neurodegeneration with brain iron accumulation type-1; PLOSL, polycystic lipomembranous osteodysplasia with sclerosing leukoencephalopathy.

a. Some familial clustering with dominant traits of variable penetrance that rarely occurs with recessive traits.

Table 4.1 Population prevalence of rare dementias

Prevalence unknown	<1 case per 100,000	1–10 cases per 100,000	>10 cases per 100,000
Lyme disease	Polycystic lipomembranous osteodysplasia with sclerosing leukoencephalopathy	Familial Alzheimer's disease	Multiple system atrophy[a]
Folate deficiency		Progressive supranuclear palsy	Frontotemporal lobar degenerations
Vitamin B_{12} deficiency		Corticobasal degeneration	
Vasculitis	Sporadic Creutzfeldt–Jakob disease	Amyotrophic lateral sclerosis	Pure hippocampal sclerosis
Sjögren syndrome		Huntington's disease	Primary progressive aphasia
Dementia pugilistica (more common in boxers)	Iatrogenic Creutzfeldt–Jakob disease	Spinocerebellar ataxias[a]	Multiple sclerosis (rate tends to increase with latitude.[a] With
Chronic subdural haematoma	New-variant Creutzfeldt–Jakob disease	Friedreich ataxia	higher rates in temperate zones and the Western hemisphere
Paraneoplastic disorder	Familial Creutzfeldt–Jakob disease	CADASIL	(e.g. Northern Europe), but there
Anoxic brain injury	Neurosyphilis	Wilson's disease	are many exceptions to this
	Herpes simplex virus encephalitis	Metachromatic leukodystrophy	gradient)
		Adrenoleukodystrophy	
		Adrenomyeloneuropathy	

[a] Prevalence varies depending on study: highest published prevalence used in this table.

clinicians in prioritizing investigations, planning treatment, and making referrals to appropriate medical colleagues.

Acknowledgements

We thank Linda Liu, librarian at Central Middlesex Hospital Library, for her assistance. We also acknowledge the input of Dr Elena Ros to one of the original articles combined in this chapter.[76] Unfortunately, it was not possible to contact her during the preparation of the chapter, for which we apologize.

For information, the original papers on which this chapter is based were:

Gupta S, Fiertag O, Warner J. Rare and unusual dementias. *Adv Psychiatr Treat* 2009; **15**: 364–371.

and

Gupta S, Fiertag O, Thanulingam T et al. Further rare and unusual dementias. *Adv Psychiatr Treat* 2012; **18**: 67–77.

References

1. Alzheimer Europe. *Rare Forms of Dementia.* Last accessed on 27 September 2019 via: www.alzheimer-europe.org/Dementia/Other-forms-of-dementia.

2. Sampson EL, Warren JD, Rossor MN. Young onset dementia. *Postgrad Med J* 2004; **80**: 125–139.

3. Jellinger K, Ala TA, Beh GO et al. Pure hippocampal sclerosis: a rare cause of dementia mimicking Alzheimer's disease. *Neurology* 2000; **55**: 735–742.

4. Honig LS, Scarmeas N, Hatanpaa KJ et al. Most cases of dementia with hippocampal sclerosis may represent frontotemporal dementia. *Neurology* 2005; **64**: 1102.

5. Mahapatra RK, Edwards MJ, Schott JM, Bhatia KP. Corticobasal degeneration. *Lancet Neurol* 2004; **3**: 736–743.

6. Yekhlef F, Ballan G, Macia F et al. Routine MRI for the differential diagnosis of Parkinson's disease, MSA, PSP, and CBD. *J Neural Transm* 2003; **110**: 151–169.

7. Rehman HU. Multiple system atrophy. *Postgrad Med J* 2001; **77**: 379–382.

8. McDermott CJ, Shaw PJ. Diagnosis and management of motor neurone disease. *BMJ* 2008; **336**: 658–662.

9. Dharmadasa T, Kiernan M. Riluzole, disease stage and survival in ALS. *Lancet Neurol* 2018; **17**: 385–386. http://dx.doi.org/10.1016/S1474-4422(18)30091-7

10. van de Warrenburg BPC, Verschuuren-Bemelmans CC, Scheffer H et al. Spinocerebellar ataxias in the Netherlands: prevalence and age at onset variance analysis. *Neurology* 2002; **58**: 702–708.

11. Schöls P, Bauer T, Schmidt T et al. Autosomal dominant cerebellar ataxias: clinical features, genetics, and pathogenesis. *Lancet Neurol* 2004; **3**: 291–304.

12. Kondo T, Takahashi K, Kohara M et al. Heterogeneity of presenile dementia with bone cysts (Nasu–Hakola disease): Three genetic forms. *Neurology* 2002; **59**: 1105–1107.

13. Di Donato I, Silvia Bianchi S, De Stefano N. Cerebral Autosomal Dominant Arteriopathy with Subcortical Infarcts and Leukoencephalopathy (CADASIL) as a model of small vessel disease: update on clinical, diagnostic, and management aspects. *BMC Med* 2017; **15**: 41. DOI:10.1186/s12916-017-0778-8.

14. Prusiner SB. Human prion diseases. *Ann Neurol* 1994; **35**: 385–395.

15. World Health Organization. *WHO Manual for Surveillance of Human Transmissible Spongiform Encephalopathies.* WHO, 2003.

16. European Centre for Disease Prevention and Control. Facts about variant Creutzfeldt-Jakob disease, 2017. Last accessed on27 September 2019 via: https://ecdc.europa.eu/en/vcjd/facts

17. European Centre for Disease Prevention and Control. *Surveillance Report – Annual Epidemiological Report for 2016: Creutzfeldt–Jakob Disease.* Last accessed on27 September 2019 via: https://ecdc.europa.eu/sites/portal/files/documents/AER_for_2016-Creutzfeldt-Jakob-disease.pdf

18. Zeidler M, Johnstone EC, Bamber RW et al. New variant Creutzfeldt-Jakob disease: psychiatric features. *Lancet* 1997; **350**: 908–910.

19. Almeida OP, Flicker L, Lautenschlager NT. Uncommon causes of dementia: rare, but not marginal. *Int Psychogeriatr* 2005; **17**: 1–2.

20. National Institute for Health and Care Excellence. *NICE Guideline – Lyme disease.* NICE, 2018. Last accessed on 27 September 2019 via: www.nice.org.uk/guidance/ng95

21. Almeida OP, Lautenschlager NT. Dementia associated with infectious diseases. *Int Psychogeriatr* 2005; **17**: 65–77.

22. Richartz E, Buchkremer G. Cerebral toxocariasis: a rare cause of cognitive disorders. A contribution to differential dementia diagnosis. *Nervenarzt* 2002; **73**: 458–462.

23. Solomon T, Hart I, Beeching N. Viral encephalitis: a clinician's guide, *Brit Med J* 2007; **7**: 288–305.

24. Grant I, Sacktor N, McArthur J. HIV neurocognitive disorders. In *The Neurology of AIDS (2nd edn)* (eds. HE Gendelman, I Grant, IP Everall, SA Lipton, S Swindells): 357–373. Oxford University Press, 2005.

25. Garg RK. Subacute sclerosing panencephalitis. *Postgrad Med J* 2002; **78**: 63–70.

26. Wills AJ, Pengiran Tengah DSNA, Holmes GKT. The neurology of enteric disease. *J Neurol Neurosurg Psychiatry* 2006; **77**: 805–810.

27. Chisolm JJ Jr. Evaluation of the potential role of chelation therapy in treatment of low to moderate lead exposures. *Environ Health Perspect* 1990; **89**: 67–74.

28. Dobson AW, Erikson KM, Aschner M. Manganese neurotoxicity. *Ann N Y Acad Sci* 2004; **1012**: 115–129.

29. Zatta P, Lucchini R, van Rensburg SJ et al. The role of metals in neurodegenerative processes: aluminum, manganese, and zinc. *Brain Res Bull* 2003; **62**: 15–28.

30. Campbell A. The potential role of aluminium in Alzheimer's disease. *Nephrol Dial Transplant* 2002; **17**(suppl 2): 17–20.

31. Kamel F, Hoppin JA. Association of pesticide exposure with neurologic dysfunction and disease. *Environ Health Perspect* 2004; **112**: 950–958.

32. Hayden KM, Norton MC, Darcey D et al. Occupational exposure to pesticides increases the risk of incident AD: the Cache County study. *Neurology* 2010; **74**: 1524–1530.

33. Pachet AK, Wisniewski AM. The effects of lithium on cognition: an updated review. *Psychopharmacol* 2003; **170**: 225–234.

34. Nunes PV, Forlenza OV, Gattaz WF. Lithium and risk for Alzheimer's disease in elderly patients with bipolar disorder. *Br J Psychiatry* 2007; **190**: 359–360.

35. Moncrieff J, Leo J. A systematic review of the effects of antipsychotic drugs on brain volume. *Psychol Med* 2010; **40**: 1409–1422.

36. Gray SL, Anderson ML, Dublin S et al. Cumulative use of strong anticholinergic medications and incident dementia. *JAMA Intern Med* 2015; **175**: 401–407.

37. Richardson K, Fox C, Maidment I et al. Anticholinergic drugs and risk of dementia: case-control study. *Brit Med J* 2018; **360**: k1315.

38. Coupland CAC, Hill T, Dening T et al. Anticholinergic drug exposure and the risk of dementia: a nested case-control study. *JAMA Intern Med* 2019; **179**: 1084–1093.

39. Wang Y-C, Tai P-A, Poly TN. Increased risk of dementia in patients with antidepressants: a meta-analysis of observational studies. *Behav Neurol* 2018,

5315098. https://doi.org/10.1155/2018/531 5098 (last accessed 30 October 2019).

40. Ruffner-Statzer S, Bernstein AL. A persistent dementia-like condition following treatment of Hepatitis C with pegylated interferon and ribavirin. *Gastroenterol Hepatol* 2008; **4**: 63–65.

41. Valentine AD, Meyers CA, Talpaz M. Treatment of neurotoxic side effects of interferon-alpha with naltrexone. *Cancer Investig* 1995; **13**: 561–566.

42. Varney NR, Alexander B, MacIndoe JH. Reversible steroid dementia in patients without steroid psychosis. *Am J Psychiatry* 1984; **141**: 369–372.

43. Wolkowitz OM, Lupien SJ, Bigler E et al. The 'steroid dementia syndrome': An unrecognized complication of glucocorticoid treatment. *Ann N Y Acad Sci* 2004; **1032**: 191–194.

44. Clarke R, Smith D, Jobst KA et al. Folate, vitamin B12, and serum total homocysteine levels in confirmed Alzheimer disease. *Arch Neurol* 1998; **55**: 1449–1455.

45. Fleminger S, Oliver DL, Lovestone S et al. Head injury as a risk factor for Alzheimer's disease. The evidence 10 years on: a partial replication. *J Neurol Neurosurg Psychiatry* 2003; **74**: 857–862.

46. Mackay DF, Russell ER, Stewart K, et al. Neurodegenerative disease mortality among former professional soccer players. *N Engl J Med* 2019; **381**:1801–1808.

47. Ernst A, Zibrak JD. Carbon monoxide poisoning. *N Engl J Med* 1998; **339**: 1603–1608.

48. Choi IS. Parkinsonism after carbon monoxide poisoning. *Eur J Neurol* 2002; **48**: 30–33.

49. Zola-Morgan S, Squire LR, Amaral DG. Human amnesia and the medial temporal region: enduring memory impairment following a bilateral lesion limited to field CA1 of the hippocampus. *J Neurosci* 1986; **6**: 2950–2967.

50. Mehta KM, Ott A, Kalmijn S et al. Head trauma and risk of dementia and Alzheimer's disease: the Rotterdam study. *Neurology* 1999; **53**: 1959–1962.

51. Fogelholm R, Waltimo O. Epidemiology of chronic subdural haematoma. *Acta Neurochir* 1975; **32**: 247–250.

52. Sahyouni R, Goshtasbi K, Mahmoodi A, Tran DK, Chen JW. Chronic subdural hematoma: a perspective on subdural membranes and dementia. *World Neurosurg* 2017; **108**: 954–958.

53. Vanderpump MP, Turnbridge WM, French JM. The incidence of thyroid disorder in the community: a twenty-year follow-up of the Whickham survey. *Clin Endocrinol* 1995; **43**: 55–68.

54. de Jong FJ, Masaki K, Chen H et al. Thyroid function, the risk of dementia and neuropathologic changes: the Honolulu-Asia Aging Study. *Neurobiol Aging* 2009; **30**: 600–606.

55. Watson LC, Marx CE. New onset of neuropsychiatric symptoms in the elderly: possible primary hyperparathyroidism. *Psychosomatics* 2002; **43**: 413–417.

56. Cheng G, Huang C, Deng H, Wang H. Diabetes as a risk factor for dementia and mild cognitive impairment: a meta-analysis of longitudinal studies. *Intern Med J* 2012; **42**: 484–491.

57. Awad N, Gagnon M, Messier C. The relationship between impaired glucose tolerance, type 2 diabetes, and cognitive function. *J Clin Exp Neuropsychol* 2004; **26**: 1044–1080.

58. McAdams-DeMarco MA, Daubresse M, Bae S et al. Dementia, Alzheimer's disease, and mortality after hemodialysis Initiation. *Clin J Am Soc Nephrol* 2018; **13**: 1339–1347.

59. Sternlieb I. Perspectives on Wilson's disease. *Hepatology* 1990; **12**: 1234–1239.

60. Estrov Y, Scaglia F, Bodamer OA. Psychiatric symptoms of inherited metabolic disease. *J Inherit Metab Dis* 2000; **23**: 2–6.

61. Jarman PR, Wood NW. Genetics of movement disorders and ataxia. *J Neurol Neurosurg Psychiatry* 2002; **73**(Suppl. 2): 22–26.

62. Scaravilli F, An SF, Groves M et al. The neuropathology of paraneoplastic syndromes. *Brain Pathol* 1999; **9**: 251–260.

63. Keime-Guibert F, Graus F, Fleury A et al. Treatment of paraneoplastic neurological syndromes with antineuronal antibodies (Anti-Hu, Anti-Yo) with a combination of immunoglobulins, cyclophosphamide, and methylprednisolone. *J Neurol Neurosurg Psychiatry* 2000; **68**: 479–482.

64. Rickards H, Jacob S, Lennox B et al. Autoimmune encephalitis: a potentially treatable cause of mental disorder. *Adv Psychiatr Treat* 2014; **20**: 92–100.

65. Kalb R, Feinstein A, Rohrig A, Sankary L, Willis A. Depression and suicidality in multiple sclerosis: red flags, management strategies, and ethical considerations. *Curr Neurol Neurosci Rep* 2019; **19**: 77.

66. Jefferies K. The neuropsychiatry of multiple sclerosis. *Adv Psychiatr Treat* 2006; **12**: 214–220.

67. Krupp LB, Christodoulou C, Melville P et al. Donepezil improved memory in multiple sclerosis in a randomized clinical trial. *Neurology* 2004; **63**: 1579–1585.

68. Wirnsberger RM, De Vries J, Wouters EF et al. Clinical presentation of sarcoidosis in the Netherlands: an epidemiological study. *Netherlands J Med* 1998; **53**: 53–60.

69. Kuker W. Cerebral vasculitis: imaging signs revisited. *Neuroradiology* 2007; **49**: 471–479.

70. Collin P, Pirttila T, Nurmikko T et al. Celiac disease, brain atrophy and dementia. *Neurology* 1991; **41**: 372–375.

71. William TH, Joseph AM, Melanie CG et al. Cognitive impairment and celiac disease. *Arch Neurol* 2006; **63**: 1440–1446.

72. Kaklamani VG, Variopoulos G, Kaklamanis PG. Behçet's disease. *Semin Arthritis Rheum* 1998; **27**: 197–217.

73. Lishman WA. *Organic Psychiatry: The Psychological Consequences of Cerebral Disorder*. Blackwell Publishing, 1998.

74. Akman-Demir G, Baykan-Kurt B, Serdaroglu P et al. Seven-year follow-up of neurologic involvement in Behçet syndrome. *Arch Neurol* 1996; **53**: 691–694.

75. Kirk A, Kertesz A, Polk MJ. Dementia with leukoencephalopathy in systemic lupus erythematosus. *Can J Neurol Sci* 1991; **18**: 344–348.

76. Ampélas JF, Wattiaux MJ, van Amerongen AP. Psychiatric manifestations of lupus erythematosus systemic and Sjogren's syndrome [article in French]. *L'Encéphale* 2001; **27**: 588–599.

Mania in Late Life

Felicity Richards and Martin Curtice

Introduction

Mania in late life is a serious disorder that demands specialist assessment and management. However, it is greatly under-researched. The mainstay of the older adult psychiatry workload will inevitably be concerned with assessing and managing dementia and depression, but the steady rise in the ageing population with longer survival means that there will be an increase in absolute numbers of older people presenting with mania. There are no specific treatment algorithms available for mania in late life. This chapter reviews mania and hypomania in late life and concentrates on diagnosis, assessment, and treatment, as well as on the management considerations associated with this important age group.

Few studies have addressed the specific difficulties faced by older-adult psychiatrists when a patient presents with mania or hypomania in late life. The numbers of patients with atypical and typical presentations of mania in later life are not insignificant and with the steady rise of the ageing population, coupled with better healthcare and greater survival, there will be increasing demands on service provision. Along with diagnostic uncertainties at presentation, mania in older adults tends to be more debilitating and severe than in the younger population, resulting in more frequent hospital admissions,[1] higher rates of psychotic symptoms,[2] with higher levels of comorbidity and polypharmacy, and no specific treatment algorithms available to address these management considerations in older adults.

The literature on mania and hypomania in late life (defined as over 65 years of age) is scant and research papers tend to use different age cut-offs, preventing easy transfer of practical information. Nevertheless, we aim here to give an overview of mania and hypomania in this important age group.

Classification of Bipolar Disorder

There are two ways available to clinicians to classify episodes of bipolar disorder. Both the ICD-11[3] and the DSM-5[4] allow for diagnoses of mania (with or without psychotic symptoms) and hypomania. It is unusual for an episode of mania or hypomania to occur in isolation.

According to ICD-11, 'Although the diagnosis can be made based on evidence of a single manic or mixed episode, typically manic or mixed episodes alternate with depressive episodes over the course of the disorder'.[3] A mixed episode 'is characterized by either a mixture or very rapid alternation between prominent manic and depressive symptoms on most days during a period of at least 2 weeks'.[3] ICD-11 also characterizes whether the current episode of bipolar affective disorder is mania or depression, and these are further divided into whether psychotic features are present or not.

DSM-5 classifies episodes into bipolar I and bipolar II disorders. Bipolar I disorder involves one or more manic or mixed episodes. The manic episode may be preceded by or may be followed by hypomanic or major depressive episodes, but are not required for diagnosis. Bipolar II disorder is characterized by one or more major depressive episodes, accompanied by at least one hypomanic episode but never having had a full manic episode.

Terms Specific to Mania in Late Life

Mania or hypomania may persist into late life as part of a lifelong affective illness, with these patients 'graduating' from the general adult services. Although mania usually presents before the age of 30, with a further peak in females in their 50s, it can present for the first time in old age, with a third peak (especially in males) in the eighth and ninth decades.[2]

Many patients are believed to convert to mania in later life, commonly following recurrent depression. This can either be a part of the natural progression of illness or be a manifestation of antidepressant-induced mania. It has been proposed that treatment with tricyclic antidepressants is twice as likely to result in a manic episode compared with treatment with selective serotonin reuptake inhibitors or placebo. Venlafaxine or other dual-action medications have also been found to increase the risk of a switch from depression into mania.[5]

Other useful concepts and subtypes have been put forward for use, especially in older adults, including 'secondary mania' (or 'disinhibition syndrome') and 'vascular mania'.

Secondary Mania

It is accepted that patients with forms of neurological illness can present with affective disorders. The concept of secondary mania, first described by Krauthammer and Klerman,[6] was used to explain late-onset presentations of mania associated with a diverse group of medical conditions. Neurologists tend to favour the term 'disinhibition syndrome', but the clinical presentation and features are similar.

Secondary manias can be seen in patients with multiple sclerosis, Parkinson's disease, temporal lobe epilepsy, AIDS, dementia, and traumatic brain injury.[7] Indeed, secondary mania is seen in 9% of patients with traumatic brain injury, with a preponderance of basal temporal lesions noted in these patients. A positive family history of affective disorder and subcortical atrophy before injury are added risk factors.[8]

A number of further studies have supported the concept of an association with neurological comorbidity. Tohen and colleagues found that patients with a first-episode mania in old age were twice as likely to have a comorbid neurological disorder compared with those who had experienced multiple episodes.[9] Many studies have suggested that secondary mania/disinhibition syndromes are associated with right-sided lesions, based on the hypothesis that disrupting connections within the orbitofrontal circuit mediates manic symptoms.[8] Indeed, Goodwin and colleagues state that any lesion involving right-sided cortical or subcortical areas may be associated with secondary mania.[5] Other examples highlighting the heterogeneous nature of the causes of secondary mania include metabolic disturbance, endocrine disorders, such as thyrotoxicosis and hydrocortisone replacement, neoplasia, and infection, all of which can also present as a delirium, often adding to diagnostic uncertainty.[8] A systematic review of 35 case reports of first-episode mania or hypomania in the over-50s found that 82% had a suspected underlying organic origin. In

28% of these cases, treatment of the organic cause contributed to successful remission of the manic episode.[10]

Vascular Mania

Steffans and Krishnan proposed vascular mania as a subtype of mania.[11] The concept is similar to that of 'vascular depression' proposed by Alexopoulous and colleagues,[12] and is used to explain the high rates of manic symptoms seen in those who have evidence of cerebrovascular disease. This concept is supported by the relatively acute onset of manic symptoms that can occur following a cerebrovascular event, the higher prevalence of silent cerebral infarcts on neuroimaging in late-onset patients, and the association of hyperintensities with risk factors such as hypertension, heart disease, and diabetes.[8, 13]

Epidemiology

There appear to be discrepancies between the reported occurrence of bipolar disorder in the older adult population and no clear consensus on mania/hypomania. A number of studies have consistently reported that the prevalence of bipolar disorder has an inverse relationship with age, with a decline in prevalence with increasing age.[14, 15] About 10% of all bipolar cases are over the age of 50 years in their first episode.[16]

One study reported an overall prevalence of late-life mania estimated to be 6% in older psychiatric inpatients, and a mean prevalence of late-onset mania of 44.2% in older inpatients with bipolar disorder.[17] Another study suggested that up to 0.5% of people over 65 will have bipolar disorder. A 1-year incidence rate of 0.1% among adults over 65 has been indicated.[18] This is lower than that for adults aged 45–65 (0.4%) and 18–44 (1.4%).[2]

Burden of Bipolar Disorder in Older People

Economic

Older patients can have a disproportionate impact on health services and some estimate that bipolar disorder accounts for approximately 8–10% of admissions to psychiatric units, similar to that of younger adults, and 6% of older adult psychiatry outpatient visits.[2] Research predicts increasing numbers of patients accessing services. A report by the King's Fund estimated the projected greatest proportional increase in the number of people with bipolar disorder and related conditions is still in those aged 65 and over.[14] However, the increase in the number of older people will not significantly affect the total number of new patients because of the lower prevalence in this group.

In the UK, the mean service costs of bipolar disorder and related conditions for those aged 65 and over are projected to be approximately four times greater than for younger age groups, owing to higher average inpatient and residential care costs.[14] In this study, the elements used to estimate total costs were prescribed drugs, inpatient care, other National Health Service (NHS) services, supported accommodation, day care, other social services, informal care, and lost employment.

Among older people, the rate of hospital admission for bipolar disorder is the same as that for schizophrenia, although the length of stay is shorter.[2] Compared with older outpatients with unipolar disorder, those with bipolar disorder use four times the amount of mental health services, including inpatient hospitalization, case management, skills training, and community support.[19] The overall cost of annual care of older adults with bipolar disorder and comorbid dementia is more than twice that for those with bipolar disorder alone.[20]

Morbidity and Mortality

According to the King's Fund report on integrating physical and mental health, people with severe mental illness such as bipolar are at a particularly high risk of physical ill health as a result of medication side effects, lifestyle-related risk factors, and socioeconomic determinants.[21] Bipolar disorders in particular are associated with higher morbidity and mortality. The increase in the number of comorbid medical conditions is directly proportional to age, and approximately 67% of over-70-year-olds who have bipolar disorder have at least one significant medical condition,[22] with another study stating that older people with bipolar disorder have an average of three to four comorbid medical conditions.[23] Patients with bipolar disorder, especially bipolar I (one or more manic episode(s) or mixed episode(s)), have increased mortality from cardiovascular causes in particular. The difference in cardiovascular mortality risk may reflect the physical health consequences of mania/hypomania because depressive symptom burden is not related to cardiovascular mortality.[24]

An increase in morbidity from obesity and type 2 diabetes mellitus has been reported in people with bipolar disorder compared with the general population. Explanations for these possible increased risks include comorbidity with substance misuse and other medical conditions, inadequate prevention of cardiovascular risk factors (such as smoking, obesity, and lack of exercise), the side effects of psychotropic medications, and poor engagement with general medical care.[25]

Suicide

Bipolar disorder is associated with a high suicide risk (lifetime risk of 8–20%),[26] especially during depressive episodes or mixed states. However, there is a lack of literature specifically concerning completed and attempted suicide in those over 65 with mania or hypomania. Factors for completed suicide in working-age patients that can be extrapolated to older people include inadequate treatment (medication) and inadequate follow-up by mental health services.[27] With the above in mind, older patients with bipolar disorder should be recognized as high risk and be provided with long-term intensive support.

Aetiology

A family history of affective illness appears to increase the risk of bipolar disorder at any age. However, older patients with first-onset mania appear to have fewer first-degree relatives with affective illness, compared with patients presenting earlier. Figures are inconclusive, with results ranging from 24% to 88% for the presence of a positive family history.[8]

As we have already discussed, physical illnesses, particularly neurological conditions, can also be associated with mania (so-called secondary mania) as can cerebrovascular incidents (i.e. 'vascular mania'). So the aetiology of mania involves genetic and other biological factors.

Diagnosis and Assessment

In the diagnosis of mania in late life, clinicians commonly use either the ICD-11 or the DSM-5 classification. However, it is important to note that rather than the classic symptoms of elevated mood and grandiosity, mania in the older person can cause initial diagnostic uncertainty, with irritability, distractibility, and disorientation being prominent presenting symptoms,[28] masking delirium, cognitive impairment, or indeed depression. The differentiation between delirium and mania or hypomania can be aided by observation over time.[1] Mania, therefore, should be included in the differential diagnosis of all older patients with a relatively acute onset of agitation and confusion, despite lack of a previous history of affective disturbance (see Box 5.1).

Taking a comprehensive history, ideally with a collateral account, is invaluable. For a first presentation of mania, the history may reveal past episodes of hypomania or depression, not severe enough to warrant referral, treatment, or intervention by mental health services. Classification of mania in later life will be helpful in deciding on management and future care.

Full investigations should include a complete physical examination, including neurological examination (see Box 5.2). Routine blood tests should be carried out and an electrocardiogram (ECG) taken, especially if antipsychotics, lithium, or valproate are being considered.

Full exploration of any causes of delirium should be excluded, to include a midstream specimen of urine. Mania in older adults is associated with a high rate of medical and neurological disease.[9] Consequently, all patients presenting with first-onset mania should be carefully screened for contributing medical disorders and brain imaging is useful in this context.

Owing to the known associations with bipolar disorder and cardiovascular risk, initial assessment should also include careful history of common cardiovascular risk factors, such as smoking, excessive alcohol use, hypertension, hypercholesterolaemia, and diabetes.[8]

Box 5.1 Differential diagnosis of mania in late life

- Delirium – hyperactive type
- Dementia – especially with frontotemporal involvement
- Stroke
- Early-onset mania, as part of coexisting bipolar affective disorder
- Secondary mania, i.e. due to medications, physical illness
- Late-onset schizophrenia-like psychosis
- Acute and transient psychotic disorders

Box 5.2 Investigations for mania in late life

- Physical examination, including neurological examination
- Blood investigations – urea and electrolytes, glomerular filtration rate, liver function tests, thyroid function tests, full blood count, vitamin B_{12} and folate, bone profile, and glucose
- Midstream specimen of urine
- ECG
- Chest X-ray
- Computed tomography (CT) and/or magnetic resonance imaging (MRI) if indicated (in the presence of neurological signs)

Considering the causes of secondary mania discussed earlier, medication(s) should be examined and any recent changes identified: antidepressants, antibiotics ('antibiomania'), in particular clarithromycin and other macrolides, steroids, and oestrogens are all examples of inducing agents for secondary mania.[28, 29]

Screening Instruments

The diagnosis of mania relies on clinical evidence and assessment. In clinical practice there are no screening tools available for easy use in psychiatric or general hospital settings. Diagnostic scales can aid in clinical diagnosis, but are mainly used in the research setting.[30] Self-report questionnaires may be more difficult to use with older people because of sensory impairments.

Psychiatric Comorbidity

Anxiety Disorders and Substance Misuse

Psychiatric comorbidity in bipolar disorder is widely documented. Reports have indicated that generalized anxiety disorder shows a lifetime prevalence of 20.5% and a 12-month prevalence of 9.5% in older patients with bipolar disorder. For panic disorder, lifetime prevalence is as high as 19%, whereas 12-month prevalence is 11.9%.[31] Similarly, comorbid post-traumatic stress disorder, substance misuse, 'other anxiety', or dementia have been found to occur in nearly 29% of older adults with bipolar disorder.[20]

Substance misuse, a significant comorbidity in younger adults with bipolar disorder, is less common in older cohorts, but nevertheless occurs more frequently than in healthy older controls. A lifetime and 20-month prevalence of 38% for comorbid alcohol use disorders has been reported,[31] and patients with bipolar disorder with a lifetime history of substance misuse appear to have a greater number of hospital admissions.[2]

Cognitive Impairment

Cognitive impairment in late-onset bipolar disorder has been widely reported and is associated with more severe cognitive impairment than in early-onset disorder.[32] Compared with age-matched controls, patients with bipolar disorder score lower on most cognitive measures and patients with late-onset disorder show more impairment in psychomotor performance and mental flexibility. Older adults whose onset of bipolar illness had been before the age of 50 were found to have impairment across a range of domains, including selective attention, verbal memory, and verbal fluency, in the euthymic state. It has been concluded that older patients with bipolar disorder may have substantial cognitive impairments, perhaps indicating a trait-like cognitive disability related to the disease.[33]

Management

Management of mania or hypomania in late life is complex. Onset is often relatively sudden and severe and individuals will therefore most likely need inpatient admission, either as informal patients or commonly under the Mental Health Act – usually as a result of the risks a manic episode can pose to the patient and to others from poor judgement and associated actions.[5] Before and following admission, the importance of good working and understanding of this disorder within multidisciplinary teams is vital. The recognition and management of concurrent physical illnesses is as much the job of the older-adult psychiatrist as of the general practitioner. Importantly, clinicians should be aware that older people can be at risk of the development of sudden-onset depressive symptoms following recovery from a manic episode.

It is not uncommon for patients to have poor engagement with primary care and contact with psychiatric services can often aid in screening for physical disorders. Issues such as adherence and the practicalities of medication prescribing in this age group need to be addressed. And clinicians need to be aware of the risks of polypharmacy and potential drug–drug interactions with a number of the psychotropics discussed later. Care planning should consider the patient's social situation and the effects that the illness can have on family members and carers.

Pharmacological Management

Treatment of older people often involves compromise because the side effects of treatment may be as harmful as the condition being treated. There continue to be no specific treatment algorithms for mania in late life,[5] with a scarcity of published controlled trials in the older population. In practice, treatment for older adults with mania or hypomania generally follows similar guidelines as for other groups. However, certain precautions should be taken because of the differences in pharmacokinetics, side effects, concomitant medication use, and comorbidity. Adherence at times can be difficult, because of the nature of acute episodes, the presence of cognitive impairment, or a reluctance to take medication.

As a general guide, medication doses are lower and should be titrated with care, owing to the reduced volume of distribution and reduced renal clearance in older people, which is especially important if thinking about lithium initiation. Pharmacotherapy can be divided into different phases of treatment: acute (manic or mixed episodes) and maintenance treatment. Comprehensive guidance is available from the British Association of Psychopharmacology,[5] and from NICE (see Box 5.3).[34]

Box 5.3 The National Institute of Health and Care Excellence (NICE) recommendations for treating bipolar disorder in older people

- When offering psychotropic medication to older people, healthcare professionals should take into account its impact on cognitive functioning in older people.
- Be aware of the need to use medication at lower doses.
- Be alert to the increased risk of drug interactions when prescribing psychotropic medication to older adults.
- Take into account negative impact that anticholinergic medications/drugs with anticholinergic activity can have on cognitive functioning and mobility.
- Ensure that medical comorbidities have been recognized and addressed.

National Institute for Health and Clinical Excellence. Bipolar Disorder. Assessment and Management. Clinical guideline [CG185] NICE, 2014 (updated 2018). Last accessed 17 October 2019 via: www.nice.org.uk/guidance/cg185

Lithium

There are few trials looking at the use of lithium treatment in late-life bipolar disorder, for acute episodes or as maintenance therapy in older adults, and very few controlled studies of the efficacy and safety of lithium in older people.[35] The GERI-BD trial (a randomized controlled trial comparing the efficacy and safety of lithium and semi-sodium valproate (Divalproex)) found that both lithium and semi-sodium valproate appear adequately tolerated and efficacious, with patients treated with lithium showing a greater reduction in mania scores over nine weeks.[36] Lithium continues to be used commonly as a mood stabilizer in older adults,[37] and is still regarded as the gold-standard treatment for older adults with bipolar disorder.[38] Advanced age, absence of a family history of bipolar disorder, mania secondary to another medical condition (e.g. stroke), or dementia predict poor response to lithium.[28] Of note, lithium treatment may protect older patients with bipolar disorder against AD,[39] and may have a potential wider neuroprotective function.[40] With regard to longer-term treatment, lithium specifically is associated with a reduced risk of suicide.[5, 26]

The impact of age-related decline in renal function is an important consideration. Renal function during chronic lithium treatment is related to age, lithium intoxication episodes, pre-existing renal disease, and treatment schedule, rather than to duration of prophylactic lithium therapy; with lithium use for more than 10 years, 10–20% of patients may display morphological kidney changes, not generally associated with kidney failure.[5, 41]

The pharmacokinetics of lithium show that the rate of excretion in older people is approximately half that in the younger population and, because of this, many older people respond to much lower doses. The doses of lithium required to achieve a given serum lithium concentration decrease threefold from middle to old age.[42] A practice guideline is available for lithium use when incidental chronic kidney disease is detected in those in whom lithium is being considered or when long-term lithium users develop chronic kidney disease.[43]

Adverse effects of lithium are not confined to the kidney and they encompass a range of systemic complaints. Lithium-induced tremor, aggravation of parkinsonian tremor, and spontaneous extrapyramidal symptoms can occur.[8] Mild tremor and nystagmus can present without functional consequences and should not be considered signs of toxicity.[28] Signs of lithium toxicity include gastrointestinal complaints, ataxia, slurred speech, delirium, or coma. They may follow periods of dehydration caused by vomiting, diarrhoea, inadequate fluid intake, or (especially pertinent in the older person) periods of immobility, development of chest infections, or sepsis. Higher rates of hypothyroidism have been found in elderly people on lithium and would need appropriate treatment.

Drug interactions are an important consideration. Concomitant use of medications that lower renal clearance can potentially increase the risk of lithium toxicity. Clinicians should always be aware of medications such as thiazide diuretics, angiotensin-converting enzyme (ACE) inhibitors, and non-steroidal anti-inflammatory medications. Serum lithium levels should be monitored more frequently in these patients.

Valproate

Valproate has been shown to be effective and well tolerated in older people, and there is evidence that it is equally well tolerated and as efficacious as lithium.[36] A positive response to valproate has been correlated to older age, increased severity of manic symptoms, neurological impairment, dysphoria, and a history of lithium non-responsiveness.[44]

When prescribing valproate, clinicians should be aware of its interactions with other anticonvulsants and the need for more careful monitoring of sedation, tremor, and gait disturbance in older people. Fully reversible cognitive impairment and parkinsonism caused by valproate have been reported with the use of sodium valproate.[45, 46] The British Association for Psychopharmacology (Goodwin 2016) recommends starting doses of 500 mg daily in older people.[5] However, starting doses of 125–250 mg at night, titrating carefully up to a maintenance dose of 500–1,000 mg/day, have also been recommended.[44]

Carbamazepine

Carbamazepine's use as a first-line treatment is not encouraged,[5] but it may be the agent of choice for secondary mania because older patients with this diagnosis have been found to respond relatively poorly to lithium.[2] Particularly concerning with carbamazepine is the risk of drug–drug interactions owing to its induction of the P450 enzyme system. Consequently, the efficacy of medications such as antipsychotics and antidepressants can be affected along with commonly prescribed drugs such as calcium channel blockers, erythromycin, and warfarin.

In older patients, serum electrolytes should be routinely checked because of the increased potential for inducing hyponatraemia,[5] and special attention should be paid to a history of blood dyscrasias or liver disease. Side effects are wide-ranging and include ataxia, confusion, diplopia, and blurred vision, as well as fatigue, gastrointestinal problems, and rare idiosyncratic effects such as Stevens–Johnson syndrome, agranulocytosis, and hepatic failure.

Antipsychotics

Mania in late life can develop quickly, potentially putting the patient and others at risk. For more severe forms, especially mania with psychotic symptoms, treatment with antipsychotics is at times unavoidable for initial stabilization.[5] For patients who present with severe mania when already taking lithium or valproate, adding an antipsychotic should be considered while gradually increasing the dose of lithium or valproate.[5, 34] If treating mania with antipsychotics, olanzapine, quetiapine, or risperidone would normally be used. Generally, patients with bipolar disorder are more likely to develop extrapyramidal side effects than patients with schizophrenia on comparable doses of antipsychotics.[5] Older patients with primary bipolar disorder have been found to have high rates of tardive dyskinesia (approaching 20%), with the prevalence increasing with age.[43] There is now convincing evidence that mortality increases with the use of antipsychotics in individuals with a dementia.[47]

Non-Pharmacological Management

Electroconvulsive Therapy

Electroconvulsive therapy may be indicated to gain rapid control and short-term improvement in a patient who is severely unwell. This is generally after all other treatment options have been considered and have failed, or when the situation is thought to be life-threatening.[48] Examples could include complications of self-neglect, dehydration, or morbid nutritional status, suicidal risk, poor medication efficacy or tolerance. Electroconvulsive therapy should be considered based on an assessment of risks and benefits. Especially in older patients, anaesthetic risk, comorbidity, and potential cognitive impairment with post-ictal confusion should be explored in detail. Care should be taken to assess consent after discussions of the risks and benefits with the patient and, where appropriate, their advocate. It would be likely (in England and Wales) that the *Mental Health Act* would need to be implemented where the patient lacked the requisite capacity to consent (and alternative jurisdictions would have similar laws, for which see Chapter 21). Any advance decision to refuse treatment should be consulted.

Psychotherapy

The Department of Health has stated that service provision should be equal among all ages.[49] Therefore, one would expect availability and access to the same type of psychotherapy as for younger adults. This guidance is mirrored by NICE 2014,[34] which states that we need to ensure older people with bipolar affective disorder are offered the same range of treatments and services as younger people with bipolar.

Psychotherapy is a valuable element in the management of bipolar disorder in general, but mainly for depressive symptoms. There is no evidence for the treatment of refractory disease with psychotherapy in the older adult population. Whereas most, if not all, advice pertains to those less than 65 years, the key areas for psychotherapy in bipolar disorder that could be pertinent to older people are discussed below.

Psychoeducation

For mania, psychoeducation has been suggested to help individuals identify signs of relapse (relapse signature), to improve adherence to treatment (adherence/compliance therapy), and to enhance general coping strategies. The maintenance of regular behavioural patterns, such as a person's daily routine and sleep, appear to be important considerations in older patients.

Cognitive-Behavioural Therapy

Cognitive-behavioural therapy (CBT) has been found to decrease relapse rates and improve mania severity and psychosocial functioning for patients with bipolar disorder when used as an adjunct with medications.[50]

Other Types of Psychotherapy

In the general adult population, family-focused therapy, group treatments (such as group psycho-education as an adjunct to pharmacotherapy), and interpersonal and social rhythm therapy all appear to have a role.[5] Their use in the older population still needs to be reviewed. Other considerations such as cognitive functioning, motivation, and sensory impairment may affect the potential efficacy in this population.

Psychosocial Interventions

Age-specific rehabilitative needs of older adults have largely been neglected,[51] and most literature on psychosocial interventions in older people with bipolar disorder has been extrapolated from mixed-age studies or based on older people with a broad range of serious mental illness.[23] A two-year randomized trial comparing the effectiveness of *Helping Older People Experience Success* (HOPES – a combined psychosocial skills training and preventive healthcare intervention) and treatment-as-usual in 183 older people with serious mental illness, 20% having a bipolar diagnosis, reported that HOPES improved social skills, self-efficacy, community functioning, leisure, and recreation skills.[51] A follow-on three-year study showed HOPES was associated with sustained long-term improvement in functioning, symptoms, self-efficacy, preventative healthcare screening, and advance care planning.[52]

The Course of Mania in Late Life

Literature on the course of mania in late life is limited. Studies indicate that older people appear to do just as well as younger adults in the acute phase of illness, achieving similar outcomes (remission and recovery).[53] However, it has been noted that overall outcome is generally worse in mania than in depression, with a higher prevalence of persistence of symptoms, cognitive decline, and greater mortality;[54] recovery in the longer term may be more difficult to maintain when compared to younger counterparts.[53]

Prevention

There is no solid evidence base for prevention of mania in late life. Primary prevention would be designed to look at influencing modifiable factors. The higher cerebrovascular and cardiovascular risk in many older patients with mania has significant management implications and would warrant close monitoring and treatment of potential risk factors, in both primary and secondary care. Treatment and maintenance care for chronic illnesses and physical disability, as well as an awareness of polypharmacy and potential drug interactions, are important.

Secondary prevention involves reducing the risk of relapse of illness by consideration of long-term medication and psychological interventions. Clinicians working with older adults should monitor treatment closely and may have to use their own judgement on the risks versus the benefits of treatment. Other strategies for preventing relapse may involve techniques such as CBT, psychotherapy, or social rhythms therapy. Social inclusion, community support, and adherence to medication may further help to reduce future recurrences of mania.

Discussion

There is a paucity of evidence on the treatment and management of mania in late life.[23] This chapter builds on the central tenets of any comprehensive older adult psychiatric assessment process, in particular providing detailed information on diagnostic and treatment issues. It is also important to consider patient and carer education. Patient.info and the Royal College of Psychiatrists provide helpful information for older patients and their carers.[55, 56]

The preponderance of work in older adult psychiatry will inevitably involve dementia and depression, but specialist knowledge in the assessment and nuances of management of mania in older adults is of equal importance.

Acknowledgement

For information, the original paper on which this chapter is based was:

Richards F, Curtice M. Mania in late life. *Adv Psychiatr Treat* 2011; 17: 357–64.

References

1. Brooks JO, Hoblyn JC. Secondary mania in older adults. *Am J Psychiatry* 2005; **162**: 2033–8.

2. Depp CA, Jeste DV. Bipolar disorder in older adults: a critical review. *Bipolar Disord* 2004; **6**: 343–67.

3. World Health Organization. *ICD-11 for Mortality and Morbidity Statistics (ICD-11 MMS)*. WHO, 2018. https://icd.who.int/browse11/l-m/en (last accessed 23 October 2019).

4. American Psychiatric Association. *Diagnostic and Statistical Manual of Mental Disorders, 5th ed. (DSM-5)*. American Psychiatric Publishing, 2013.

5. Goodwin GM, Haddad PM, Ferrier IN et al. Evidence-based guidelines for treating bipolar disorder: revised third edition recommendations from the British Association for Psychopharmacology, *J Psychopharmacol* 2016; **30**: 495–553.

6. Krauthammer C, Klerman GL. Secondary mania. Manic syndromes associated with antecedent physical illness or drugs. *Arch Gen Psychiatry* 1978; **35**: 1333–9.

7. Schneck CD. Bipolar disorder in neurologic illness. *Curr Treat Options Neurol* 2002; **4**: 477–86.

8. Shulman KI, Herrmann N. Manic syndromes in old age. In *Oxford Textbook of Old Age Psychiatry* (eds. R Jacoby, C Oppenheimer, T Dening, A Thomas): 557–62. Oxford University Press, 2008.

9. Tohen M, Shulman KI, Satlin A. First episode mania in late life. *Am J Psychiatry* 1994; **151**: 130–2.

10. Sami M, Khan H, Nilforooshan R. Late onset mania as an organic syndrome: a review of case reports in the literature. *J Affect Disord* 2015; **188**: 226–31.

11. Steffans DC, Krishnan KRR. Structural neuroimaging and mood disorders. Recent findings, implications for classification, and future directions. *Biol Psychiatry* 1998; **43**: 705–12.

12. Alexopoulous GS, Meyers BS, Young RC et al. Clinically defined vascular depression. *Am J Psychiatry* 1997; **154**: 562–65.

13. Tamashiro JH, Zung S, Zanetti MV et al. Increased rates of white matter hyperintensities in late-onset bipolar disorder. *Bipolar Disord* 2008; **10**: 765–75.

14. McCrone P, Dhanasiri S, Patel A et al. *Paying the Price. The Cost of Mental Health Care in England to 2026*. King's Fund, 2008.

15. Byers AL, Yaffe K, Covinsky KE et al. High occurrence of mood and anxiety disorders among older adults. *Arch Gen Psychiatry* 2010; **67**: 489–96.

16. Almeida OP, Fenner S. Bipolar disorder: similarities and differences between patients with illness onset before and after 65 years of age. *Int Psychogeriatr* 2002; **14**: 311–22.

17. Dols A, Kupka RW, van Lammeren et al. The prevalence of late-life mania: a review. *Bipolar Disord* 2014; **16**:113–18.

18. Hirschfeld RM, Calabrese JR, Weissman MM et al. Screening for bipolar disorder in the community. *J Clin Psychiatry* 2003; **64**: 53–9.

19. Bartels S, Forester B, Miles K et al. Mental health service use by elderly patients with bipolar disorder and unipolar major depression. *Am J Geriatr Psychiatry* 2000; **8**: 160–6.

20. Sajatovic M, Blow FC, Ignacio RV. Psychiatric comorbidity in older adults with bipolar disorder. *Int J Geriatr Psychiatry* 2006; **21**: 582–7.

21. Naylor C, Das P, Ross S et al. *Bringing Together Physical and Mental Health: A New Frontier for Integrated Care*. The King's Fund, 2016. Last accessed 17 October 2019 via: www.kingsfund.org.uk/publications/physical-and-mental-health

22. Beyer J, Kuchibhatla M, Gersing K et al. Medical comorbidity in a bipolar outpatient clinical population. *Neuropsychopharmacology* 2005; **30**: 401–4.

23. Sajatovic M, Strejilevich SA, Gildengers AG et al. A report on older-age bipolar disorder from the International Society for Bipolar Disorders Task Force. *Bipolar Disord* 2015; **17**: 689–704.

24. Fiedorowicz JD, Solomon DA, Endicott J et al. Manic/hypomanic symptom burden and cardiovascular mortality in bipolar disorder. *Psychosom Med* 2009; **71**: 598–606.

25. Morriss R. Metabolism, lifestyle and bipolar affective disorder. *J Psychopharmacol* 2005: **19**: 94–101.

26. Aizenberg D, Olmer A, Barak Y. Suicide attempts amongst elderly bipolar patients. *J Affect Disord* 2006; **91**: 91–4.

27. Keks NA, Hill C, Sundram S et al. Evaluation of treatment in 35 cases of bipolar suicide. *Aust N Z J Psychiatry* 2009; **43**: 503–8.

28. Kennedy GJ. Bipolar disorder in late life: mania. *Prim Psychiatry* 2008; **15**: 28–33.

29. Abovesh A, Stone C, Hobbs WR. Antimicrobial induced mania (antibiomania). A review of spontaneous reports. *J Clin Psychopharmacol* 2002; **22**: 71–81.

30. Scottish Intercollegiate Guidelines Network. *Bipolar Affective Disorder. A National Clinical Guideline.* SIGN, 2005. Last accessed on 17 October 2019 via: www .sign.ac.uk/pdf/sign82.pdf

31. Goldstein BI, Herrmann N, Shulman KI. Comorbidity in bipolar disorder among the elderly. Results from an epidemiological community sample. *Am J Psychiatry* 2006; **163**: 319–21.

32. Schouws SNTM, Comijs HC, Stek ML et al. Cognitive impairment in early and late bipolar disorder. *Am J Geriatr Psychiatry* 2009; **17**: 508–15.

33. Schouws SN, Zoeteman JB, Comijs HC et al. Cognitive functioning in elderly patients with early onset bipolar disorder. *Int J Geriatr Psychiatry* 2007; **22**: 856–61.

34. National Institute for Health and Clinical Excellence. *Bipolar Disorder. Assessment and Management. Clinical guideline [CG185]* NICE, 2014 (updated 2018). Last accessed 17 October 2019 via: www .nice.org.uk/guidance/cg185

35. De Fazio P, Gaetano R, Caroleo M et al. Lithium in late-life mania: a systematic review. *Neuropsychiatr Dis Treat* 2017; **13**: 755–66.

36. Young RC, Mulsant BH, Sajatovic M et al. GERI-BD: a randomized double-blind controlled trial of lithium and divalproex in the treatment of mania in older patients with bipolar disorder. *Am J Psychiatry* 2017; **174**: 1086–93.

37. Shulman KI, Rochon P, Sykora K et al. Changing prescription patterns for lithium and valproic acid in old age. Shifting practice without evidence. *Brit Med J* 2003; **326**: 960–1.

38. Fotso Soh J, Klil-Drori S, Rei S. Using lithium in older age bipolar disorder: special considerations. *Drugs Aging* 2019; **36**: 147–54.

39. Nunes PV, Forlenza OV, Gattaz WF. Lithium and risk for Alzheimer's disease in elderly patients with bipolar disorder. *Br J Psychiatry* 2007; **190**: 359–60.

40. Diniz BS, Machado-Vieira R, Forlenza OV. Lithium and neuroprotection: translational evidence and implications for the treatment of neuropsychiatric disorders. *Neuropsychiatr Dis Treat* 2013; **9**: 493–500.

41. Hetmar O, Povlsen UJ, Ladefoged J et al. Lithium: long-term effects on the kidney. A prospective follow-up study ten years after kidney biopsy. *Br J Psychiatry* 1991; **158**: 53–8.

42. Rej S, Beaulieu S, Segal M et al. Lithium dosing and serum concentrations across the age spectrum: from early adulthood to the tenth decade of life. *Drugs Aging* 2014; **31**: 911–6.

43. Kripalani M, Shawcross J, Reilly J et al. Lithium and chronic kidney disease. *BMJ* 2009; **339**: 166–70.

44. Sajatovic M. Treatment of bipolar disorder in older adults. *Int J Geriatr Psychiatry* 2002; **17**: 865–73.

45. Walstra G. Reversible dementia due to valproic acid therapy. *Ned Tijdschr Geneeskd* 1997; **141**: 391–93.

46. Schreur L, Middeljans-Tijssen C, Hengstman G et al. Cognitive impairment

and parkinsonism due to the use of sodium valproate. *Tijdschr Gerontol Geriatr* 2009; **40**: 29–33.

47. Livingston G, Sommerlad A, Orgeta V et al. The Lancet Commissions. Dementia prevention, intervention, and care. *Lancet* 2017; **390**: 2673–734.

48. National Institute for Health and Care Excellence. *Guidance on the Use of Electroconvulsive Therapy*, TA59. NICE, 2003. Last accessed 17 October 2019 via: www.nice.org.uk/guidance/ta59

49. Department of Health. (2009) *New Horizons: A Shared Vision for Mental Health.* Department of Health, 2009. Last accessed on 17 October 2019 via: www.ndti.org.uk/uploads/files/New_Horizons_A_Shared_Vision_For_Mental_Health_PDF.pdf

50. Chiang K-J, Tsai J-C, Liu D et al. Efficacy of cognitive-behavioral therapy in patients with bipolar disorder: a meta-analysis of randomized controlled trials. *PLoS ONE* 2017; **12**(5): e0176849. https://doi.org/10.1371/journal.pone.0176849 (last accessed 23 October 2019).

51. Mueser KT, Pratt SI, Bartels SJ et al. Randomized trial of social rehabilitation and integrated health care for older people with severe mental illness. *J Consult Clin Psychol* 2010; **78**: 561–73.

52. Bartels SJ, Pratt SI, Mueser KT et al. Long-term outcomes of a randomized trial of integrated skills training and preventive health care for older adults with serious mental illness. *Am J Geriatr Psychiatry* 2014; **22**: 1251–61.

53. Oostervink F, Nolen WA, Kok RM. Two years' outcome of acute mania in bipolar disorder: different effects of age and age of onset, *Int J Geriatr Psychiatry* 2015; **30**: 201–9.

54. Shulman KI, Herrmann N. The nature and management of mania in old age. *Psychiatr Clin North Am* 1999; **22**: 649–65.

55. Patient.info. *Bipolar Disorder*. Patient Information Publications. Patient.info, 2017. Last accessed on 17 October 2019 via: https://patient.info/health/bipolar-disorder-leaflet

56. Royal College of Psychiatrists. *Bipolar Disorder*. RCPsych, 2019. Last accessed on 17 October 2019 via: www.rcpsych.ac.uk/mental-health/problems-disorders/bipolar-disorder

Alcohol Misuse in Older People

Rahul Rao and Ilana B Crome

Introduction

The clinical and public mental health aspects of alcohol misuse in older people (both men and women) have increasing relevance for both old age and addiction psychiatrists. Clinical presentations are often complex and involve a number of different psychiatric, physical, and psychosocial factors. The assessment, treatment, and aftercare of alcohol-related and other comorbid mental disorders will also involve a broad range of interventions from a wide range of practitioners. Given its growing clinical relevance, there are particular areas such as alcohol-related brain damage and drug interactions with alcohol that deserve special attention.

In 2011, the Royal College of Psychiatrists published its first report on substance misuse and older people, *Our Invisible Addicts*.[1] This set out key recommendations at the levels of policy, public health, service delivery, and treatment, as well as training and education. As a result of growing recognition of the nature and scale of the issues for policy relating to service development, workforce planning, and research, this report was extensively revised in 2018.[2] Translating these needs into guidance is a key step in the process of achieving integrated care for older people with alcohol misuse and comorbid psychiatric disorder.[3] This chapter details the rationale for nurturing this area of clinical practice in psychiatry by expanding on the main areas for development, with a clinical focus. These areas comprise the epidemiology of alcohol misuse in older people; assessment (including screening); psychosocial interventions; supporting families and carers; legal and ethical aspects; acute psychiatric presentations; drug interactions; alcohol-related brain damage; and the relevance of multi-agency working.

Epidemiology

There has been seen a sharp escalation in morbidity and mortality from alcohol misuse in older people. Between 2005 and 2013, the percentage of men in the UK drinking 8 or more units of alcohol on any 1 day in the past week fell by only 5% in those aged 65 and over, compared with a reduction of at least 12% in all other age groups.[4] In the over-65s, the percentage of people who reported not drinking at all has fallen from 29.4% in 2005 to 24.2% in 2017.[5] Risky drinking, which is falling in all other age groups, is increasing in the over-50s.[5] This rise in drinking in 'baby boomers' (those born between 1946 and 1964) is of concern.[6] The highest mortality rate for alcohol-related deaths was in men aged between 55 and 74.[1] The number of people between the ages of 60 and 74 admitted to hospitals in England with mental and behavioural disorders associated with alcohol use has risen by over 50% since

2006, more than in the 15–59 age group. People aged 75 years and over with mental and behavioural disorders associated with alcohol experienced longer hospital admissions than their younger counterparts.[7]

These overall findings cannot be explained purely by rising numbers of older people in the general population, given that the population of people aged 65 and above in England and Wales increased by 11% between 2001 and 2011.[8]

Assessment

The assessment of an older person with alcohol misuse requires careful consideration (Box 6.1), taking into account age-specific factors that may influence the approach to interviewing, clinical presentation, and risks from the misuse. It is important to recognize that even low levels of alcohol use in older people can be harmful, so that dependence criteria do not necessarily have to be met to form a judgement as to whether alcohol is partly or wholly responsible for the clinical presentation.

In late-onset drinking the bias is towards women, whose problem drinking in later life is usually in reaction to a life crisis.[9] Women are a particularly vulnerable group, as alcohol

---

Box 6.1 Assessment of an older person with alcohol misuse

General Principles

Respect dignity, individuality, values, and experiences

Take into account sensory and cognitive impairment

Be aware that atypical presentations and under-reporting are common

Use additional information from other sources

Be aware of psychiatric comorbidity, functional abilities, and loss events

Consider the influence of other substances, physical disorders, and social support

Special Areas for Consideration

Living arrangements

Other substance use and misuse (nicotine/over-the-counter/prescribed/illicit drugs)

Access to alcohol (e.g. relatives/formal carers/home delivery)

Drinking 'environment' (e.g. home drinking, drinking partners)

Medical history (physical complications from alcohol)

Mental capacity

Drug interactions (including other substances)

Risk of falls, social/cultural isolation, and elder abuse (including need for safeguarding vulnerable adults)

Level of nutrition

Social support from informal carers and friends

Social pressures from debt and alcohol-using carers

Comorbid psychiatric illness (mostly depression and alcohol-related brain damage)

misuse is associated with depression and social isolation, both of which are more common in older women than in older men.[10]

Screening for Alcohol Misuse

The CAGE questionnaire screens for the core features of alcohol dependence, but it is insensitive to harmful and hazardous drinking in older people (it is further discussed in Chapter 7).[11] The Alcohol Use Disorders Identification Test (AUDIT) has been validated in some older populations,[12] with greatest sensitivity and specificity being shown with a cut-off point of 5 for older men and 3 for older women.

Shorter versions of the AUDIT include the AUDIT-5 (5 items) and the AUDIT-C (3 items). A cut-off point of 4 has been suggested for both the AUDIT-5[13] and the AUDIT-C.[14] However, these studies have not undergone extensive replication in older people. The Short Michigan Alcoholism Screening Test – Geriatric version (SMAST-G) has shown the greatest validity and use in older populations.[15]

Given the lack of sensitive screening tools for alcohol problems in older people, tools for working-age adults need to be combined with quantity/frequency measures and a comprehensive assessment that incorporates the approach taken in Box 6.1.

Psychosocial Interventions

Only 6–7% of high-risk substance misusers over the age of 60 receive the treatment that they require.[16] However, since older people are likely to be in contact with the healthcare system, there are significant opportunities to identify problems associated with substance misuse.

Recent studies have shown positive outcomes from psychosocial interventions. Although there is relatively little research in this age group, consistently positive findings emerged from those studies in which psychosocial treatment for alcohol problems in the older patient was investigated. The studies demonstrated that older people want to abstain; have the capacity to change; can be successfully offered help by physicians; respond well to brief advice and motivational enhancement therapy; do not necessarily need age-specific treatment programmes; can achieve improvement in outcomes across a range of domains (mental and physical health, relationships, legal, occupational, and financial issues) comparable to that in younger adult populations; and have the prospect of long-term recovery. Although more research needs to be done, older adults should not be barred from treatment because of age.

The Brief Intervention and Treatment for Elders (BRITE) project reported a reduction in alcohol use and problems from 80% to 18%, but there was no control group in this study.[17] The Healthy Living as You Age (HLAYA) study found improvement in both controls (advice only) and intervention (integrated care) groups at 12 months.[18] This is in keeping with the Primary Care Research in Substance Abuse and Mental Health for the Elderly (PRISM-E) study, which found that patients did better in integrated mental health and substance misuse care in primary care compared with referral to specialist providers.[19]

Box 6.2 outlines some of the challenges to recovery faced by people with alcohol misuse.

Supporting Families and Carers

Little is known about formal interventions for supporting families and carers affected by the lives of older people with alcohol misuse.[20] Families often take a long time both to identify

> **Box 6.2** Challenges to recovery from alcohol misuse
>
> *Recovery can be a lengthy process and its particular challenges include:*
>
> Supporting access to specialist services (e.g. overcoming stigma)
>
> Mobilising personal and social resources (e.g. contact with family and friends, buddying and befriending, attendance at Alcoholics Anonymous)
>
> Changing social contacts (e.g. avoiding drinking partners)
>
> Achieving controlled drinking, rather than abstinence
>
> Patient's ownership of the care plan
>
> Emotional factors (e.g. bereavement, loss, sexuality, history of abuse, relationship problems, past traumatic experiences)
>
> Practical considerations (e.g. diet, sleep, hazardous prescribed drug interactions, physical health, drinking and driving, fall hazards, safe storage of medications)
>
> Managing setbacks and not seeing them as failures
>
> Managing harm reduction using the community reinforcement approach

drinking problems and to seek help.[21] Fewer than 1% of alcohol services in England provide a service specifically for older people.[22]

Ageism from family members not appreciating the likelihood of alcohol problems in later life, together with the stigma of being labelled an 'alcoholic' and subsequent under-reporting of alcohol intake, can both influence the detection of alcohol misuse.[23] Concern from carers (commonly family members and friends) is the most common factor motivating older people to seek treatment for alcohol problems.[24] Receiving help from family and friends to cut down drinking lowers the likelihood of alcohol problems in older people.[25]

The Stress-Strain-Coping-Support (SSCS) model offers a practical approach to understanding the effects of substance misuse on family and carers,[26] with interventions centred on building resilience in individuals and a family/social structure.

Legal and Ethical Aspects

Alcohol misuse in older people can present unique legal and ethical challenges. The complexity of dependence accompanied by age-related impaired decision-making results in a conflict between encouraging controlled drinking or abstinence and continuous alcohol misuse that is influenced by a lack of mental capacity. Using the core feature of harm awareness, an assessment of mental capacity in substance use can help to distinguish an unwise decision from a lack of mental capacity per se.

Capacity can also vary over time and change in relation to different decisions. In alcohol misuse, mental incapacity may fluctuate according to level of intoxication or delirium and may be associated with a revolving-door phenomenon of hospital discharge and re-admission. This is further complicated by the observation that cognitive impairment may improve within the first 60 days of abstinence.[27] Capacity should be seen as decision-specific. If a person is deemed to be 'lacking capacity', it means that they lack capacity to make a particular decision or take a particular action for themselves at the time the decision or action needs to be taken.

Although older people with alcohol-related brain damage can often be treated under the Mental Capacity Act 2005, it should be acknowledged that the Mental Health Act 1983, as amended in 2007, can also be used if there is evidence of a mental disorder such as dementia and if the criteria for using this Act are satisfied (for further discussion of capacity and mental health legislation, see Chapters 21 and 22).

Acute Presentations of Alcohol Misuse

As signs and symptoms of alcohol misuse can be very non-specific, under-reported, and under-recognized, alcohol misuse may remain undetected in many patients in an acute setting.

Alcohol Withdrawal Syndrome

The clinical response to symptoms of alcohol withdrawal will depend on the extent of alcohol use, the degree of dependence (if any), general health, and social circumstances. Treatment may include supervised care by health and social care staff or family, and home visits. However, if older people do demonstrate alcohol withdrawal syndrome, the threshold for admission to hospital may have to be lower because of the greater seriousness of medical complications such as neurological and hepatic disorders in this age group. Furthermore, a clinical judgement needs to be made about the patient's ability to make decisions about detoxification, since this may be impaired owing to cognitive dysfunction directly as a result of substance misuse or indirectly as part of a co-occurring mental or physical disorder.

Although long-acting benzodiazepines are the treatment of choice for alcohol withdrawal syndrome in adults, older people should start with a lower dose. It is important to strike a balance between a dose sufficient to alleviate the symptoms but not enough to result in intoxication. It may be preferable to consider shorter-acting medications such as lorazepam or oxazepam, especially if there is hepatic dysfunction. It is important to ensure that the dose takes account not only of the patient's age (older people should have roughly half the dose given to a working-age adult), but also physical conditions (e.g. if the patient has liver disease, accumulation may be more likely) and mental state (the patient may have a co-occurring depression, anxiety, or psychosis).

An effect on memory can be detected even within the normal dose range of prescribed benzodiazepines and a dependence syndrome may result from low-dose prescription, so withdrawal with confusion may further complicate the clinical picture.

The starting dose is often related to the score on the Severity of Alcohol Dependence Questionnaire (SADQ), although this scale has been developed in younger people and should be translated cautiously. The regime consists of medication in 3 or 4 doses divided over 24 hours and, following stabilization over 3 or 4 days, reduction usually takes place over 7–10 days. Other prescribed and over-the-counter medication, illicit drugs, and existing health conditions must be considered when formulating the dosage regime. Patients may already be on benzodiazepines or be using medications (including opiate analgesia) that are not prescribed.

Convulsions and the possibility of Wernicke–Korsakoff syndrome should be considered, but patients should routinely be treated with vitamins B and C by intramuscular or even intravenous administration to avoid malabsorption. Emergency treatment for anaphylaxis *must* be available as, although this is very rare, it can be fatal. Anti-craving agents (such as acamprosate and naltrexone) and aversive medications (such as disulfiram) should be considered, but the evidence base in older people is sparse and a clinical decision needs to be based on the condition of the patient and the adverse effects profile.

Wernicke's Encephalopathy

Acute intoxication may mask the development of the potentially life-threatening Wernicke's encephalopathy, which can present during alcohol withdrawal or can be misdiagnosed as alcohol withdrawal. Wernicke's encephalopathy is a spectrum of disease resulting from thiamine deficiency, usually caused by alcohol misuse. There is a greater risk in those who drink continuously rather than binge drink, and the condition has a peak onset in men aged 40–59 and in women aged 30–49. It is usually described in terms of the classic triad of confusion, ataxia, and ophthalmoplegia and is a medical emergency.[28] It is important to maintain a high level of suspicion for the possibility of Wernicke's encephalopathy, particularly if the person is intoxicated.

The condition can be reversed if detected and treated promptly with parenteral (intramuscular or intravenous) thiamine. Untreated Wernicke's encephalopathy may lead to Korsakoff's psychosis, in which there is lasting damage to areas of the brain involved with memory.[29] It is important to differentiate Wernicke–Korsakoff syndrome from delirium and from other conditions that cause a thiamine deficiency, including thyrotoxicosis, metastatic cancer, long-term dialysis, and congestive heart failure.

Delirium Tremens

Delirium may be associated with intoxication or withdrawal states. Recognizing delirium tremens in acute hospital settings is especially important as it has a high morbidity and mortality but is treatable. It is characterized by hallucinations, disorientation, tachycardia, hypertension, fever, agitation, convulsions, and diaphoresis (sweating) and typically sets in following acute reduction and/or cessation of alcohol. It typically begins 48–96 hours after the last drink and, in the absence of complications, can last for up to 7 days.[30]

Elderly patients and those with concurrent medical conditions, both acute and chronic, are at higher risk of complications. Concurrent medical conditions are common and may include dehydration, unrecognized head trauma, electrolyte abnormalities, infections (including meningitis), gastrointestinal haemorrhage, pancreatitis, liver disease, and myocardial infarction. These conditions may neither be obvious nor self-reported in delirious patients. Close monitoring by nursing staff is critical for the patient's protection. A quiet room for rehydration and nursing is essential.

Physical Presentations

Older people are more sensitive to the effects of alcohol because of reduced liver metabolism and also because the typically lower water:fat ratio in their bodies results in higher circulating levels of alcohol. Common acute physical presentations of alcohol misuse in older people are falls, memory problems, and motor or sensory problems caused by a stroke. There is also an increased risk of subarachnoid haemorrhage. The aetiology of falls, like many of the common presentations described here, is multifactorial. Physiological changes associated with age, sensory deficits, postural imbalance, chronic health problems, and substance misuse, as well as environmental hazards, have all been identified as risk factors. Loss of balance, coordination, and judgement, risk-taking, autonomic neuropathy, peripheral neuropathy, cardiac disease, osteoporosis, and myopathy may all be related to alcohol misuse and make a fall more likely.

Structural and functional alcohol-related damage of the gastrointestinal system can be both acute and chronic and includes the following:

- acute gastric mucosal damage from peptic ulceration or trauma (Mallory–Weiss syndrome);
- fatty infiltration of the liver, which can progress to alcoholic hepatitis and then to cirrhosis;
- weight loss from malnutrition because of reduced food intake owing to abdominal discomfort from liver damage;
- portal hypertension from liver damage, associated with bleeding oesophageal varices;
- increased risk of gastrointestinal cancer caused by reduced levels of available vitamin A and the common concurrent use of tobacco.

Self-Harm

Alcohol reduces anxiety and inhibitions, as well as increasing impulsivity. These factors facilitate self-harm and suicide in elderly people, who as a group are already at greater risk of suicide. Reducing suicide risk in older people with depression and alcohol misuse therefore requires both a thorough assessment and a comprehensive alcohol history.

Suicide rates increase with age up to the highest rate for 45–49 year olds after which rates then fall, rising again over the age of 80.[31] Suicide rates in older people have been falling in the UK; however, this may change as the 'baby boomers' move into old age since this cohort have had higher suicide rates at any given age than earlier or later cohorts. The upper end of this cohort is already over 65 and the over-65 population will expand further over the next few decades.[32]

The relationship between per capita alcohol consumption and suicide in older people in the UK is not as strong as in countries such as Sweden, Belgium, and Portugal,[33] but there are risk factors common to all age groups that need to be taken into consideration for those at risk of suicide. These often cluster together in risk profiles and they include male gender, family history of psychiatric disorder, previous attempted suicide, more severe depression, hopelessness, and comorbid anxiety and alcohol misuse.[34]

The PRISM-E study found that heavy drinking (more than 21 UK units of alcohol per week) was positively associated with symptoms of depression and/or anxiety, as well as with perceived poor physical health.[35] The risk of suicide associated with alcohol dependence increases with age;[36] both mood disorder and physical illness are associated with completed suicide in older men with alcohol dependence.[37]

Drug Interactions

People over 65 years take more prescribed and over-the-counter drugs than younger people, and women are more likely to take these drugs than men. This means that any alcohol use may be even more problematic. Women are at particular risk of drug interactions with alcohol.

Overall, women have a lower proportion of body water (in which alcohol is distributed before it leaves the body) than men. Women have a higher blood alcohol concentration after drinking the same amount of alcohol as men, so a woman of the same weight as a man would end up with a 50% higher blood alcohol level.[38] Alcohol also suppresses the drive to breathe, which can be fatal when taken with high doses of opiates.

The most common drugs implicated in adverse interactions with alcohol are benzodiazepines and amitriptyline.[39] However, antibiotics, analgesics, anti-allergy drugs, anticoagulants, anti-emetics, anticonvulsants, antihypertensives, nicotine, aspirin, paracetamol, and many other psychotropic drugs (clozapine, mirtazapine, olanzapine, quetiapine, trazodone, and zuclopenthixol) all interact with alcohol.

Disulfiram is sometimes used in the treatment of alcohol dependence (under specialist supervision). It produces an unpleasant reaction after drinking just a small amount of alcohol. The reaction, which includes flushing of the face, throbbing headache, palpitations, nausea, and vomiting, can last for several hours. In view of this, it is rarely used in older people.

Alcohol-Related Brain Damage

Alcohol-related brain damage (ARBD) is a term used to cover a spectrum of disorders affecting memory, executive functioning, and judgement induced by chronic and heavy alcohol consumption that results in some degree of brain damage or dysfunction. Alcohol-related brain damage accounts for between 10% and 12.5% of cases of dementia in the UK.[40, 41] Only 16% of people with evidence of brain damage on post-mortem examination have been found to have any clinical presentation of the problem while alive.[42]

Commonly used screening instruments for cognitive function do not assess the frontal lobe, which is known to be more sensitive than other brain areas to the initial effects of alcohol toxicity.[43] If a more comprehensive assessment of cognitive function is required, the Addenbrooke's Cognitive Examination offers such a screen.[44]

Alcohol-related brain damage does not fall into any specific diagnostic classification and appropriate criteria for diagnosis have not been widely accepted, although alcohol-related dementia has been defined according to the following criteria: deterioration of memory and of one other higher cortical function, not explained by delirium, other substance misuse, or alcohol withdrawal syndrome.[27]

Short-term management should include immediate measures for detoxification and general nutrition (with use of parenteral thiamine as necessary), and treatment of any comorbid physical or psychological conditions or complications.

Long-term management depends on the person's recovery during rehabilitation. Once ARBD is established, the prognosis for recovery can be split broadly into quarters: 25% make a complete recovery, 25% make a significant recovery, 25% make slight recovery, and 25% make no recovery.[45] If patients make a complete or significant recovery they can be cared for in the community with the help of the family and local services, depending on the degree of disability. If they make only slight or no recovery during rehabilitation then institutional care in care homes may be the only viable option.

Alcohol-related brain damage presents a particular challenge to recovery in older people with alcohol misuse, because those with ARBD are less likely to move to controlled drinking or abstinence than those who are cognitively intact.[46]

There remains considerable scope for service development to meet the needs of older people with ARBD,[47] particularly in the delivery of such a service within limited resources. This will require a seamless approach from health and social care professionals, policy makers, educationalists, and researchers.[48] In particular, there is a need to develop care pathways in order to improve behavioural, neuropsychological, and social aspects of ARBD.

Multi-Agency Working

Multi-agency working is key to improving outcomes for older people with alcohol misuse (Box 6.3). At the level of primary care, there is an opportunity for screening and brief intervention. Links can also be forged with social services if there is a need for day care or for

---

Box 6.3 Case history: A (fictitious) example of multi-agency working with an older person with alcohol misuse

AH is a 67-year-old widower referred by his general practitioner (GP) following a routine consultation. His wife had died 3 months previously. Over the past 2 months, he had escalated his alcohol intake from 4 units to 12 units per day in the form of normal-strength beer. He had also started to feel 'fed up' and had lost interest in going to the pub, drinking at home instead.

AH was assessed 2 weeks later on a home visit by the local community mental health team (CMHT). At assessment, his flat was cluttered, with no food in the refrigerator, and the living room was strewn with beer cans. He had been asking a neighbour to buy bread and milk, as well as alcohol. His drinking day started at around 10:00 a.m., but he did not report any morning sweats or shakes on waking.

AH was born in Ireland and came to live in the UK in his 20s, working mainly in the construction industry. He got married in his 30s and continued to work until he retired in his 60s. There were two children from the marriage, but they both lived abroad and there had been no contact with them since his wife died. He had had a single episode of depression in his 40s, treated by his GP with antidepressants.

In his substance misuse history, he started drinking alcohol socially at the age of 16, consuming 4 units of normal-strength beer every day. This drinking pattern continued until he married, when it fell to 2 units per day. There had been no history of marital or occupational problems associated with alcohol misuse and no history of dependence. AH had smoked 20 medium-tar filtered cigarettes per day since the age of 16. There was no history of illicit drug misuse or misuse of prescribed drugs or over-the-counter medication.

In his medical history, AH had chronic obstructive pulmonary disease, hypertension, and gastro-oesophageal reflux.

A diagnosis of depressive disorder was made. He was started on a selective serotonin reuptake inhibitor and both brief and extended interventions to reduce drinking were delivered over the following 2 weeks. This was supplemented by CMHT support and attendance at a day centre for older Irish people. After successfully cutting down his alcohol intake to 2 units per day, AH was discharged after 6 months of CMHT support, but was re-referred 18 months later after escalating his alcohol intake following a diagnosis of diabetes mellitus. At the point of referral, he was found to show features of alcohol dependence, had stopped his antidepressant 6 months previously, and was expressing suicidal thoughts.

Following a 3-month inpatient admission that involved detoxification and re-starting antidepressants, he was taken on by the older adult home treatment team and also received psychological therapy that involved motivational interviewing techniques. This was supplemented by the community reinforcement approach from community (district) nurses and medical care by the CMHT. After 12 months of CMHT support, he was discharged, again returning to controlled drinking.

Two years later, AH was referred by his GP following placement in a nursing home. He had reportedly developed cognitive decline and there had been several inpatient medical admissions and failed home leave (even with a package of care). At assessment, there was evidence of moderate dementia, with prominent frontal lobe impairment.

addressing issues around the protection of vulnerable adults. The voluntary (third) sector can also support patients, as well as their families and carers.

At the level of secondary care, there is further scope for providing services that can implement both treatment and harm reduction. For example,

- substance misuse services might offer psychological interventions (e.g. motivational interviewing) and detoxification;
- old age psychiatry services might offer the community reinforcement approach (see below) and, through their occupational therapists, can intervene to improve the quality of the living environment; they can also offer psychological treatment for comorbid mood disorders and neuropsychological testing for ARBD;
- geriatric services might offer a comprehensive assessment that includes physiotherapy;
- specialist housing might provide 'wet hostels' (staffed community facilities where any level of drinking is permitted, with no therapeutic focus on reducing alcohol intake) to reduce vulnerability, and there is also scope for specialized residential units that can provide an environment of controlled drinking.

The community reinforcement approach to treating alcohol and other drug problems is designed to make changes in the individual's environment, to reduce substance misuse. Community reinforcement approach addresses multiple problems by utilizing community resources such as family, social, recreational, and occupational supports to effect change in an individual's drinking or drug-using behaviour so that reduction of substance use becomes more rewarding than substance misuse.

The development of integrated care to manage alcohol misuse and comorbid psychiatric disorder in older people is one of the most important challenges to workforce development in the twenty-first century.[49] Older people require a greater focus on physical disorders, depression, organic brain disorders, and social factors such as social isolation, bereavement, activities of daily living, mental capacity, safeguarding, and carer support.

The first UK training course for health professionals on improving knowledge, skills, and attitudes regarding alcohol misuse and comorbid psychiatric disorder in older people shows promise in improving competencies in screening and brief intervention and has marked a turning point in the development of a competent workforce.[50]

Conclusions

The number of older people is rising rapidly, with a concomitant increase in rates of comorbid mental and physical disorders, for which they inevitably take numerous prescription drugs and over-the-counter medications.[51] In this context of polypharmacy, an older person's clinical presentation can be transformed by alcohol use, misuse, and dependence.

It is incumbent on medical practitioners to lead and manage teams that can assess, detect, treat, and refer to relevant services. With older patients, this demands awareness of their distinctive attributes, appreciation of the complex interrelationship between addiction and other medical and psychiatric conditions, confidence in the implementation of effective interventions, a grasp of legal and ethical factors, meticulous support of teams, and perceptive appreciation of the needs of families and carers.

Detailed knowledge is needed not only of the acute effects, adverse actions, and chronic consequences of alcohol use, misuse, and dependence, but also of their interactions and impact on medical and mental illnesses. There is also the need to be gentle, tolerant, and soothing with patients and families who are struggling with sometimes harrowing situations. A sense of hope and optimism is justified because the evidence suggests that many older people want to stop misuse and that success among people who receive treatment to curtail or contain their use is as high among older people as among younger adults. Addiction practitioners need to be aware of the special issues involved in treating older people and know how to offer an age-sensitive service, so that older people are not barred from the opportunities for improvement that are available to younger people. This involves considering the needs of older people at every point of service delivery, including availability, accessibility, intelligent adaptation of facilities, and sympathetic modification of treatment options. In short, specialists can work together to value older substance misusers so that they can achieve a healthy, active future.

Acknowledgements

For information, the citation for the original paper on which this chapter is based is:

Rao R, Crome I. Alcohol misuse in older people. *Adv Psychiatr Treat* 2016; **22**: 118–26.

References

1. Crome, I, Dar, K, Janikiewicz, S et al. *Our Invisible Addicts* (College Report CR165). Royal College of Psychiatrists, 2011.

2. Royal College of Psyhciatrists. *Our Invisible Addicts*, 2nd edition (College Report CR211). Royal College of Psychiatrists, 2018. Last accessed 1 October 2019 via: www.rcpsych.ac.uk/docs/default-source/improving-care/better-mh-policy/college-reports/college-report-cr211.pdf?sfvrsn=820fe4bc_2

3. Rao, RT, Crome, I, Crome, P et al. *Substance Misuse in Older People: An Information Guide* (Cross-Faculty Report OA/AP/01). Royal College of Psychiatrists, 2015.

4. Office for National Statistics. *Drinking Habits among Adults 2012*. ONS, 2013. Last accessed 25 September 2019 via: www.ons.gov.uk/ons/dcp171778_338863.pdf

5. Office for National Statistics. *Adult Drinking Habits in Great Britain: 2005 to 2016*. ONS, 2017. Last accessed 25 September 2019 via: www.ons.gov.uk/releases/adultdrinkinghabitsingreatbritain2015

6. Rao R. Substance misuse in older people. *BMJ* 2017; **358**: j3885.

7. Alcohol Concern. *Alcohol and the Mental Health of Older People*. Alcohol Concern, 2013.

8. Office for National Statistics. *2011 Census, Population and Household Estimates for the United Kingdom*. ONS, 2012. Last accessed 25 September 2019 via: www.ons.gov.uk/ons/publications/re-reference-tables.html?edition=tcm%3A77-270247

9. Schonfeld L, Dupree LW. Antecedents of drinking for early- and late-onset elderly alcohol abusers. *J Stud Alcohol* 1991; **52**: 587–92.

10. Van den Berg JF, Kok RM, van Marwijk HW et al. Correlates of alcohol abstinence and at-risk alcohol consumption in older adults with depression: the NESDO study. *Am J Geriatr Psychiatry* 2014; **22**: 866–74.

11. Ewing JA. Detecting alcoholism: the CAGE questionnaire. *JAMA* 1984; **252**: 1905–7.

12. Roberts AME, Marshall J, Macdonald AJD. Which screening test for alcohol consumption is best associated with 'at risk' drinking in older primary care attenders? *Prim Care Ment Health* 2005; **3**: 131–8.

13. Philpot M, Pearson N, Petratou V et al. Screening for problem drinking in older people referred to a mental health service: a comparison of CAGE and AUDIT. *Aging Ment Health* 2003; **7**: 171–5.

14. Aalto M, Alho H, Halme J et al. The Alcohol Use Disorders Identification Test (AUDIT) and its derivatives in screening for heavy drinking among the elderly. *Int J Geriatr Psychiatry* 2011; **26**: 881–5.

15. Blow FC, Gillespie BW, Barry KL. Brief screening for alcohol problems in elderly

populations using the Short Michigan Alcoholism Screening Test–Geriatric Version (SMAST-G). *Alcohol Clin Exp Res* 1998; **22** (Suppl. 3): 131A.

16. Alcohol Concern. *15:15 The Case for Better Access to Treatment for Alcohol Dependence in England.* Alcohol Concern, 2013.

17. Schonfeld L, King-Kallimanis BL, Duchene DM et al. Screening and brief intervention for substance misuse among older adults: the Florida BRITE project. *Am J Public Health* 2010; **100**: 108–14.

18. Borok J, Galier P, Dinolfo M et al. Why do older unhealthy drinkers decide to make changes or not in their alcohol consumption? Data from the Healthy Living as You Age Study. *J Am Geriatr Soc* 2013; **61**: 1296–302.

19. Oslin D, Grantham S, Coakley E et al. PRISM-E: comparison of integrated care and enhanced specialty referral in managing at-risk alcohol use. *Psychiatr Serv* 2006; **57**: 954–8.

20. Copello A, Orford J. Addiction and the family: is it time for services to take notice of the evidence? *Addiction* 2002; **97**: 1361–3.

21. AdFam. *Parental Substance Misuse: Through the Eyes of the Worker.* AdFam, 2013.

22. Wadd S, Lapwort K, Sullivan M et al. *Working with Older Drinkers.* University of Bedfordshire, 2011.

23. Rockett IR, Putnam SL, Jia H et al. Declared and undeclared substance use among emergency department patients: a population-based study. *Addiction* 2006; **101**: 706–12.

24. Finlayson R, Hurt R, Davis L et al. Alcoholism in elderly persons: a study of the psychiatric and psychosocial features of 216 inpatients. *Mayo Clin Proc* 1988; **63**: 761–8.

25. Moos RH, Schutte K, Brennan P et al. Ten-year patterns of alcohol consumption and drinking problems among older women and men. *Addiction* 2004; **99**: 829–38.

26. Orford J, Copello A, Velleman R et al. Family members affected by a close

relative's addiction: the stress-strain-coping-support model. *Drugs (Abingdon Engl)* 2010; **17** (Suppl. 1): 36–43.

27. Oslin D, Atkinson R, Smith D et al. Alcohol related dementia: proposed clinical criteria. *Int J Geriatr Psychiatry* 1998; **13**: 203–12.

28. Sechi G, Serra A. Wernicke's encephalopathy: new clinical settings and recent advances in diagnosis and management. *Lancet Neurol* 2007; **6**: 442–55.

29. So YT, Simon RP. Deficiency diseases of the nervous system. In *Bradley's Neurology in Clinical Practice* (6th ed.) (eds. RB Daroff, GM Fenichel, J Jankovic, JC Mazziotta): 1340–52. Saunders, 2012.

30. Mayo-Smith MF. Pharmacological management of alcohol withdrawal: a meta-analysis and evidence-based practice guideline. *JAMA* 1997; **278**: 144–51.

31. Office for National Statistics. *Suicides in the UK: 2017 Registrations.* ONS, 2017. Last accessed 26 September 2019 via: www .ons.gov.uk/peoplepopulationandcommu nity/birthsdeathsandmarriages/deaths/bul letins/suicidesintheunitedkingdom/ 2017registrations

32. Conwell Y, van Orden K, Caine ED. Suicide in older adults. *Psychiatr Clin North Am* 2011; **34**: 451–68.

33. Ramstedt M. Alcohol and suicide in 14 European countries. *Addiction* 2001; **96**: 59–75.

34. Hawton K, Casañas I, Comabella C et al. Risk factors for suicide in individuals with depression: a systematic review. *J Affect Disorders* 2013; **147**: 17–28.

35. Kirchner JE, Zubritsky C, Cody M et al. Alcohol consumption among older adults in primary care. *J Gen Intern Med* 2007; **22**: 92–7.

36. Conner KR, Beautrais AL, Conwell Y. Moderators of the relationship between alcohol dependence and suicide and medically serious suicide attempts: analyses of Canterbury Suicide Project data. *Alcohol Clin Exp Res* 2003; **27**: 1156–61.

37. Conner KR, Conwell Y. Age-related patterns of factors associated with

completed suicide in men with alcohol dependence. *Am J Addict* 1999; **8**: 312–8.

38. Pharmaceutical Press. *Stockley's Drug Interactions*. Pharmaceutical Press, 2012.

39. Gallagher P, O'Mahony D. STOPP (Screening Tool of Older Persons' potentially inappropriate Prescriptions): application to acutely ill elderly patients and comparison with Beers' criteria. *Age Ageing* 2008; **37**: 673–9.

40. Lishman WA. Alcohol and the brain. *Br J Psychiatry* 1990; **156**: 635–44.

41. Harvey RJ, Rossor MN, Skelton-Robinson M et al. *Young Onset Dementia: Epidemiology, Clinical Symptoms, Family Burden, Support and Outcome*. Dementia Research Group, Imperial College, 1998.

42. Harper CG, Sheedy D, Halliday GM et al. Neuropathological studies: the relationship between alcohol and aging. In *Alcohol Problems and Aging* (eds. ESL Gomberg, AM Hegedus, RA Zucker) NIAAA Research Monograph no. 33: 117–34. National Institute on Alcohol Abuse and Alcoholism, 1998.

43. Zahr NM, Kaufman KL, Harper CG. Clinical and pathological features of alcohol-related brain damage. *Nat Rev Neurol* 2011; **7**: 284–94.

44. Mioshi E, Dawson K, Mitchell J et al. The Addenbrooke's Cognitive Examination Revised (ACE-R): a brief cognitive test battery for dementia screening. *Int J Geriatr Psychiatry* 2006; **21**: 1078–85.

45. MacRae R, Cox S. *Meeting the Needs of People with Alcohol Related Brain Damage: A Literature Review on the Existing and Recommended Service Provision and Models of Care*. Dementia Services Development Centre, University of Stirling, 2003.

46. Rao R. Outcomes from liaison psychiatry referrals for older people with alcohol use disorders in the UK. *Ment Health Subst Use* 2013; **6**: 362–8.

47. Rao R, Shanks A. Development and implementation of a dual diagnosis strategy for older people in south east London. *Adv Dual Diagn* 2011; **4**: 28–35.

48. Rao R, Draper B. Alcohol related brain damage in older people. *Lancet Psychiatry* 2015; **2**: 674–45.

49. Academy of Medical Royal Colleges. *Alcohol and Other Drugs: Core Medical Competencies* (Occasional Paper OP85). Royal College of Psychiatrists, 2012.

50. Saxton L, Lancashire S, Kipping C. Meeting the training needs of staff working with older people with dual diagnosis. *Adv Dual Diagn* 2011; **4**: 36–46.

51. Crome I, Wu LT, Rao RT, Crome P. (eds.) *Substance Use and Older People*. John Wiley & Sons, 2014.

Chapter

7

Drug Misuse in Older People
Old Problems and New Challenges

Ajay Wagle and Vellingiri Raja Badrakalimuthu

Introduction

An increase in the population of older people, associated with the increasing demand for holistic care to meet their complex needs, has focused attention on substance misuse in older adults. There is growing awareness among health and social care professionals of the challenges that older adults face in accessing and receiving appropriate treatment for substance misuse and the need for policy revisions to define an inclusive substance misuse service that will be able to address addiction and the impact on physical, mental and social well-being of vulnerable and frail older people.

Historically, substance misuse among older adults has received little attention because of misguided suppositions such as 'substance misuse is seldom seen after middle-age', 'long-term drug addicts die prematurely or recover spontaneously', 'late-onset addiction is rare' or 'late-onset addiction is restricted to a small group of aging criminals'.[1] But evidence from 1990 onwards has confirmed that this population will not necessarily die, go away or 'mature out of it'! Meanwhile, the UK Office for National Statistics Study of Psychiatric Morbidity showed, as early as 2002, lifetime experience of any illicit drug use as 24 per 1,000 in 65–69 age group and 34 per 1,000 in the 70–74 age group with drug use in the previous year being 10 and 6 per 1,000 respectively.[2]

Many in this population will themselves not recognize substance misuse as a condition that needs treatment; and it may only be assessed when a crisis impacts on the physical or mental health, or the social well-being of the individual. An understanding of substance misuse in older adults has to focus on psychological aspects of addiction as those who have had long-term substance misuse from an earlier age have different characteristics to those who start their misuse in later life. For example, those who start in later life most likely misuse alcohol and rarely return to illicit drugs. The lack of diagnostic certainties in this population with complex physical and mental health comorbidities, along with the lack of rigorous training and exposure of healthcare professionals to these situations, suggests that services may ultimately fail to resolve substance misuse in this vulnerable population. As an example, McInnes and Powell report that junior doctors identify only 3 out of 88 medical inpatients as having harmful use of benzodiazepines.[3]

Healthcare professionals, psychiatrists in particular, have to be aware of atypical presentations caused by physical health comorbidities, the limited reliability of questionnaires and diagnostic tools, domestic and social precipitants, all of which need in-depth assessment. This is difficult where time has become an expensive commodity within primary and secondary care services. This chapter provides insights to the extent of the problems in older adults, their impact and consequences, and evidence-based treatments available for clinicians and their patients.

For the purposes of this chapter, older adults are defined as the population over 60 years of age; and misuse will be used in the wider context of occasional use, including (a) intoxication without complications not amounting to harmful use, abuse or dependence, (b) harmful use, (c) abuse and (d) dependence (as defined in ICD-10), as well as 'abuse' as defined by authors in their studies. This chapter does not deal with alcohol misuse and its related disorders except in passing, since these have already been dealt with in Chapter 6.

Extent of Substance Misuse and Risk Factors

In an English sample of over 4,000 people over the age of 50 years, lifetime cannabis abuse of 11.4%, past-year cannabis abuse of 1.8%, lifetime tranquilisers abuse of 2.3%, and past-year tranquilisers abuse of 0.4% was reported in the 50–64 years age group; and it was 1.7%, 0.4%, 1.5% and 0.4% respectively, for the 65 years and above population.[4] In an American population, a higher proportion of abuse was reported in 2006 compared to 1985, with cannabis being the most commonly abused substance (1.6% vs 0.3%), followed by cocaine (0.3% vs 0.1%) and inhalants (0.1% vs 0%).[5] In a sample of over 8,000 people 65 years and above, lifetime prevalence of the abuse of sedatives was reported as 1.1%; for tranquilisers it was 0.7%, opioids 1.1%, amphetamines 0.4%, cannabis 1.4%, crack cocaine 0.2%, hallucinogens 0.1%, inhalants 0.06% and heroin 0.01%.[6]

In terms of risk factors associated with substance misuse in this population, Lin et al. report divorce or separation.[7] Blazer and Wu report major depression for cannabis and cocaine users, with male Afro-Caribbeans abusing cannabis and Caucasians abusing cocaine.[8] Johnson et al. report older users have later onset of cannabis, cocaine and crack use, have earlier onset of heroin use and are more likely to have histories of sexually transmitted disease than young users.[9] Finally, Lofwall et al. report admissions to hospitals increasing for comorbid substance and alcohol abuse compared to decreases in admissions for alcohol abuse only.[10] Table 7.1 provides a summary of risk factors for substance misuse in older adults.

Misused Substances

Benzodiazepines and Hypnotics

Improvement in recognition of anxiety disorders and reduction in use of antipsychotics have led to increase in use of benzodiazepines. As early as 1988, Morgan reported a prevalence of 16% for hypnotic drug use from a British sample of over-65-year-olds with a higher proportion over 75 years, 25% abusing benzodiazepines for more than 10 years and 71% reporting daily use.[11] The National Survey on Drug Use and Health, an annual survey of over 70,000 respondents in the United States, reports that in the age group of 50 years and over, females use tranquilisers (benzodiazepines, meprobamate and muscle relaxers used non-medically) and sedatives (temazepam, flurazepam, triazolam and barbiturates used non-medically) more than males: 74.5% female vs 25.5% male, with a higher prevalence of tranquilisers amongst Caucasians and sedatives amongst Hispanics.[12] For those who might think the Z-drugs are safer than benzodiazepines from the perspective of addiction, Cimolai has cautioned that there is emergence of addiction amongst those prescribed Zopiclone for insomnia.[13]

In older adults, physical dependence on benzodiazepines can arise without dose escalation owing to pharmacokinetic properties, duration of treatment, shorter half-lives and

Table 7.1 Risk factors for substance misuse in older adults

Predisposing factors
- Family history
- Previous substance misuse or dependence
- Personality traits
- Social norms

Factors that may increase substance exposure and consumption level
- Gender (men: alcohol, illicit drugs; women: sedative hypnotics, anxiolytics)
- Chronic illnesses associated with pain (opioid analgesics, cannabis), insomnia (hypnotic drugs), anxiety (anxiolytics)
- Long-term prescribing (sedative hypnotics, anxiolytics)
- Caregiver overuse of medication (institutionalised elderly)
- Life-stress, social isolation
- Negative effects (depression, demoralisation, anger)
- Family collusion
- Bereavement (male widowers)
- Boredom and disposable income

Factors that may increase the effects and abuse potential of substances
- Age-associated drug sensitivity (pharmacokinetic and pharmacodynamic factors)
- Chronic medical illnesses
- Other medications (drug–drug interactions)

Adapted from Atkinson MR. Substance abuse in elderly, In *Psychiatry in the Elderly* (eds. Jacoby R, Oppenheimer C) 799–834 Oxford University Press, 2002.

higher milligram potency of particular agents.[14] Non-benzodiazepine factors for misuse include prior or concurrent alcohol or sedative drug dependence, chronic insomnia and/or pain, personality disorder, depression, anxiety and regular use of at least three non-psychotropic drugs.[15] Fernandez and Cassagne-Pinel have suggested that drug addiction in older people cannot be reduced simply to a physiological addiction to a particular drug, but must be understood in terms of a complex process (which would require a detailed analysis to understand) of a psychological addiction to a particular drug too. With regard to benzodiazepine addiction in older people, multiple pathologies, as well as changes induced by the ageing process itself, are involved. Old age can engender a depression that results in addictive behaviour.[16]

Opioids and Cocaine

Pain relief, an essential part of the treatment of chronic illnesses, has led to varying degrees of opiate or opioid misuse ranging from inappropriate use to dependency. There has to be a distinction between dependence on prescribed and non-prescribed opiates, with prescribed opiate dependence starting with increasing doses made necessary for pain relief. In terms of heroin abuse though, it is more the case that the people dependent have commenced abuse of heroin at a younger age and present with polysubstance misuse (see below). Woo and Chen reported opiate use prevalence in psychiatric emergency patients at 3.3%.[17] Moore et al. reported past-year prevalence for opioids as 0.5%,[6] whilst Rajaratnam et al. gave past-month opioid use among people aged more than 55 years as 27% in a sample of 156 patients.[18] Beynon et al., in a study of more than 1,000 substance misusers, showed that the proportion of 50–74 year olds in contact with syringe exchange programmes rose from 0.2% in 1998 to 3.8% in 2004.[19] The majority of those receiving treatment in this group were aged 50–54, and there was an increasing number of both male and female drug users aged 55–59 years and of males between 60 and 64 years.[19]

Rivers and colleagues in a study amongst adults over 60 years reported 2% testing positive for cocaine in emergency departments and found rates of older adults entering treatment for cocaine use at 0.1%.[20] There is anecdotal evidence to suggest increasing prevalence of cocaine use among the baby boomer generation as they get older.

Atkinson has stated that opioid misusers are often men who have survived their addiction for years, have led socially isolated lives and have been secretive about their drug use having avoided law enforcement agencies and supported their drug habits through legal employment.[1] There have been observations of younger family members influencing older adults to misuse drugs. Alcohol dependence and childhood abuse are associated with opioid misuse and male gender, relatively young age (66 years) and alcohol/drug misuse with cocaine misuse.

Other Drugs

Fahmy et al. reported a 10-fold increase in lifetime use for cannabis, amphetamine and LSD from 1993 to 2007.[4] White et al. found a significant increase in misuse of cannabis and inhalants,[5] whilst Lin et al. reported lifetime prevalence of amphetamines at 0.11%.[7] Blazer and Wu[8] and Moore et al.[6] reported past-year use of hallucinogens as 0.1% and methamphetamine as 0.1%.

Chronic and painful diseases increase the drive to misuse euphoric drugs such as cannabis, with men at the highest risk of abusing stimulants, sedatives and tranquilisers.[21] Simoni-Wastila and Stricker associated misuse of illicit substances with misuse of prescription drugs.[22]

Inappropriate and Over-The-Counter Medications

Older adults are significant self-medicators. They purchase 40% of all over-the-counter medications. Commonly misused medications include analgesics, laxatives, and cough and cold products. On average older people are prescribed twice as many medications as working-age adults. One in ten older people is prescribed potentially inappropriate drugs.[23] Prescribing is often less rational, with less stringent monitoring, particularly in institutional settings, and there is increased complexity around hoarding and drug sharing. Psychotropic drug misuse is four times higher in women compared to men and is associated with lower levels of education, income, health, social support as well as widowhood. Other risk factors for abuse in older adults include personality disorders, somatoform conditions, anxiety, adjustment and sleep disorders.[24]

Polysubstance Misuse

Polysubstance misuse usually takes the form of coexisting dependence on alcohol and either prescribed sedatives or opioid analgesics. Amongst prescription drug users, 77% were on drugs that interacted with alcohol and 19% reported concomitant alcohol misuse. Of all emergency department visits by older people involving opioid analgesics, 72% have been associated with multiple drug misuse.[25]

Diagnostic Challenges

Clinical services, including geriatric inpatient units and older adults' community mental health settings, are still ill-equipped to provide the knowledge, skills and attitudes required for assessment and treatment of substance misuse in older adults.

There are several age-related factors that tend to reduce the likelihood of diagnosing substance misuse in older adults. Some of these factors are:

- lack of recognition of urges as cravings
- misattributions
- lack of awareness that a previously safe situation has now become physically hazardous because negative effects might occur at relatively low doses
- failure to connect symptoms to substance misuse
- cognitive impairment interfering with monitoring.
- failure by family members to acknowledge that substance misuse is a problem
- reduced social contact leading to lack of opportunity for peer recognition of drug abuse.

An audit in Norfolk conducted in 2005 found that 60% of older patients admitted to an acute psychiatric ward had no documented notes on drug or alcohol history. The same audit reported that junior doctors felt it was inappropriate to ask older adults about their drug or alcohol histories, believing that it would only be a negative finding or it may cause offence. They also reported a lack of focused training in assessing and treating substance misuse in older adults.

Symptoms and signs of substance misuse can be mistaken for depression or dementia. Delirium from substance withdrawal during admissions to acute medical hospitals can be misattributed to other physical illnesses. Substance misuse in older adults amongst ethnic minorities remains a much understudied area.

There are several ways to improve screening for substance misuse in older adults (see Table 7.2). It is necessary to be vigilant when assessing high-risk populations including the homeless, those with a history of substance misuse, depression or bereavement, retirement, social isolation and immobility. The eight-question NM-ASSIST (www.drugabuse.gov/nmassist/step/0) is a simple tool for exploring substance misuse. Apart from scored questions, it also includes questions about intravenous drug use. However, this tool is only one indicator of an older adult's potential substance misuse problem.

A modified form of the CAGE questionnaire (see Box 7.1), omitting the first question about cutting down, has been trialled for use in older adults and has been shown to have improved sensitivity and specificity compared with the full CAGE questionnaire.[26] The Drug Abuse Screening Test (DAST) is available in 10-, 20- and 28-item versions and has moderate to high levels of validity, sensitivity and specificity.

Good history-taking skills using motivational interview technique, the ability to apply diagnostic criteria in complex presentations with physical and psychiatric sequelae of substance misuse and appropriate involvement of specialists in other medical specialties will undoubtedly increase the chances of accurate diagnosis.

Impact of Substance Misuse

The ageing body with its altered pharmacokinetics, sensory impairment and, in particular, the ageing brain with its cognitive impairment can lead to significant and rapid biopsychosocial deterioration in older adults, leading to imminent death (see Table 7.3).

Table 7.2 Improving diagnosis

- Vigilance and high degree of suspicion in high-risk groups
- Review of regular medications
- Monitoring of prescriptions in primary care and pharmacy
- Routine screening during history-taking

Further drug/alcohol assessment if any of the following are observed:
- Unexplained cognitive impairment and neurological symptoms
- Fluctuating motor activity
- Autonomic symptoms on physical examination
- Sudden changes in social and financial situation
- Unexplained abnormal liver function tests

Corroboration by:
- Home visits
- Third-party information with consent

Table 7.3 Drug-poisoning deaths per 100,000 aged 55–64

	White	Black	Hispanic	Male	Female
Natural and semi-synthetic opioids	5.2	2.5	2.3	5.1	3.9
Synthetic opioids	1.5	0.8	Not available	1.2	2.2
Benzodiazepines	2.9	0.8	1	2.7	2.2
All drug poisoning	18	20.2	9.8	20	14.1

SAMHSA Treatment Episodes Data Set-Admissions (TEDS-A)-Concatenated, 1992–2010. Office of Applied Studies, Substance Abuse and Mental Health Services Administration (SAMHSA). ICPSR25221-v5. Inter-university Consortium for Political and Social Research, Ann Arbor, MI (2012).

Box 7.1 The CAGE questionnaire (see also Chapter 6)

1. Have you ever felt you needed to **C**ut down on your drinking?
2. Have people **A**nnoyed you by criticising your drinking?
3. Have you ever felt **G**uilty about drinking?
4. Have you ever felt you needed a drink first thing in the morning (**E**ye-opener) to steady your nerves or to get rid of a hangover?

Substance Misuse and Mental Health

Frischer and colleagues reported a 27% increase in comorbid psychiatric illness and substance misuse in older adults attending primary care, benzodiazepine use with confusion being the commonest presentation.[28] Dual diagnoses have also been reported in 37% of elderly psychiatric hospital patients, of whom 29% were misusing alcohol and substances, 17% had attempted suicide and 5% had overdosed on a substance of misuse.[29] Among older adults admitted to hospital with prescribed drug dependence, a third to a tenth present with mood disorder, organic mental disorder, personality disorder, somatoform disorder or anxiety.

Substance Misuse and Physical Health

In the USA, high rates of sexually transmitted diseases, liver diseases and stroke have been reported in those misusing substances, with injecting drug users reporting worse health status than national samples.[31] Older adults with substance misuse disorders make greater use of healthcare resources than those without and tend to use emergency departments frequently. In comparison with a younger cohort, older adults who start substance misuse in late life have significantly more medical problems and worse general health.[10]

Physiological alterations influence the serum levels of drugs and in some instances natural progression of liver diseases, such as that caused by Hepatitis C, will mean that effects of drug use become evident only in old age. In older people, impairment produced by benzodiazepines can be more severely compromising than the same dose given to younger people. Falls, elevated liver enzymes, pancreatitis, hepatitis, hypertension, arrhythmia, urinary incontinence, lung disease and arthritis, as well as drug–drug inter-actions including interactions with antibiotics and diabetic medications, are common in older adults with substance misuse.[30] Hip fractures and road traffic accidents are asso-ciated with benzodiazepine misuse in older adults. Serious discontinuation symptoms occur in up to 90% on low-dose benzodiazepines and grand mal seizures occur in 20–30% untreated for benzodiazepine withdrawal. Cannabis use has been demonstrated to have adverse neurological effects including impaired perceptuo-motor coordination and motor performance.

Substance Misuse and Cognition

Cognitive functioning is influenced by type, quantity, duration, intoxication and with-drawal effects, as well as sensory impairment and comorbid physical and mental illnesses in older adults. Older adults can often be overlooked or misdiagnosed. Long-term memory, psychomotor speed, learning and retention of new information, verbal memory and visuo-spatial ability have all been observed to be impaired by substance misuse including opioids, benzodiazepines and cannabis.[32] Evidence exists to suggest that benzodiazepine use in the elderly population is associated with cognitive decline, dementia and AD. Stronger links have emerged from studies examining longer-acting benzodiazepines, longer durations of use and earlier exposure to benzodiazepines.[36] Cognition may improve when benzodiaze-pines are discontinued. Cognitive impairment impacts on engagement with a treatment plan for managing substance misuse and interferes with psychosocial interventions.

Treatment and Outcomes

A significant proportion of older adults does not seek treatment for substance misuse and they are typically excluded from clinical trials. Despite these shortcomings, the general principles of treatment are to stabilize, reduce consumption, treat comorbidities and organize psychosocial interventions aimed at relapse prevention. Inpatient units, especially when detoxification can be complex in the context of comorbid physical ailments, have to be considered for frail older adults.

Table 7.4 Drug services for older adults

What should services look like?

- Accessible through multiple referral routes
- Well networked with community resources
- Strong links with older persons' mental health services
- Able to provide targeted information for older adults
- Have sites for consultation in primary and secondary care centres

What should they do?

- Improve detection and engage in treatment
- Provide pragmatic and optimistic management
- Encourage harm reduction
- Oversee detox and maintenance treatments
- Provide psychological assessments and therapies
- Liaise with primary and secondary care to provide physical and mental healthcare
- Provide social interventions including family work
- Teach, train and research
- Reduce prejudice and stigma

Characteristics associated with better outcomes when addressing substance abuse in older adults using age-sensitive treatments include a supportive and non-confrontational approach with flexibility, sensitivity to gender, cultural differences and client functioning, with a holistic focus and emphasis on coping and social skills. Age-sensitive management should include biopsychosocial assessment, a treatment plan, attention to co-occurring conditions, referrals and care co-ordination and empirically supported psychosocial interventions. Older adults are more likely to have abstinence as a goal and they do better than younger cohorts especially long term. Success of treatments depends on having appropriate services for older adults (Table 7.4).

As there is very little study on treatment for individual substances, this section will focus on benzodiazepines and opioid misuse treatment. However, it needs to be said that pharmacists and primary care physicians have an important role to play in over-the-counter and prescribed medication misuse. One has to be aware, too, of comorbid alcohol misuse and the place of motivational interviewing, brief alcohol directed interventions in opportunistic settings, guided self-management, as well as psychosocial interventions focusing on social circumstances and networks – all of which have been trialled successfully. Miller et al. in a systematic review (albeit not confined to older people) showed that although treatment effects were modest, medications for alcohol dependence, in conjunction with either brief support or more extensive psychosocial therapy, could be effective in primary and specialty care medical settings.[35]

Opioids

Elderly methadone-dependent patients are more likely to be seen in geriatric settings, are less likely to request detoxification and often prefer higher doses. They tend to face a variety of physical and psychosocial obstacles in accessing treatment. Sartre et al. reported that patients between 55 and 77 years stay in treatment longer, are less likely to report friends or family encouraging drug use, are more likely to report abstinence in the past month or year, but are less likely to be members of 12-step programmes and more likely to have worse health.[33] Lofwall et al. have reported similarly high rates of retention in treatment alongside fewer positive urine screens for substances, but poorer physical health and poor quality of life in terms of physical functioning and pain.[10] Similar statistics showing poor physical health as well as an increase in the prevalence of mental illness in older adults in methadone maintenance treatment have been reported.[30]

Completers compared to non-completers of treatment programmes are more likely to decrease their use of non-medical prescription drugs, show improved cognitive functioning, increased vitality and decreases in bodily pain along with improvements in mental health.[34]

Treatment for older adults can include expert medical advice, given that there are frequently comorbid conditions, especially in the sub-group with analgesic dependence. Assessment for pain and depression will be important. A change to long-acting opioids may allow for easier reduction in use.

Benzodiazepines

It is well recognized that it is difficult to dissuade older adults from persisting with sedatives. Treatment plans have to focus on addressing psychosocial factors. There is a significant need for education about physiological and psychological dependence. Successful treatment plans have emphasized the importance of tailoring reduction guidelines to individual needs, especially when using long-acting benzodiazepines. And each step in the reduction programme needs to be for a longer time than might be the case in a younger adult.

Conclusion

Substance misuse in older adults is a major health and social care challenge. Policy recommendations need to address issues around the fragmentation of services and should aim at specialist multidisciplinary teams able to access multiple health and social care agencies. Education and training of clinicians who care for older adults, irrespective of specialties and professions, will play an important role in identifying and signposting older adults to access timely and appropriate treatment for substance misuse. Awareness of substance misuse problems in older adults has to be increased through public education initiatives. Social and healthcare services must work collaboratively with substance users through robust care pathways for better outcomes in terms of health and well-being.

Acknowledgement

For information, the original paper on which this chapter is based was:

Badrakalimuthu VR, Rumball D, Wagle A. Drug misuse in older people: old problems and new challenges. *Adv Psychiatr Treat* 2010; **16**: 421–429.

Dr Daphne Rumball was a co-author on that paper and both she and Dr Wagle had supervised its preparation, for which Dr Badrakalimuthu remains grateful. However, Dr Rumball gracefully declined the invitation to co-author the current chapter. We (JCH and PL) remain appreciative to Dr Rumball for her support.

References

1. Atkinson MR. Substance abuse in elderly, In *Psychiatry in the Elderly* (eds Jacoby R, Oppenheimer C) 799–834 Oxford University Press, 2002.

2. Coulthard M, Farrell M, Singleton N et al. *Tobacco, Alcohol and Drug Use and Mental Health*. TSO (The Stationery Office) 2002.

3. McInnes E, Powell J. Drug and alcohol referrals. Are elderly substance abuse diagnosis and referrals missed? *BMJ* 1994; **308**; 444–446.

4. Fahmy V, Hatch SL, Hotopf M and Stewart R. Prevalence of illicit drug use in people aged 50 years and over from two surveys. *Age Ageing* (2012); **41**, 553–556.

5. White JB, Duncan DF, Bradley D et al. Generational shift and drug abuse in older Americans. *J Soc Behav Health Sci* (2011); **5**; 58–66.

6. Moore AA, Karno MP, Grella CE et al. Alcohol, tobacco, and non-medical drug use in older US adults: data from the 2001/02 National Epidemiological Survey of Alcohol and Related Conditions. *J Am Geriatr Soc* (2009); **57**; 2275–2281.

7. Lin JC, Karno MP, Grella CE et al. Alcohol, tobacco, and non-medical drug use in US adults aged 65 and older: Data from the 2001/02 National Epidemiological Survey of Alcohol and Related Conditions. *Am J Geriatr Psychiatry* (2011); **19**; 291–299.

8. Blazer DG and Wu LT. The epidemiology of substance use and disorders among middle aged and elderly community adults: National Survey on Drug Use and Health (NSDUH). *Am J Geriatr Psychiatry* (2009); **17**;237–245.

9. Johnson SD, Striley C and Cottlet LB. Comorbid substance use and HIV risk in older African American drug users. *J Aging Health* (2007); **19**; 646–658.

10. Lofwall MR, Schuster A and Strain SK. Changing profile of abused substances by older persons entering treatment. *J Nerv Ment Dis* (2008); **196**; 898–905.

11. Morgan K, Dallosso H, Ebrahim S et al. Prevalence, frequency, and duration of hypnotic drug use among elderly living at home. *BMJ (Clinical Research Edn* 1988); **296**; 601–602.

12. *Centre for Behavioral Health Statistics and Quality Results from the 2011 National Survey on Drug Use and Health: Mental Health Detailed Tables*. Substance Abuse and Mental Health Services Administration, Rockville MD (2012).

13. Cimolai N. Zopiclone: is it a pharmacological agent for abuse? *Canadian Family Physician* (2007); **53**; 2124–2129.

14. Higgitt AC. Indications for benzodiazepine prescriptions in the elderly. *Int J Geriatr Psychiatry* (1988); **3**; 239–243.

15. Lechevallier N, Fourier A, Berr C. Benzodiazepines in the elderly. The EVA study [In French] *Revuew d'Epidemiologieet de Sante Publique* (2003); **51**; 317–326.

16. Fernandez L, Cassagne-Pinel C. Benzodiazepine addiction and symptoms of anxiety and depression in elderly subjects. *L'Encephale* (2001); **27**; 459–474.

17. Woo BKP, Chen W. Substance misuse among older patients in psychiatric emergency service. *Gen Hosp Psychiatry* (2010); **32**; 99–101.

18. Rajaratnam R, Sivesind D, Todman M et al. The aging methadone maintenance patient: treatment adjustment, long-term success, and quality of life. *J Opioid Mang* (2009); **5**; 27–37.

19. Beynon CM, McVeigh J and Roe B. Problematic drug use, ageing and older people: trends in the age of drug users in northwest England, *Ageing Soc* (2007); **27**; 799–810.

20. Rivers E, Shirazi E, Aurora T et al. Cocaine use in elderly patients presenting to an inner-city emergency department. *Acad Emergency Med*(2004); **11**; 874–877.

21. Trafton JA, Olivia E, Horst D et al. Treatment needs associated with pain in substance use disorder patients. Implications of concurrent treatment. *Drug and Alcohol Dependence* (2004); **73**; 23–31.

22. Simoni-Wastila L, Stricker G. Risk Factors associated with problem use of prescription drugs. *Am J Pub Health* (2004); 94; 266–268.

23. Gottlieb S. Inappropriate drug prescribing in elderly people is common. *BMJ* (2004); 329; 367.

24. Mossley JM Shapiro E. Physician use by elderly over an eight year period. *J Pub Health* (1985); 75; 133–134.

25. Gfroerer J, Penne M, Pemberton M et al. Substance abuse treatment among older adults in 2020. The impact of aging baby-boom cohort. *Drug and Alcohol Dependence* (2003); 69; 127–135.

26. Hinkin CH, Castellon SA, Dickson-Fuhrman E et al. Screening for drug and alcohol abuse among older adults using modified version of CAGE. *Am J Addict* (2001); 10; 319–326.

27. SAMHSA Treatment Episodes Data Set-Admissions (TEDS-A)-Concatenated, 1992–2010. Office of Applied Studies, Substance Abuse and Mental Health Services Administration (SAMHSA). ICPSR25221-v5. Inter-university Consortium for Political and Social Research, Ann Arbor, MI (2012).

28. Frischer M, Crome I, Macleod J et al. Substance misuse and psychiatric illness: prospective observational study using the general practice database. *J Epi Comm* (2005); 59; 847–850.

29. Blixen CE, McDougall GJ, Suen LJ. Dual diagnosis in elders discharged from a psychiatric hospital. *Int J Geriatr Psychiatry* (1997); 12; 307–313.

30. Rosen D, Smith ML, Reynolds CF. The prevalence of mental and physical health disorders among older methadone patients. *Am J Geriatr Psychiatry* (2008); 16; 488–497.

31. Torres LR, Kaplan C, Valdez A. Health consequences of long-term injection heroin use among aging Mexican American men. *J Aging Health* (2011); 23; 912–932.

32. McMorn S, Schoedel KA, Sellers EM. Effects of low-dose opioids on cognitive dysfunction. *JCO* (2011); 29; 4342–4343.

33. Sartre DD, Blow FC, Chi Fw, Weisner C. Gender differences in seven-year alcohol and drug treatment outcomes among older adults. *Am J Addict* (2007); 16; 216–221.

34. Outlaw FH, Marquart JM, Roy A et al. Treatment outcomes for older adults who abuse substances. *J Appl Gereontol* (2012); 31; 78–100.

35. Miller PM, Brooks SW & Stewart SH. Medical treatment of alcohol dependence: a systematic review. *Int J of Psychiatry Med* (2011); 42; 227–66.

36. Picton JD, Marino AD & Nealy KL. Benzodiazepine use and cognitive decline in the elderly. *Am J of Health-Sys Pharm* (2018); 75; e6–e12

Mental Health in Parkinson's Disease

Shoned Jones, Kelli M Torsney, Lily Scourfield, Katie Berryman, and Emily J Henderson

Introduction

Idiopathic Parkinson's disease (PD) is the second most common neurodegenerative disorder after Alzheimer's disease (AD), and motorically it is characterized by tremor, ridigity, bradykinesia, and postural instability. Whilst it was historically considered to be a movement disorder there are multiple non-motor symptoms, which often precede the motor symptoms by years or even decades.[1] These include dysautonomia, sleep disturbances, neuropsychiatric disturbances, pain, and sensory problems. These have a negative effect on quality of life and are associated with overall higher carer burden and, potentially, higher care costs whilst being frequently undeclared by patients.[2,3]

The motor syndrome is increasingly recognized as reflecting the 'tip of the iceberg' and, furthermore, Parkinson's has been described as the 'quintessential neuropsychiatric disorder'.[4]

This accurately reflects both commonality of neuropsychiatric symptoms (Figure 8.1) as well as the negative impact these disorders have on patients' social functioning and ability to work.[5] Alpha synuclein pathology and disruption of neurochemical pathways underlie some of the symptomatology, whereas adverse effects of treatments can precipitate other manifestations such as impulse control disorders and psychosis. Adequate recognition and a robust evidence base for management of these troublesome symptoms remain an urgent need; however, the literature in the field is expanding (Figure 8.2).

Depression

In his original essay on the 'Shaking Palsy', James Parkinson noted that 'A more melancholy object I never beheld'.[6] Nowadays, depression is still recognized as a common non-motor feature of PD, with the prevalence of clinically significant symptoms being 35%.[7] A multi-centre study demonstrated that half the study patients were depressed according to the Beck Depression Inventory (BDI) whilst only 1% had self-reported symptoms.[8,9] There are particular diagnostic challenges which arise from patients' under-reporting of their depressive symptoms,[10] hypomimia (lack of facial expression), concurrent mood disturbances such as anxiety or apathy,[11] psychomotor slowing, as well as from under-recognition by clinicians.[12] There are a number of validated screening tools available which may be used to identify depression in people with PD including the Hamilton Depression Rating Scale (HAM-D), BDI, Hospital Anxiety and Depression Scale (HADS), Montgomery Asberg Depression Rating Scale (MADRS), and the Geriatric Depression Scale (GDS). A working group on depression in Parkinson's recommended that an inclusive approach be taken to

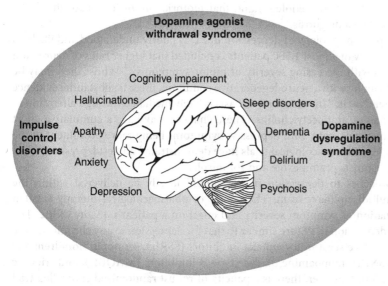

Figure 8.1 The spectrum of neuropsychiatric disorders in Parkinson's disease

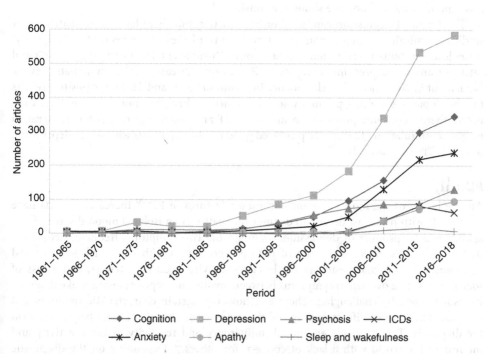

Figure 8.2 Graph showing number of articles published in each neuropsychiatric domain

symptoms (i.e. regardless of the aetiology) and that motoric 'on' or 'off' state should be considered when making a diagnosis.[13]

The underlying pathophysiology of depression in PD is poorly understood and likely to be multifactorial. A study of almost 1,500 patients concluded that higher rates of depression were seen in patients with increasing severity of motor symptoms.[14] Whilst there may be a reactive element to living with a neurodegenerative condition, there is substantial evidence of a neurotransmitter deficit. This biochemical basis is likely mediated through alteration in serotonin, noradrenaline, and acetylcholine. These changes may have a cumulative effect with the hypodopaminergic state, with depressive symptoms being more prominent in the motorically 'off' state.[15] Pharmacological trials have demonstrated an antidepressant effect with the dopamine agonists pramipexole and ropinirole.[16]

Treatment approaches to depression in PD should ideally be delivered within the framework of a multidisciplinary team. The choice of pharmacological therapy is often driven by determination of symptom severity and effect on a patient's quality of life. The options in treating depression in PD are similar to that for depression in any chronic disease state and include selective serotonin reuptake inhibitors (SSRIs), serotonin noradrenaline uptake inhibitors (SNRI), monoamine oxidase type B inhibitors (MAOBIs), and tricyclic antidepressants (TCAs). However, there is a paucity of robust randomized controlled trial (RCT) evidence. Selective serotonin reuptake inhibitors are most commonly prescribed because of their more favourable side effect profile and lower potential for drug–drug and drug–disease interactions. The use of MAOBIs for the motor treatment of PD increases the risk of developing serotonin syndrome through the addition of an antidepressant, although this is rare in clinical practice.[17] Whilst the use of TCAs have a potential advantage in promoting sleep in patients who suffer insomnia, the anticholinergic effects of this drug class and daytime somnolence should be considered.

Treatment of depression can be a complex matter, but there have been relatively few studies specifically on depression in PD and many of these have been of poor quality. A Cochrane systematic review ten years ago found 'Insufficient data on the effectiveness and safety of any antidepressant therapies in Parkinson's disease…'.[18] A systematic review carried out in 2016 showed weak evidence in favour of SSRIs and TCAs; the positive results for the dopamine agonist pramipexole (mentioned earlier), but not for rotigotine, were noted; there were some promising results for CBT and conflicting results for transcranial magnetic stimulation (TMS); ECT produced good results in patients with severe depression, but no RCTs were available.[19]

Apathy

Apathy is one of the most common non-motor features of PD.[20] Increasing efforts have been made within the last decade to distinguish apathy as an isolated mood disorder from apathy as a by-product of depression, although the two symptoms frequently coexist.[20] Apathy may be defined as a 'state of reduced motivation with decreased goal-directed behaviours'.[21] This may result in low levels of activity, reduced interests, and a loss of socialization. The overlap in symptoms between apathy and depression can make diagnosing isolated apathy challenging. There are, however, certain characteristic thoughts and symptoms that are specific to apathy and the presence or absence of these help to confirm the diagnosis. These include emotional indifference and reactivity, reduced activity and interest in the world with a lack of concern for others.[22] Depending on the diagnostic criteria used, and the concurrent symptoms of depression and cognitive impairment, the prevalence of apathy ranges from 17% to 70% in PD[23] and, similarly to depression, the symptoms may precede the motor symptoms of PD. The pathophysiology is poorly understood, but may be associated with a neuronal disruption in areas that regulate goal-directed behaviour: mainly dopaminergic projections between the frontal cortex and the ventral tegmentum.[21,24]

The development of diagnostic criteria for apathy has advanced significantly with the establishing of a task force, commissioned in 2008 by the International Parkinson's and Movement Disorder Society, to assess the clinimetrics of the available rating scales.[25] Subsequent review of the clinimetric properties of 13 scales suggested that the five-item WHO Well-being Index (WHO-5) and Neurastenia Scale detect apathy severity, and the 33-item Lille Apathy Rating Scale (LARS) is valid in the diagnosis of 33 items, while the Starkstein Apathy Scale (SAS) has utility in the exclusion of apathy.[26]

There is a range of therapeutic approaches to treating apathy including dopaminergic medications.[13,27] A double-blind RCT comparing the cholinesterase inhibitor rivastigmine with placebo showed a significant improvement in the symptoms of apathy at 6 months.[28]

Anxiety

It is estimated that a third of people with PD experience symptoms of anxiety, which is considered to be a group of disorders consisting of generalized anxiety disorder (GAD), obsessive compulsive disorder, agoraphobia, social phobia, and panic disorder. It can be difficult to distinguish symptoms of anxiety from those of depression or even somatic PD (e.g. sleep disturbances, apathy), which can also be present simultaneously, so the identification of one should lower the threshold of clinical suspicion for the other. Classification of these conditions varies in studies, therefore the reported prevalence rates vary, ranging from 3.6% to 55%.[29,30] A systematic review reported the average prevalence of all anxiety disorders in PD to be 31%, with GAD, panic disorder, and social phobia being the most common.[30] This wide difference in prevalence may be accounted for by the under-reporting of symptoms by patients and under-recognition by clinicians.

Researchers will often rely on established criteria, for example from the DSM-IV, to make a diagnosis; however, diagnosis in a clinical setting can remain challenging. A study of 42 patients with PD in a university-based movement disorders clinic found that 29% had DSM-III-R anxiety disorder diagnoses, but an additional 40% had anxiety symptoms that did not meet the diagnostic threshold.[31] Self-reported anxiety scales have been tested in PD, but their clinical utility is uncertain owing to the lack of consensus regarding appropriate cut-off scores.[32] A detailed patient history and a collateral history are essential but often omitted because of time constraints in clinic. Furthermore, identification can be complicated by the presence of an underlying cognitive impairment. Specific symptoms of anxiety in PD include panic attacks during off periods, excessive worry, and increased subjective motor symptoms. The timing of symptoms can mirror motor fluctuations or manifest in an unrelated pattern.[23]

Similarly to depression in PD, the aetiology of anxiety is multifactorial. There are neurobiological changes resulting in the development of anxiety and a proposed reactive model of anxiety secondary to the underlying burden of PD. Social anxiety is especially common in the context of the reactive model, with people with PD expressing concern over being negatively perceived in public leading to social withdrawal. Patients may also fear the progression of the disease, disability, institutionalization, and issues surrounding their death. With the high falls risk in the disease, an associated fear of falling can be very prominent.[33]

The role of dopaminergic neurotransmission in the context of anxiety is poorly understood but has been linked to both social phobia and anxiety symptoms in animal models.[33] Seratonergic and noradrenergic systems also have a role in PD anxiety owing to their widespread distribution in the structures involved in emotional modulation. Research demonstrates that people with PD who score higher on anxiety questionnaires have a shorter serotonin transporter allele, highlighting the potential role of neuropsychiatric genetics in this group.[34]

Anxiety in PD has a huge impact on quality of life, not only for the patient but also for their family and carers. Social anxiety can lead to isolation in the community which further exacerbates anxiety, creating a self-perpetuating cycle. It can also precipitate loneliness, particularly in older people, which can contribute to the subsequent development of depression. This can in turn affect treatment plans, hindering motivation and engagement in rehabilitation and healthcare services.[33]

There is a paucity of evidence on the management of anxiety in PD. There are no robust clinical trials of either pharmacological or psychological strategies. Anxiety has been assessed as a secondary outcome in clinical trials for depression but because of the selection criteria used, any therapeutic effects on anxiety were diluted.[35]

Guidance for managing anxiety in older adults with chronic physical health conditions[35] can be extrapolated, which places initial emphasis on lifestyle modification, focusing on optimal sleep, exercise, nutrition, and socializing in addition to eliminating any exacerbating medical causes for anxiety such as metabolic anomalies, nutritional deficiencies, and drug reactions. Pharmacological approaches are then advised with the introduction of SSRIs and SNRIs. The use of benzodiazepines is discouraged because of their side effect profile. Behavioural therapies in the form of cognitive behavioural therapy, mindfulness, and desensitization are also of benefit but are reliant on adequate motivation and adherence.[35]

Psychosis

Psychosis in PD is a spectrum of neuropsychiatric manifestations consisting of 'positive' symptoms, namely illusions, hallucinations, and delusions.[36] Definitions of psychotic symptoms in the context of PD are consistent with the definitions in the wider psychiatric literature. The prevalence of psychosis also varies depending on the diagnostic tool used. In 2007, the combined National Institute of Neurological Disorders and Stroke (NINDS) and National Institute of Mental Health (NIMH) work group proposed a unifying diagnostic criterion for PD psychosis which includes the presence of at least one psychotic symptom.[36] Longitudinally, prevalence increases with disease duration,[37] and, at 12 years, 60% of patients from a community cohort reported hallucinations or delusions.[38]

Proposed risk factors for the development of psychosis in PD include duration and severity of PD, and cognitive impairment. The development of these symptoms at a time when demands associated with caring for people with PD are already high results in a greater sense of burden for the carer in comparison with caring for those without psychosis and is also a predictive factor for nursing home placement.[39] Additional risk factors for psychosis include treatment with dopaminergic and anticholinergic medications.

The relationship between the use of PD medication and development of PD psychosis remains controversial. Anecdotally, an association between PD psychosis and the use of dopaminergic therapies and duration of treatment has been observed. Psychotic symptoms can develop on initiation of medication with a subsequent improvement with reduction or withdrawal and this is most potently seen with the use of dopamine agonists. None the less, a causal effect of dopaminergic medications has not been established and psychotic symptoms have been described in recently diagnosed patients who have not yet started treatment.[40]

The initial management of PD psychosis involves the identification and treatment of any precipitating factors. Psychosis may be the manifestation of an acute illness or change in medication and a thorough clinical evaluation is imperative. If the patient is tolerating the symptoms of psychosis with no adverse features, the best approach may be to watch and wait. Many patients with PD do not find hallucinations distressing and retain insight.

Where intervention is warranted, there are a number of approaches. In patients with significant cognitive impairment rivastigmine has good efficacy.[41] Clozapine and pimavanserin (a 5-HT2A inverse agonist, not yet licensed for use in the UK)[42] are efficacious. There are barriers for the routine use of clozapine in the clinical setting, namely the regular blood tests required to monitor for agranulocytosis and the registration required for prescribing the drug. Other atypical antipsychotics used in clinical practice include quetiapine, olanzapine, and risperidone, but these can cause worsening of motor symptoms and other side effects including QT prolongation on the electrocardiogram (ECG), sedative effects, metabolic syndrome, and a potential deterioration in cognition. The most recent NICE guidance advocates the use of low-dose quetiapine and clozapine as the most appropriate medications in PD psychosis,[43] and in clinical practice at present, quetiapine is commonly used.

Cognitive Impairment

Cognitive impairment is a common non-motor manifestation in PD and is heterogeneous in terms of its severity, rate of progression, and the cognitive domains affected. It has a significant negative impact on patients and their carers and is associated with increased disability, mortality,[44] carer burden,[45] and need for nursing home placement.[46]

Cognitive impairment ranges from subjective cognitive decline, to mild cognitive impairment (MCI), to dementia, but does not necessarily progress linearly. Longitudinal studies suggest MCI in PD increases the risk of developing Parkinson's disease dementia (PDD). Janvin et al. showed, whilst controlling for age, disease stage, education, and gender, that MCI was strongly associated with PDD development (odds ratio 5.1; 95% CI, 1.51–16.24, $p = 0.005$) over a 4-year follow-up.[47] However, this study included relatively small numbers. More recently, evidence suggests MCI may not always progress to PDD, with some patients remaining stable on longitudinal assessments or even reverting back to normal cognition.[48] The prevalence of MCI in PD ranges from 15% to 53%[49] but this large variation in prevalence is likely caused by differences in study settings (hospital versus community patients), variable clinical characteristics, and inconsistent definitions of MCI in PD. The Movement Disorders Society published a unifying set of diagnostic measures in 2012 to standardize practice across clinical trials.[50] From a clinical perspective, MCI and PDD can best be differentiated by determining whether the cognitive impairment significantly impacts activities of daily living.

Several longitudinal studies have demonstrated that approximately 50% of patients develop PDD ten years after initial PD diagnosis.[51,52] The Sydney Multicenter Study, the largest follow-up study of newly diagnosed patients, showed 83% of patients with PD developed PDD at 20 years post diagnosis and 75% developed PDD before death.[53] Additionally, not only does the progression of cognitive impairment in PD vary, so too does the pattern affected. Cognitive deficits may affect executive function, attention, processing speed, and/or visuospatial function.[54] The CamPaIGN (Cambridgeshire Parkinson's Incidence from GP to Neurologist) cohort study assessed cognition at 3.5 and 5.5 years post diagnosis and found a decline in mini-mental state examination (MMSE) scores at a rate of 0.3 ± 0.1 points per year over 5.2 years.[55] In addition, they showed that deficits in semantic fluency and visuospatial function at baseline were associated with a greater risk for developing PDD whereas deficits in executive function were not.[54,55] This finding, in addition to other studies, led to the 'dual syndrome hypothesis' which suggests that patients with primarily executive dysfunction, driven by changes in dopaminergic pathways, are less likely to develop PDD, whereas those with memory and visuospatial functional deficits, caused predominantly by deficits in acetylcholine (ACh), are more prone to rapid cognitive decline and progression to PDD.

The heterogeneity of both the presentation and progression of cognitive impairment in PD is not fully understood and is clearly a complex interplay between genetic and environmental factors. Risk factors associated with an increased risk for PDD include patient age, older age of disease onset, and the presence of hallucinations. In addition, the Parkinson's phenotype with a more predominant gait dysfunction is associated with more rapid cognitive decline than those with a tremor-dominant phenotype.[55] Genetic factors also play a role with mutations in the alpha-synuclein (SCNA)[56] and glucocerebrosidase (GBA1) genes[57] being associated with more rapid cognitive decline, in addition to an earlier onset of PDD. One retrospective longitudinal study found that 56% of GBA1 mutation carriers had dementia at age 70, compared with 15% of sporadic PD patients.[57] Interestingly, patients with a PARKIN mutation, which accounts for 50% of autosomal recessive PD, are less likely to develop PDD, with one review finding PDD in fewer than 3% of cases.[58]

The only drug currently licensed for PDD is rivastigmine, a cholinesterase inhibitor, with memantine, an NMDA receptor antagonist used as second treatment line if the patient is intolerant to rivastigmine.[43] However, a meta-analysis including three RCTs comparing memantine 20 mg daily to placebo concluded it only had a mildly beneficial effect on the global impression of change assessment, with no significant change on cognitive function assessed using the MMSE.[59] There is currently no proven treatment for MCI in PD, and given the limited pharmacological options, it is important to consider non-pharmacological options including physical exercise programmes, cognitive training and stimulation using pharmacological and non-pharmacological approaches.

A systematic review of eight studies including 158 patients suggested that physical exercise had beneficial effects on global cognition.[60] Physical activity intervention studies have historically recruited small numbers of patients and utilized heterogeneous interventions with varying degrees of exercise intensity, mode, and duration.

Cognitive training is a structured teaching programme designed to target specific cognitive domains. A meta-analysis involving seven studies (272 patients) showed a small but statistically significant improvement compared with controls.[61] Overall, given the heterogeneity of cognitive impairment in PD and the impact it has on the patient's quality of life and carer burden, the primary aim of management should be to apply an individualized approach whilst addressing patient and carer concerns and expectations.

Delirium

Given the propensity to develop dementia and the high degree of cognitive vulnerability it is proposed that people with PD are at increased risk of developing delirium in the setting of acute illness.[62] The features of delirium such as cognitive fluctuation, somnolence, and hallucinations (see Chapter 19 for a fuller discussion of delirium) can overlap with those seen particularly in PDD, which can confound the diagnosis. There is a lack of evidence as to the long-term motor and cognitive outcomes for people with PD who have experienced delirium, although there is a suggestion that both domains can worsen, albeit the studies were relatively small.[63,64] Whilst antipsychotics can worsen motor symptoms, clinically quetiapine is most commonly used where pharmacological strategies are required in addition to treating any underlying precipitants and using conservative strategies such as one-to-one nursing and environmental optimization.

Treatment-Related Disorders

Impulse Control Disorders

Impulse control disorders (ICDs) are addictive behaviours manifesting as binge eating, pathological gambling, compulsive shopping, or abnormal sexual behaviours.[65] These can occur in isolation or together. In PD, they are associated with dopamine agonist therapy, and all patients initiated on this treatment should be counselled as to the risk and proactive enquiry at subsequent appointments should be used to ascertain whether these symptoms are arising. Left unrecognized and untreated, ICDs can have very significant ramifications on personal relationships and finances. Individuals at higher risk of developing ICDs are men, those with certain personality traits or psychiatric disturbance (such as impulsivity, novelty-seeking, anxiety, and depression), younger patients, smokers, and those taking higher doses of DA (dopamine agonists) for a longer duration. Management consists of down-titration of DA therapy supported by cognitive behavioural therapy with careful management of worsening motor symptoms.[66]

Dopamine Agonist Withdrawal Syndrome

Dopamine agonist withdrawal results from the rapid down-titration or withdrawal of a dopamine agonist drug. Clinically it is recognized by a cluster of symptoms including autonomic instability (fatigue, orthostatic hypotension, nausea, vomiting, diaphoresis), psychological symptoms (anxiety, panic attacks, dysphoria, depression, fatigue, agitation, irritability, suicidal ideation) as well as generalized pain, and drug cravings.[67] The cessation or rapid reduction of dopamine agonist drugs is a major factor in the development of the syndrome and patients should be monitored closely in case this occurs.

Dopamine Dysregulation Syndrome

Dopamine dysregulation syndrome refers to the compulsive (mis)use of dopaminergic therapy. The combination of dopamine replacement therapy, coupled with predisposing individual risk factors and PD pathology, yield an addictive syndrome.[68] This manifests as mood fluctuations and addictive behaviour. Management consists of careful down-titration of dopamine agonist therapy and fractionation of levodopa therapy. Intrajejunal levodopa infusion therapy or deep brain stimulation can be considered in refractory cases.

Conclusion

Neuropsychiatric manifestations of PD are common and have a devastating effect on patients' quality of life and cause significant carer strain. Assessment and active management of the neuropsychiatric symptoms encountered in people with PD are essential to mitigate these very distressing sequelae and the resultant negative impact these conditions can have on functioning. The overlap of symptoms can make the diagnosis of a mental health disorder in the context of PD challenging, but proactive enquiry is the first step in better defining and treating these syndromes. In this brief review we have sought to give an overview of the spectrum of conditions, current understanding of pathophysiology, criteria for diagnosis, and management strategies.

Acknowledgements

The authors would like to thank the anonymous reviewers of the original paper and the helpful comments of an anonymous reviewer of the book chapter.

For information, the original paper on which this chapter is based was:

Jones S, Torsney K, Scourfield L, Berryman K, Henderson E. Neuropsychiatric symptoms in Parkinson's disease: Aetiology, diagnosis and treatment. *BJPsych Adv*, 1–10. doi:10.1192/bja.2019.79.

References

1. Klingelhoefer L, Reichmann H. Pathogenesis of Parkinson disease: the gut-brain axis and environmental factors. *Nat Rev Neurol* 2015; **11**: 625–36.

2. Chaudhuri KR, Prieto-Jurcynska C, Naidu Y et al. The nondeclaration of nonmotor symptoms of Parkinson's disease to health care professionals: an international study using the nonmotor symptoms questionnaire. *Mov Disord* 2010 30; **25**: 704–9.

3. Politis M, Wu K, Molloy S et al. Parkinson's disease symptoms: the patient's perspective. *Mov Disord* 2010; **25**: 1646–51.

4. Weintraub D, Burn DJ. Parkinson's disease: the quintessential neuropsychiatric disorder. *Mov Disord* 2011; **26**: 1022–31.

5. Perepezko K, Hinkle JT, Shepard MD et al. Social role functioning in Parkinson's disease: a mixed-methods systematic review. *Int Journal Geriatr Psychiatry* 2019; **34**: 1128–38.

6. Parkinson J. *An Essay on the Shaking Palsy.* London: Sherwood, Neely and Jones; 1817.

7. Reijnders JSAM, Ehrt U, Weber WEJ, Aarsland D, Leentjens AFG. A systematic review of prevalence studies of depression in Parkinson's disease. *Mov Disord* 2008; **23**: 183–9.

8. Huse D, Schulman K, Orsini L et al. Factors impacting on quality of life in Parkinson's disease: results from an international survey. *Mov Disord* 2005; **20**: 1449–54.

9. Findley L, Eichhorn T, Janca A et al. Factors impacting on quality of life in Parkinson's disease: results from an international survey. *Mov Disord* 2002; **17**: 60–7.

10. Dissanayaka NNW, Sellbach A, Silburn PA et al. Factors associated with depression in Parkinson's disease. *J Affect Disord* 2011; **132**: 82–8.

11. Pagonabarraga J, Kulisevsky J, Strafella AP, Krack P. Apathy in Parkinson's disease: clinical features, neural substrates, diagnosis, and treatment. *Lancet Neurol* 2015; **14**: 518–31.

12. Shulman L, Taback R, Rabinstein A, Weiner W. Non-recognition of depression and other non-motor symptoms in Parkinson's disease. *Park Relat Disord* 2002; 8: 193–7.

13. Marsh L, McDonald WM, Cummings J et al. Provisional diagnostic criteria for depression in Parkinson's disease: report of an NINDS/NIMH Work Group. *Mov Disord* 2006; 21: 148–58.

14. Riedel O, Klotsche J, Spottke A et al. Frequency of dementia, depression, and other neuropsychiatric symptoms in 1,449 outpatients with Parkinson's disease. *J Neurol* 2010; 257: 1073–82.

15. van der Velden RMJ, Broen MPG, Kuijf ML, Leentjens AFG. Frequency of mood and anxiety fluctuations in Parkinson's disease patients with motor fluctuations: a systematic review. *Mov Disord* 2018; 33: 1521–7.

16. Barone P, Poewe W, Albrecht S et al. Pramipexole for the treatment of depressive symptoms in patients with Parkinson's disease: a randomised, double-blind, placebo-controlled trial. *Lancet Neurol* 2010; 9: 573–80.

17. Richard IH, Kurlan R, Tanner C et al. Serotonin syndrome and the combined use of deprenyl and an antidepressant in Parkinson's disease. Parkinson Study Group. *Neurology* 1997; 48: 1070–7.

18. Ghazi-Noori S, Chung TH, Deane K, Rickards HE, Clarke CE. Therapies for depression in Parkinson's disease. *Cochrane Database Syst Rev* 2003; Issue 2. Art. No.: CD003465. [Republished in 2010 with no changes to the conclusions.]

19. Starkstein SE, Brockman S. Management of depression in Parkinson's Disease: a systematic review. *Mov Disord Clin Pract* 2017; 4: 470–7.

20. den Brok MGHE, van Dalen JW, van Gool WA, Moll van Charante EP, de Bie RMA, Richard E. Apathy in Parkinson's disease: a systematic review and meta-analysis. *Mov Disord* 2015; 30: 759–69.

21. Marin RS. Apathy: a neuropsychiatric syndrome. *J Neuropsychiatry Clin Neurosci* 1991; 3: 243–54.

22. Pagonabarraga J, Kulisevsky J, Strafella AP, Krack P. Apathy in Parkinson's disease: clinical features, neural substrates, diagnosis, and treatment. *Lancet Neurol* 2015; 14: 518–31.

23. Aarsland D, Brønnick K, Alves G et al. The spectrum of neuropsychiatric symptoms in patients with early untreated Parkinson's disease. *J Neurol Neurosurg Psychiatry* 2009; 80: 928–30.

24. Carlson JM, Foti D, Mujica-Parodi LR, Harmon-Jones E, Hajcak G. Ventral striatal and medial prefrontal BOLD activation is correlated with reward-related electrocortical activity: a combined ERP and fMRI study. *Neuroimage* 2011; 57: 1608–16.

25. Shulman LM, Armstrong M, Ellis T et al. Disability rating scales in Parkinson's disease: critique and recommendations. *Mov Disord* 2016; 31: 1455–65.

26. Carrozzino D. Clinimetric approach to rating scales for the assessment of apathy in Parkinson's disease: a systematic review. *Prog NeuroPsychopharmacology Biol Psychiatry* 2019; 94: 109641.

27. Chaudhuri KR, Martinez-Martin P, Antonini A et al. Rotigotine and specific non-motor symptoms of Parkinson's disease: post hoc analysis of RECOVER. *Park Relat Disord* 2013; 19: 660–5.

28. Devos D, Moreau C, Maltête D et al. Rivastigmine in apathetic but dementia and depression-free patients with Parkinson's disease: a double-blind, placebo-controlled, randomised clinical trial. *J Neurol Neurosurg Psychiatry* 2014; 85: 668–74.

29. Dissanayaka NNW, Sellbach A, Matheson S et al. Anxiety disorders in Parkinson's disease: prevalence and risk factors. *Mov Disord* 2010; 25: 838–45.

30. Broen MPG, Narayen NE, Kuijf ML, Dissanayaka NNW, Leentjens AFG. Prevalence of anxiety in Parkinson's disease: a systematic review and meta-analysis. *Mov Disord* 2016; 31: 1125–33.

31. Pontone GM, Williams JR, Anderson KE et al. Prevalence of anxiety disorders and anxiety subtypes in patients with

Parkinson's disease. *Mov Disord* 2009; 24: 1333–8.

32. Leentjens AFG, Dujardin K, Marsh L et al. Anxiety rating scales in Parkinson's disease: critique and recommendations. *Mov Disord* 2008; 23: 2015–25.

33. Prediger RDS, Matheus FC, Schwarzbold ML, Lima MMS, Vital MABF. Anxiety in Parkinson's disease: a critical review of experimental and clinical studies. *Neuropharmacology* 2012; 62: 115–24.

34. Menza MA, Sage J, Marshall E, Cody R, Duvoisin R. Mood changes and 'on-off' phenomena in Parkinson's disease. *Mov Disord* 1990; 5: 148–51.

35. Koychev I, Okai D. Cognitive–behavioural therapy for non-motor symptoms of Parkinson's disease: a clinical review. *Evid-Based Ment Health* 2017; 20: 15–20.

36. Ravina B, Marder K, Fernandez HH et al. Diagnostic criteria for psychosis in Parkinson's disease: report of an NINDS, NIMH Work Group. *Mov Disord* 2007; 22: 1061–8.

37. Gibson G, Mottram PG, Burn DJ et al. Frequency, prevalence, incidence and risk factors associated with visual hallucinations in a sample of patients with Parkinson's disease: a longitudinal 4-year study. *Int J Geriatr Psychiatry* 2013; 28: 626–31.

38. Forsaa EB, Larsen JP, Wentzel-Larsen T et al. A 12-year population-based study of psychosis in Parkinson disease. *Arch Neurol* 2010; 67: 996–1001.

39. Marsh L, Williams J, Rocco M, Grill S, Munro C, Dawson T. Psychiatric comorbidities in patients with Parkinson disease and psychosis. *Neurology* 2004; 63: 293–300.

40. Aarsland D, Marsh L, Schrag A. Neuropsychiatric symptoms in Parkinson's disease. *Mov Disord* 2009; 24: 2175–86.

41. Burn D, Emre M, McKeith I et al. Effects of rivastigmine in patients with and without visual hallucinations in dementia associated with Parkinson's disease. *Mov Disord* 2006; 21: 1899–907.

42. Cummings J, Isaacson S, Mills R et al. Pimavanserin for patients with Parkinson's disease psychosis: a randomised, placebo-controlled phase 3 trial. *Lancet* 2014; 383: 533–40.

43. National Institute for Health and Care Excellence. *Parkinson's Disease in Adults. NICE Guideline (NG71).* London: NICE; July 2017. www.nice.org.uk/guidance/ng71/evidence/full-guideline-pdf-453846 6253 [last accessed 6th February 2020.]

44. Levy G, Tang M-X, Louis ED et al. The association of incident dementia with mortality in PD. *Neurology* 2002; 59: 1708–13.

45. Aarsland D, Larsen JP, Karlsen K, Lim NG, Tandberg E. Mental symptoms in Parkinson's disease are important contributors to caregiver distress. *Int J Geriatr Psychiatry* 1999; 14: 866–74.

46. Aarsland D, Larsen J, Tandberg E, Aake K. Predictors of nursing home placement in Parkinson's disease: a population-based, prospective study. *J Am Geriatr Soc* 2000; 48: 938–42.

47. Janvin CC, Larsen JP, Aarsland D, Hugdahl K. Subtypes of mild cognitive impairment in Parkinson's disease: progression to dementia. *Mov Disord* 2006; 21: 1343–9.

48. Lawson RA, Yarnall AJ, Duncan GW et al. Stability of mild cognitive impairment in newly diagnosed Parkinson's disease. *J Neurol Neurosurg Psychiatry* 2017; 88: 648–52.

49. Yarnall AJ, Rochester L, Burn DJ. Mild cognitive impairment in Parkinson's disease. *Age Ageing* 2013; 42: 567–76.

50. Litvan I, Aarsland D, Adler CH et al. MDS Task Force on mild cognitive impairment in Parkinson's disease: critical review of PD-MCI. *Mov Disord* 2011; 26: 1814–24.

51. Williams-Gray CH, Mason SL, Evans JR et al. The CamPaIGN study of Parkinson's disease: 10-year outlook in an incident population-based cohort. *J Neurol Neurosurg Psychiatry* 2013; 84: 1258–64.

52. Auyeung M, Tsoi T, Mok V et al. Ten year survival and outcomes in a prospective cohort of new onset Chinese Parkinson's

disease patients. *J Neurol Neurosurg Psychiatry* 2012; **83**: 607–11.

53. Hely MA, Reid WGJ, Adena MA, Halliday GM, Morris JGL. The Sydney multicenter study of Parkinson's disease: the inevitability of dementia at 20 years. *Mov Disord* 2008; **23**: 837–44.

54. Williams-Gray CH, Foltynie T, Brayne CEG, Robbins TW, Barker RA. Evolution of cognitive dysfunction in an incident Parkinson's disease cohort. *Brain* 2007; **130**: 1787–98.

55. Williams-Gray CH, Evans JR, Goris A et al. The distinct cognitive syndromes of Parkinson's disease: 5 year follow-up of the CamPaIGN cohort. *Brain* 2009; **132**: 2958–69.

56. Waxman EA, Giasson BI. Molecular mechanisms of α-synuclein neurodegeneration. *Biochim Biophys Acta – Molecular Basis of Disease* 2009; **1792**: 616–24.

57. Cilia R, Tunesi S, Marotta G et al. Survival and dementia in GBA-associated Parkinson's disease: the mutation matters. *Ann Neurol* 2016; **80**: 662–73.

58. Grünewald A, Kasten M, Ziegler A, Klein C. Next-generation phenotyping using the Parkin example: time to catch up with genetics. *JAMA Neurol* 2013; **70**: 1186–91.

59. Wang HF, Yu JT, Tang SW et al. Efficacy and safety of cholinesterase inhibitors and memantine in cognitive impairment in Parkinson's disease, Parkinson's disease dementia, and dementia with Lewy bodies: systematic review with meta-analysis and trial sequential analysis. *J Neurol Neurosurg Psychiatry* 2015; **86**: 135–43.

60. Murray DK, Sacheli MA, Eng JJ, Stoessl AJ. The effects of exercise on cognition in

Parkinson's disease: a systematic review. *Transl Neurodegener* 2014; **3**: 5. https://translationalneurodegeneration.biomedcentral.com/articles/10.1186/2047-9158-3-5 [last accessed on 6th February 2020].

61. Leung IH, Walton CC, Hallock H et al. Cognitive training in Parkinson disease: a systematic review and meta-analysis. *Neurology* 2015; **85**: 1843–51.

62. Vardy ERLC, Teodorczuk A, Yarnall AJ. Review of delirium in patients with Parkinson's disease. *J Neurol* 2015: **262**: 2401–10.

63. Serrano-Dueñas M, Bleda MJ. Delirium in Parkinson's disease patients. A five-year follow-up study. *Park Relat Disord* 2005; **11**: 387–92.

64. Umemura A, Oeda T, Tomita S, et al. Delirium and high fever are associated with subacute motor deterioration in Parkinson disease: a nested case-control study. *PLoS One* 2014; 9(6): e94944. https://journals.plos.org/plosone/article?id=10.1371/journal.pone.0094944 [last accessed on 6th February 2020].

65. Weintraub D, Koester J, Potenza MN et al. Impulse control disorders in Parkinson disease: a cross-sectional study of 3090 patients. *Arch Neurol* 2010; **67**: 589–95.

66. Okai D, Askey-Jones S, Samuel M et al. Trial of CBT for impulse control behaviors affecting Parkinson patients and their caregivers. *Neurology* 2013; **80**: 792–9.

67. Nirenberg MJ. Dopamine agonist withdrawal syndrome: implications for patient care. *Drugs Aging* 2013; **30**: 587–92.

68. Béreau M, Fleury V, Bouthour W et al. Hyperdopaminergic behavioral spectrum in Parkinson's disease: a review. *Rev. Neurol. (Paris)* 2018; **174**: 653–63.

Chapter

The Home Assessment in Old Age Psychiatry
A Practical Guide

Bradley Ng and Martin Atkins

Introduction

The psychiatric assessment of older people can be carried out in many environments, including outpatient clinics, hospital wards, care facilities for the elderly and the individual's own home. Each presents advantages, disadvantages and challenges. An initial assessment conducted in the patient's home remains an important aspect of many old age psychiatric services in high-income countries. This chapter explores and discusses the clinical aspects of conducting an initial psychiatric assessment of an older person in their home. It aims to be neither prescriptive nor exhaustive, but hopes to increase the awareness of the reader to certain themes and considerations in such assessments. We draw on the literature in old age psychiatry, geriatric medicine and other disciplines as well as our own, and our colleagues', clinical experience.

The Advantages and Disadvantages of a Home Assessment

There are several potential advantages of a home assessment. One witnesses first-hand how the person mobilizes and operates in their environment, with less reliance on the patient's or collateral accounts, which may be incomplete, biased or misleading.[1] The patient, their caregivers and family may be present and be more at ease and forthcoming in their own home.[2–4] Relevant environmental and psychosocial factors, family strengths and resources, and the role of other services may become more apparent.[3, 5] Home assessments have the potential to detect previously unnoticed or underappreciated problems, psychiatric or otherwise, as seen in Box 9.1.[1, 6–10] It may become apparent that the referred psychiatric issue may not be the most pressing matter.[11–12] Physical disabilities, deteriorating cognition, poor insight, immobility, no driver's licence or driving ability, the lack of family to assist with travel, unfriendly public transport or a bewildering hospital system may be practical factors that favour a home assessment.[13]

There are disadvantages with home assessments as well. Some patients may be very uncomfortable with health personnel visiting their home. An explanation for the visit must, therefore, be given at initial contact, as well as the option of an outpatient appointment. The ability and equipment to conduct a physical examination are limited in a home visit. Finding a mutually convenient time for all involved may lead to delays. Home assessments do require more time for travel and potentially could be longer than outpatient assessments, because more issues may be uncovered. On clinical grounds, however, we believe this is an advantage and well worth any extra time spent.

Box 9.1 Potential problems identified by home assessments

Psychiatric/medical
- Depression
- Cognitive impairment or dementia
- Behavioural and psychological symptoms of dementia (BPSD)
- Psychosis
- Alcohol misuse
- Acute medical illness
- Pain problems
- Polypharmacy issues

Geriatric
- Falls and other safety issues
- Incontinence issues
- Sensory impairment
- Poor nutrition
- Caregiver and family stress/conflict/burnout
- Neglect and abuse
- Medication errors
- Need for ongoing placement or care

Environmental
- Neglected household or squalor
- Inadequate utilities/heating
- Poor food availability
- Mobility challenges

Scanameo A, Fillit H. A practical guide to seeing the patient at home. *Geriatrics* 1995; 50: 33–7.
Levine SA, Barry PP. Home care. In *Geriatric Medicine: An Evidence-Based Approach* (eds. CK Cassel, RM Leipzig, HJ Cohen, EB Larson, DE Meier DE) 4th ed: 121–131. Springer, 2002.

Preparation

The Referral and Allocation

Although many old age psychiatric services accept and encourage referrals from a variety of sources, including patients and carers,[14] we believe the involvement or approval of the patient's general practitioner (GP) is essential. The GP is the primary healthcare provider and frequently has an intimate and long-standing relationship with the patient. There are occasions when a referral is received from a source other than the GP while the GP is already managing the situation well and views specialist input as unnecessary or inappropriate. The GP is the practitioner most likely to have an overall understanding of co-morbid physical illnesses, long-standing psychiatric disorders and current prescription medications. This information is invaluable in services where non-medical clinicians are required to triage or respond to the referral.

The reason for the referral and perceived urgency must be as clear as possible. Other information includes the details of involvement of other mental health services or practitioners, government or non-government agencies, and formal and informal social supports. Contact details for family and/or carers should be obtained as well as any known risk factors or dangers to the patient, family, carers or health and community personnel.

Which, and how many, staff respond to a referral will depend on several factors, including service policy, staffing levels, the patient's history with the service and transport availability. If a patient was previously known to a service or has accepted the referral and has no identifiable risk factors, it may be appropriate for only one staff member to respond. If there are potential risks and complexity, two clinicians have the advantages of mitigating safety concerns, gathering more information and developing an initial multidisciplinary formulation. Whether or not a doctor needs to go on every home assessment is debatable[15] and often dictated by availability. Studies have shown non-medical staff to be equally skilled at providing initial assessments in old age psychiatry.[16] Depending on availability, allocation by profession may have benefits in an initial assessment. For example, a referral indicating significant social stresses might be allocated to a social worker in the multidisciplinary team, while cognitive impairment or falls might prompt an occupational therapy perspective.

Initial Contact

Telephone contact with the patient should be made beforehand to obtain consent for a home assessment, to obtain permission to gather collateral history and to facilitate participation in the assessment, if appropriate, of family, carers or other parties involved.[17] Alternative approaches will need to be considered when the patient cannot be contacted by phone, including writing to the patient or visiting unannounced. Culturally and linguistically diverse populations may require a clinician who speaks the patient's language, interpreter services or, as a last resort, a family member to assist with the assessment.

Issues of informed consent are influenced by the referrer's assessment of the patient's presentation. If the patient has significant cognitive impairment, it may be considered appropriate to contact family or carers without consent, or to visit without prior notification. Sometimes the patient is unaware of the referral, or even the referrer. How much is disclosed to the patient may depend on the referrer, their relationship with the patient and the apparent willingness of the patient to engage in assessment. It may prove necessary to go back to the referrer for clarification of some issues following initial telephone contact with the patient.

The clinician should try to find out whether there are family members who may be able to assist the assessment, to clarify the patient's own perceptions of their circumstances and to identify the patient's own priorities and concerns. An appointment date can be confirmed, necessary directions elicited and any problems regarding access discussed (e.g. bad roads, access to gated communities, building security controls).

Identified Risks and Safety Issues

Potential risks to staff should be identified prior to any home assessment with strategies implemented to reduce or minimize them. These factors will dictate the arrangements and timing of the assessment, including the number and mix (professional background, gender) of staff and the potential role of any emergency services and police.

Morning appointments may be preferable in neighbourhoods that are violent or have illicit drug problems. Any vehicles should not be ostentatious or contain valuables and be parked to ensure rapid egress if this proves necessary. A 'doctor's bag' may also attract the attention of individuals with drug-seeking behaviour, and a nondescript bag or rucksack may be preferable in such areas. Mobile telephone reception needs to be monitored.

Owners should be asked to restrain or isolate potentially aggressive animals. This can be done by telephone from the front gate, if necessary. The general layout of the property should be considered, including routes of egress, alternative exits and barriers such as secured doors or excessive household items and refuse. Consideration of the situation of stairwells and functionality of lifts (elevators) is necessary in multi-storey residential blocks. This may be necessary owing to issues with the patient's partner or family, including hostility, violence and drug and alcohol issues.

Safety issues include the availability of mobile phones or other telecommunications, ready access to relevant phone numbers (home base, crisis response team, ambulance and police) and sufficient fuel (a major issue in more rural areas). Visits should be planned in accordance with service safety policies, including staff working alone and with an effective system in place for tracking where staff have gone and their expected return time.[19] Equipment that might be taken on home assessments is detailed in Box 9.2.

Awareness and re-evaluation of such risk issues should be ongoing throughout a home visit. Any signs of aggression, anger or intoxication from substances in the patient or others should be monitored closely and note taken of any potential weapons in the environment. While de-escalating confrontational situations is an option, assessments should be politely terminated if there is evidence of escalation that poses a threat to staff, or indeed to the patient or any other people in the household. If it proves necessary to terminate the home visit, the degree and urgency of the situation, as well as risks to the person and healthcare staff, will dictate what subsequent response is required.

Box 9.2 Home assessment equipment

- Patient records and stationery
- Medical equipment such as blood pressure cuff, stethoscope and thermometer
- Blood test request forms, radiological request forms and prescription pad
- Medication samples
- Antipsychotic depots and syringes (e.g. if a previously known patient is known to have defaulted on a depot antipsychotic)
- Relevant mental health legislation paperwork
- Spare clothing, especially trousers, are always worth consideration if squalid home circumstances are anticipated
- Patient education materials and brochures introducing the service
- Dictaphone
- Introduction/business card

Scanameo A, Fillit H. A practical guide to seeing the patient at home. *Geriatrics* 1995; 50: 33–7.
Unwin BK, Jerant AF. The home visit. *Am Fam Physician* 1999; 60: 1481–8.

Commencing the Assessment

Before the Front Door

The cleanliness and general milieu of the neighbourhood, proximity of other houses or apartments, evidence of crime, lighting and the extent of local noise and disturbance will usually be evident. The availability of local resources, such as shops, bus stops, public transport and medical services, may be identified in passing. Is the house hard to find and is it clearly identified with a number? [4]

Valuable information can be gathered before approaching the front door. Uncollected mail in the post box may indicate cognitive, mood, or mobility concerns. Refuse and recycling bins may point to the patient's overall level of organization, alcohol use and functioning. The derelict state of the building and garden may raise similar concerns or point to financial issues. Potential accessibility (stairs, ramps, handrails and lifts) and mobility risks (uneven, overgrown or slippery paths, and lighting) can be assessed. Is there a car? What is its state and has it been used recently?

The general security of the home may give clues to cognitive problems (doors left open inappropriately) or delusion-based modifications (barricades or excessive numbers of locks) and contributes to the risk assessment. Unexpected safety concerns include evidence of intrusion by others (graffiti, dumped rubbish) or the presence of apparently inappropriate persons in the dwelling. A delay in opening the front door may be caused by patient frailty, deafness, poor mobility, fear or apathy.[19]

Starting the Interview

How the interview commences depends on the circumstances and the individuals involved, especially their interpersonal skills and experience in putting the patient at ease and in establishing a rapport. As a 'guest' in their house, staff should informally and continually ask the patient's permission for their actions during a home assessment. Observations of the home are gently raised with the patient or other parties to allow explanation.

The patient may indicate a preference as to where the assessment should occur, though some prompting may be required: 'Where would you like us to sit?' Occasionally the patient will not want strangers entering the home and may prefer to speak on the doorstep or in the garden. This should be respected to allow the patient to develop sufficient confidence to grant voluntary access into the home later to continue the assessment. If there are risk concerns, assessments conducted near exits or in relatively open spaces are advised.

A judgement will have to be made quickly about whether to interview the patient alone, with family/carers or both. Joint assessments by two clinicians have several advantages in this regard, including the opportunity to 'split forces' and interview the patient and family/carers separately and simultaneously, thus saving time. This is valuable when the parties are uncomfortable speaking in front of each other. Consent to obtain collateral history is important, and in our experience, it is rarely withheld by patients. Such information is essential to corroborate the patient's account, especially when significant cognitive impairment is suspected.

The Home Assessment

General Observations

An examination of the patient's home needs to have flexibility and respect for the patient's privacy. With an empathic and non-confrontational approach, most patients are very

---

Box 9.3 Environmental risk factors for falls

- Slippery or uneven pathways, floors or stairs
- Very steep or narrow steps
- Loose carpets, mats and rugs
- Clutter, pets, cords or spilt liquid on the floor
- No handrails or bathroom/toilet grab rails
- Unsuitable furniture
- Shelves or cupboards too high or low
- Use of ladders or step ladders
- Broken or rotting floorboards
- Poor lighting

Scanameo A, Fillit H. A practical guide to seeing the patient at home. *Geriatrics* 1995; 50: 33–7.
Lord SR, Sherrington C, Menz HB, Close JCT. *Falls in Older People*, 2nd ed. Cambridge University Press, 2007.
Lowery K, Buri H, Ballard C. What is the prevalence of environmental hazards in the homes of dementia
sufferers and are they associated with falls. *Int J Geriatr Psych* 2000; 15: 883–6.

---

agreeable to a quick walk around the home and it allows an opportunity for non-clinical discussions that many welcome. An overenthusiastic or intrusive approach may jeopardize any initial rapport developed with the patient.

Home environments can range from extreme tidiness, to hoarding, or gross squalor. Are there piles of newspapers, magazines or refuse? Are there unpleasant or rank odours from poor hygiene, squalor, toileting issues or pets? If there are pets, what is the standard of care? What are the reasons for the extra security measures? Are there cigarette burns on the carpet? What is the general state of lighting, electricity, heating, water and ventilation? There may be evidence of unpaid utility bills. Unsecured valuables or cash and offers of such or other payments may highlight risks of exploitation. What are the potential fall hazards (Box 9.3)? The general condition of the home may reflect the financial circumstances of the occupant, but this can be misleading, especially in individuals with cognitive impairment or delusions of poverty.[20]

The Living Room

The living room or lounge is usually the starting place for an assessment. Family photos are a good way of breaking the ice, demonstrating a personal interest in the patient, providing an initial idea of family relationships and acting as a useful cognitive screen. Can they remember the names and ages of family members? Where do they live? Hobbies and interests may also be starting points for developing rapport and allow an assessment of any changes in interest, enthusiasm or cognition.

The television provides a useful cue to enquire about the latest reality TV show, drama cliff-hanger or sports results. Is it functional and can the patient use the remote control and DVD, or even video, player? Or is there evidence that the patient now uses a computer, tablet device or mobile phone for such entertainment? A decline in the usual level of interest in television programmes may be related to cognitive decline or an affective disorder.

The presence of computers, smart phones and tablet devices can provide a discussion point for clinicians. How adept is the patient at using such devices? Have they learnt how to use them before and are now struggling? Is this a new interest? Are they worried about scams? Can they take photos on their phones? Do they prefer to be contacted by text message? Do they use apps? One can gather a large amount of information on the patient's capabilities, strengths and any challenges faced, but this has to be balanced by not being too intrusive.

The Kitchen

A detailed kitchen assessment may be very revealing. What is the general state of cleanliness and hygiene? Are there rodents or cockroaches? Is there a working smoke alarm? Are there burnt pots or pans, or plumbing problems? Is the stove, oven, microwave or dishwasher operational?

Insufficient or inadequate food in the fridge or pantry is of obvious concern and leads to questions about eating habits, shopping and cooking abilities. Is there evidence of poorly prepared meals or dietary quirks? If meals are being delivered, a quick glance in the fridge will reveal if they are being consumed and their expiry dates. Delivered meals are no longer exclusively from non-governmental organizations – *Uber Eats* and other apps deliver meals and alcohol. There may be evidence of high levels of alcohol consumption. Offers of cups of tea should not be refused, as they allow immediate and meaningful insights into cognitive impairment and functional abilities.[19] It is easy to find an excuse not to drink the tea if hygiene levels appear worrying.

The Bathroom and Bedroom

Access to the toilet, bath and shower may reveal falls risks, access problems and hygiene issues. Blocked toilets or drains can rapidly lead to squalor. A failure to keep plumbing in working order may reflect cognitive decline. Similar issues may also be seen in the laundry, resulting in the gradual accumulation of dirty clothing.

Except for a possible quick glance, we often choose not to enter bedrooms out of respect for the patient's privacy. Occasionally, patients are interviewed in their bed, because of physical infirmity, social withdrawal in the case of depression or temporal disorientation or apathy in dementia. Malodorous conditions and unwashed bedding are readily identifiable. Mobility issues may lead to alternative sleeping arrangements. Occasionally there may be a more bizarre explanation, such as psychosis, and gentle enquiry will generally reveal the motivation.

The Garden

The state of the garden, if there is one, may indicate the patient's functioning and leisure interests. The degree of upkeep can contribute to the impression of physical abilities and limitations. In the case of physically able patients who express an interest in gardening but whose garden shows evidence of neglect, possibilities include cognitive decline, avolition or anergia related to depression, or avoidance of the garden associated with paranoid ideation related to neighbours.

Medications

A home assessment allows a more comprehensive medication list and history. Patients often fail to bring all, or even any, of their medications to an outpatient clinic, despite specific instructions to do so.

The medications prescribed by a GP are not necessarily taken by the patient. A filled prescription does not mean it is being taken. The patient may not be prescribed opioids but may be using their spouse's supply. Sometimes a medication container may be filled with a completely different medication! [17] Over-the-counter medications, vitamins and herbal and dietary supplements are some examples of other medications being omitted from lists provided by patients and carers. Some medications may be kept in other parts of the house, for example, hypnotics in the bedroom. [4] In some countries, medications may have multiple trade names leading to many patients inadvertently duplicating their medications.

The mode of dispensing medications varies considerably, including boxes, bottles, dosette boxes and blister packs. Can the arthritic patient open medication bottles or read the print? How does the patient administer their medications and is there any supervision? Dispensing and expiry dates can be checked, and compliance can be approximated using these factors and an estimate of the number of tablets remaining.

Gathering all of the patient's medication during an assessment may identify many of the highlighted issues. [18] Asking why the patient takes each particular medication provides clues to their insight into their medical conditions. Multiple prescriptions or an excess of medications raises the issue of 'doctor shopping' [20] by deliberately consulting a variety or doctors, their import by family members from overseas or the use of the internet to obtain medications. Overuse of opioids and benzodiazepines has to be considered. This may also be a good time to enquire gently about other substances such as marijuana.

Finally, after any home assessment, the patient and their families should be encouraged to dispose of any expired, unnecessary or ceased medications.

Home Help and Family Support

At some point it is routine to enquire about domestic support. The frequency and perceived quality of support, as well as the relationship with carers, should be explored. Patients may point out practical examples of their dissatisfaction.

There will also be an initial impression of how the patient interacts with any family members and vice versa. Are some family members sympathetic or understanding? What are the non-verbal cues? Who has the power? Is there hostility or aggression? Is the nominated caregiver more frail or unwell than the patient? Legal issues, such as an enduring power of attorney, can also be raised. The patient's relationship with their neighbours could be invaluable or fraught. If the patient identifies certain neighbours as supportive, consider obtaining permission to collect collateral history from them. Angry or hostile neighbours sometimes 'give' history, even when not approached, if one is easily identified as coming from a 'health service'.

Finally, the clinician does need to consider exploitation and elder abuse. There may also be evidence of scams, either by phone or mail, or even the purchase of unwanted or unnecessary services, renovations or house upgrades.

After the Visit

Obtaining a corroborative history, as necessary, from informants such as the GP, other medical specialists, family members who were not available for the assessment and home service providers will help to fill any gaps in the assessment. Often family members will provide an alternative perspective or emphasis that can substantially alter impressions gained from an unaccompanied patient, especially where cognitive impairment is significant. Family members are often also more forthcoming if they are not speaking in front of the patient.

Conclusions

This chapter has briefly highlighted the clinical challenges and strategies in conducting a home assessment in old age psychiatry. A home visit has the potential to provide a comprehensive and holistic overview of the patient and allows psychiatric services to provide individualized interventions, despite the associated costs and risks, in comparison with an outpatient assessment. The final decision on whether or not a service undertakes home assessment ultimately depends on the resources and experience of the clinical team.

Acknowledgement

For information, the original paper on which this chapter is based was:

Ng Bradley, Atkins M. Home assessment in old age psychiatry: a practical guide. *Adv Psychiatr Treat* 2012; **18**:400–7.

References

1. Levy MT. Psychiatric assessment of elderly patients in the home: a survey of 176 cases. *J Am Geriatr Soc* 1985; **33**: 9–12.

2. Benbow SM. The community clinic: its advantages and disadvantages. *Int J Geriatr Psych* 1990; **5**: 119–21.

3. Anderson DN, Aquilina C. Domiciliary clinics I: effects of non-attendance. *Int J Geriatr Psych* 2002; **17**: 941–4.

4. Scanameo A, Fillit H. A practical guide to seeing the patient at home. *Geriatrics* 1995; **50**: 33–7.

5. Koenig HG. The physician and home care of the elderly patient. *Gerontology Geriatr Educ* 1986; **7**: 15–24.

6. Arcand M, Williamson J. An evaluation of home visiting of patients by physicians in geriatric medicine. *Brit Med J* 1981; **283**: 718–20.

7. Currie CT, Moore JT, Friedman SW, Warshaw GA. Assessment of elderly patients at home: a report of fifty cases. *J Am Geriatr Soc* 1981; **29**: 398–401.

8. Ramsdell JW, Swart JA, Jackson JE, Renvall M. The yield of a home visit in the assessment of geriatric patients. *J Am Geriatr Soc* 1989; **37**: 17–24.

9. Ramsdell JW, Jackson JE, Renvall Guy HJB, Renvall MJ. Comparison of clinic-based home assessment to a home visit in demented elderly patients. *Alz Dis Assoc Dis* 2004; **18**: 145–53.

10. Levine SA, Barry PP. Home care. In *Geriatric Medicine: An Evidence-Based Approach* (eds. CK Cassel, RM Leipzig, HJ Cohen, EB Larson, DE Meier) 4th ed: 121–131. Springer, 2002.

11. Simon A. Some observations of a geropsychiatrist on the value of house calls. *Gerontologist* 1984; **24**: 458–64.

12. Grauer H, Kravitz H, Davis E, Rodriguez C. Homebound aged: the dilemma of psychiatric intervention. *Can J Psychiat* 1991; **36**: 497–501.

13. Burton JR. The house call: an important service for the frail elderly. *J Am Geriatr Soc* 1985; **33**: 291–3.

14. Richardson B, Orrell M. Home assessments in old age psychiatry. *Adv Psychiatr Treat* 2002; **8**: 59–65.

15. Orrell M, Katona C. Do consultant home visits have a future in old age psychiatry? *Int J Geriatr Psych* 1998; **13**: 355–7.

16. Draper B. The effectiveness of old age psychiatry services. *Int J Geriatr Psych* 2000; **15**: 687–703.

17. Zebley JW. Geriatric follow-up: what only a home visit can tell you. *Geriatrics* 1986; **41**: 100–104.

18. Byrne G, Neville C. *Community Mental Health for Older People*. Churchill Livingstone, 2010.

19. Fottrell E. A personal view of psychogeriatric domiciliary visits. *Geriatrics* 1989; **2**: 22–5.

20. Unwin BK, Jerant AF. The home visit. *Am Fam Physician* 1999; **60**: 1481–8.

21. Lord SR, Sherrington C, Menz HB, Close JCT. *Falls in Older People*, 2nd ed. Cambridge University Press, 2007.

22. Lowery K, Buri H, Ballard C. What is the prevalence of environmental hazards in the homes of dementia sufferers and are they associated with falls. *Int J Geriatr Psych* 2000; **15**: 883–6.

Driving in Dementia
A Clinician's Guide

Sarah Wilson and Gill Pinner

Introduction

With an ageing population and more drivers on the road, the number of drivers with dementia is due to grow exponentially over the next 50 years. Although decisions regarding possession of a driving licence in the UK are made by the Driver and Vehicle Licensing Agency (DVLA), psychiatrists need to consider the DVLA guidance and inform patients and their carers of their responsibility to remain safe and legal on the roads. Doctors have a duty of care to advise patients who are unfit to drive to cease driving and to inform the DVLA of patients who pose a risk to the general public by continuing to drive when advised not to. This chapter offers a review of the literature on dementia and driving and sum-marizes the evidence and advice for navigating this minefield, including the recently published consensus guidelines for driving with dementia or mild cognitive impairment (MCI). We shall discuss the use of psychological test batteries in clinical practice, along with the most useful questions to ask in memory clinics. We shall consider legal guidance for various countries, as well as the important (but often overlooked) issue of helping older people prepare for retirement from driving.

Driving and dementia is a relatively new field of research. The subject first appeared in the literature in the 1980s and since then the number of studies exploring this issue has exploded. Given the ageing population and that the number of drivers around the world is increasing, the larger number of people driving with dementia will pose significant demands on licensing agencies and on clinicians about how best to protect individuals and the wider public.

Driving is not a right. A car is a lethal weapon and drivers are granted a licence provided the strict criteria set by licensing agencies are met. Driving is not safe, nor even possible in more advanced dementias, but as awareness and diagnostic techniques improve and diagnoses are made earlier, clinicians must be fully informed when advising people with early dementia on how their driving might be affected as their condition progresses.

How Can Clinicians Assess Driving Risk?

There are many difficulties in developing universal guidelines for people driving with dementia, although Consensus Guidelines for the UK have recently been published.[1] There is no question that drivers with dementia pose a risk to themselves and other road users as their illness progresses. The challenge is assessing the level of risk and identifying at what stage the risk becomes untenable. The symptoms of dementia can vary greatly between individuals depending on the type of dementia. This is very important when assessing driving ability.

Use of Self-Reporting

Studies looking at self-reports of crashes and abnormal driving behaviour have found problems with recall bias. Holland showed that most drivers perceived their own chance of having a road accident to be significantly lower, and their own skill to be greater, than that of their peers.[2] When this is enhanced by the forgetfulness and lack of insight found in dementia, there are obvious shortcomings with using self-report alone as a method of risk assessment.

Use of Carer Reporting

A commonly used source of information on a patient's fitness to drive is an interview with carers, but Johnson noted that friends and relatives do not always give a true picture.[3] This may be because they do not wish to take away the patient's independence, or because they do not wish to become burdened by a relative who can no longer drive but wishes to remain sociable. Partners may overestimate driving ability if they rely on their loved one to get around or have memory impairment themselves. Informants are also wary of being blamed for a patient's licence being taken away.

Adler et al. found drivers with dementia had a greater risk than controls of crashes and getting lost, and relatives often took over responsibility for the transportation needs of older family members.[4] They also found that concerned relatives tried to stop individuals with dementia from driving, but long-standing family dynamics often interfered with the sensitive negotiation required. Older people are more likely to accept a recommendation to stop driving from a doctor or authority figure than from a relative or friend.

A study by Brown et al. suggested that both patient and informant perception of driving ability did not relate well to actual driving ability.[5] Participants (with mild, very mild or no dementia), informants and an experienced neurologist were asked to rate participants' driving ability as safe, marginal or unsafe. The participants then underwent an on-road driving assessment with a professional driving instructor. Only the neurologist's ratings correlated with the on-road driving assessment.

However, Croston et al. reported that informants often observed drivers with Alzheimer's dementia (AD) having difficulty with traffic awareness, maintaining appropriate speeds and staying in their own lane.[6] This suggests informants may be reliable sources of information if asked appropriate and relevant questions about driving safety.

Use of Other Collateral Information

It may be useful to enquire whether the patient has been involved in any recent accidents, or indeed a community psychiatric nurse may report seeing dents and scratches appearing on the car. Collecting data from police records and insurance companies poses difficulties as diagnoses of dementia may be unknown, especially in the early stages, and minor bumps and offences often go unnoticed or unreported.

Two studies from the United States have looked at state-recorded crash details and found that the crash and violation rates of individuals with dementia were not significantly different to those of age-matched controls.[7, 8] Both studies found, however, that patients with dementia did not drive as frequently or as far as controls and the crash characteristics between the two groups differed, with the dementia group having more at-fault crashes.

The Importance of the Clinical Presentation

It is really important to consider the nature of the symptom profile and natural history of the patient's specific dementia. Establishing the dementia subtype is important, as some sub-types are associated with higher risk than others. DLB (dementia with Lewy bodies) and FTD (frontotemporal dementia) are the riskiest dementias in relation to driving.[9] The hallucinations associated with DLB are likely to have an impact on attention when driving, and any parkinsonian symptoms will affect reaction times.[10] The changes in impulsivity, forward planning and shifting attention found in FTD mean driving skills can be affected very early in the disease.

Studies looking at specific types of dementia have mostly focused on people with AD. Most individuals with moderate to severe AD are unsafe or unable to drive, so studies have focused on the mild to very mild end of the spectrum,[5, 11] with very mild dementia being equivalent to MCI.

Drivers with a mild dementia were found to have an increased risk of crashes and abnormal driving behaviours and a faster rate of decline than those with very mild dementia.[11] It has been suggested, therefore, that those individuals with mild AD have their driving status reviewed every six months, while those with MCI should be reviewed every year.

The general consensus is that it is usually safe to continue driving for around 3 years after the onset of AD.[7, 12, 13] Other dementias, such as the vascular type, may remain stable for longer, although the cognitive decline is far more unpredictable. As discussed earlier, FTD and DLB usually require individuals to stop driving much earlier. Sleep disturbance, anxiety and low mood associated with dementia may also affect driving ability by reducing concentration.[14]

Consider Comorbidities

Older people with dementia often have multiple physical comorbidities that can affect driving ability and may require the individual to stop driving. Medications prescribed for physical comorbidities, as well as antidepressants and antipsychotics, can affect sensorimotor and perceptual abilities that might have a further detrimental effect on driving ability.

Retirement from Driving

As driving with dementia is dangerous and inevitably requires individuals to cease driving, it could be argued that drivers with dementia should have their licences revoked as soon as the diagnosis is made. However, a number of important factors need to be taken into account.

Modification of Driving Behaviour

It is important to appreciate that many older people begin to modify their driving behaviour with time, avoiding busy roads at busy times, using familiar routes and not driving in bad weather or at night. When comparing driving safety statistics and age, this needs to be taken into account. Previous perceived wisdom that older people as a group have more crashes has been disproven, as studies have established this is on account of low mileage and not increasing age.[15] Evidence suggests that patients with AD usually modify their driving behaviour, but this is often not enough to reduce their crash risk completely.[4, 16]

Impact of Available Alternative Transport

Around the world there are clear differences in vehicle use between rural and urban areas. Across all age groups, people are less likely to drive in cities than in the country, because of readily available public transport systems and overcrowded roads. In rural areas, a car can be a lifeline for individuals where alternative transport is non-existent and travel is required to access food and other services.[3]

Declining mobility and physical disability associated with ageing has been shown to lead to a reliance on private vehicles, as other forms of transport such as walking and public transport are no longer realistic options.[17] There is also evidence that older people do not feel public transport is adequate, efficient or safe enough for their needs.[13]

Driving Cessation

A number of studies have looked at driving retirement and found that very few people even consider making plans for when they are no longer able to drive.[4, 6] This is an inevitable stage of life for most people, Foley et al. showed that men tend to outlive their driving ability by 6 years and women by 10 years.[18] Even when given a diagnosis of dementia, many individuals do not make plans for complete driving cessation.[3, 13] This may in part be caused by individuals not recognizing they have impairment as a result of their cognitive state, which is quite different to people with physical illnesses such as epilepsy or visual problems when insight is not impaired.

Making the decision to retire from driving will have significant psychosocial consequences that may have a negative impact on people with dementia. Marottoli et al. have shown that cessation of driving leads to a significant reduction in out-of-home activity levels, as well as an increase in depressive symptoms.[17, 19] It is increasingly clear that to stop driving is a life-altering decision, reducing independence and limiting access to family, friends and services.[13]

Legislation

The legal requirements for doctors to report potentially dangerous drivers to licensing authorities vary around the world. Rosser explained how in The Netherlands, patient confidentiality takes precedence over reporting, while Danish doctors are obliged to inform the police authority if someone poses a risk.[20] Hungary provides very specific guidance on psychometric testing for people with dementia wishing to acquire or retain a driving licence, whilst other countries still do not specifically refer to dementia in driving guidelines. In Portugal, the neurologist is the named specialist for permitting driving, while in Estonia it is the psychiatrist who makes decisions about driving with dementia.

In the United States and Canada, guidelines and obligations vary between states, provinces and territories. Physicians in all areas are permitted to report medically at-risk drivers, although this is a requirement in only 16 of the 64 states, provinces and territories. One major difference between the United States and Canada and the UK and Europe is that many US and Canadian states and provinces can apply conditions or restrictions to a licence, rather than refusing to issue one at all.

Box 10.1 DVLA guidance

(This applies to Group 1 – car and motorcycle licences. Dementia precludes drivers from holding a Group 2 – bus and lorry licence – and such licences should be surrendered or will be revoked when a diagnosis is made.)

'It is difficult to assess driving ability in people with dementia. The DVLA acknowledges that there are varied presentations and rates of progression, and the decision on licensing is usually based on medical reports.

Considerations include:

- poor short-term memory, disorientation, and lack of insight and judgement almost certainly mean no fitness to drive
- disorders of attention cause impairment
- in early dementia, when sufficient skills are retained and progression is slow, a licence may be issued subject to annual review.

A formal driving assessment may be necessary'

Driver and Vehicle Licensing Agency. *Assessing Fitness to Drive: A Guide for Medical Professionals*. DVLA, 2019.

DVLA and the Law

In the UK, driving licences are provided by the DVLA. Since the agency was set up in 1972, it has developed medical guidance for many illnesses that can adversely affect driving ability. Dementia has only been recognized as a specific condition in recent years. Prior to this, dementia and cognitive impairment were grouped under 'neurological conditions'. Over time, guidelines for many medical conditions have become clearer and tighter; however, the current guidance for drivers with dementia remains necessarily nebulous (see Box 10.1).[21]

The responsibility for renewing or revoking driving licences in the UK ultimately falls to the DVLA, but it is recognized that decisions are usually based on medical reports from doctors who care for these patients. A Canadian report by Hopkins et al. noted that the responsibility for identifying drivers with dementia has fallen on the healthcare system, a role for which it was neither designed nor equipped to handle. They also noted that placing this responsibility on clinicians can be detrimental to the doctor–patient relationship.[21]

Naidu and McKeith surveyed old age psychiatrists who completed DVLA medical reports in 2006 and concluded that the current system for determining driving ability in people with cognitive impairment was unsatisfactory.[22] The DVLA addressed this by developing a medical questionnaire specifically for cognitive impairment and dementia, but this still relies heavily on psychiatrists' clinical opinions, requiring yes/no answers to statements such as 'Does your patient lack insight and/or judgement to a degree that would make driving dangerous?'

All drivers are required to inform the DVLA of any diagnosis or disability which may affect their driving; it is prudent for doctors to advise patients of this. With dementia, however, a definitive diagnosis may not be made until the illness is well established, especially if the patient does not recognize the symptoms, does not have insight or is in a state of denial. Once a diagnosis is made, the same factors may still be relevant, as the patient may dispute the diagnosis or may neither understand nor recall the advice.[9]

> **Box 10.2** GMC guidance
>
> 'If you become aware that a patient is continuing to drive when they may not be fit to do so, you should make every reasonable effort to persuade them to stop. If you do not manage to persuade the patient to stop driving, or you discover that they are continuing to drive against your advice, you should consider whether the patient's refusal to stop driving leaves others exposed to a risk of death or serious harm. If you believe that it does, you should contact the DVLA or DVA promptly and disclose any relevant medical information, in confidence, to the medical adviser.
>
> Before contacting the DVLA or DVA, you should try to inform the patient of your intention to disclose personal information. If the patient objects to the disclosure, you should consider any reasons they give for objecting. If you decide to contact the DVLA or DVA, you should tell your patient in writing once you have done so, and make a note on the patient's record.'
>
> *'DVA' refers to the Driver and Vehicle Agency (DVA) in Northern Ireland.
>
> General Medical Council (GMC). *Confidentiality: Patients' Fitness to Drive and Reporting Concerns to the DVLA or DVA*. GMC, 2019.

Patients with MCI may not need to notify the DVLA if there is no likely driving impairment, but notification and medical reports may be required if there is any possible impact on driving (such as disorders of attention, lack of judgement or lack of insight).[21] The General Medical Council (GMC) provides specific guidance on confidentiality (see Box 10.2), with the reason to break this being if the risks and interests of public safety outweigh the interests of the patient.[23]

Driving Ability Tests

On-road Testing

The gold standard of fitness to drive is an on-road assessment, but this is not a readily available test. There are 19 main mobility test centres across the UK. As well as providing driving assessments to people with dementia, they offer assessments to people of all ages with medical conditions or disabilities affecting driving skills. They also assess and advise carers who need to transport individuals with restricted mobility in their vehicles and make recommendations on vehicle modifications (see www.drivingmobility.org.uk).

Logistically, these centres do not have the capacity to offer one-off tests to every driver with dementia, let alone repeated tests as the condition deteriorates. In any case, many people being diagnosed with dementia have either already stopped driving or else are quite happy to do so without further assessment. It would also be impractical and costly to co-ordinate repeated on-road tests with follow-up appointments in memory clinics scattered around the region.

Regular testing may also be detrimental to the patient with early dementia, as the added stress and anxiety of getting to the centre (which could be up to 50 miles away) and being tested could lead to false failures. For this reason, research has focused on finding a simple test or battery of tests which can be carried out in memory clinics.

In-office Testing

Researchers have been trying to develop batteries of so called 'in-office tests' to evaluate driving safety and ability better in dementia, bringing together more specific psychometrics with effective probing collateral reports.

Molnar et al. completed a systematic review of simple in-office cognitive tests which claimed to differentiate drivers with dementia as 'safe' or 'unsafe'.[24] They found that commonly recommended tests, such as the MMSE or Trail Making Test B, did not demonstrate robustly positive findings across studies and that the Clock Drawing Test was not evaluated in any study. Cut-off scores were only reported in one study, making any meaningful comparison of studies impossible and preventing the creation of evidence-based guidelines to allow clinicians to identify patients as safe or unsafe to drive. Molnar et al. explored this further and suggested alternative solutions. The most commonly employed technique currently is stratification, where rather than a dichotomous pass/fail outcome, there is a third 'indeterminate' outcome, which can suggest the need for further assessment such as the on-road driving test.

Current Tests That Have Been Developed

The United States and Canada

Office-based tests in the United States and Canada include the SAFE DRIVE checklist, the Canadian Driving Research Initiative for Vehicular Safety in the Elderly (CanDRIVE) assessment algorithm, and the Ottawa Driving and Dementia Toolkit.[25,26,27] The SAFE DRIVE and CanDRIVE are prompts to ask questions about driving, while the Ottawa Driving and Dementia Toolkit is a whole assessment package that starts with a 10-minute checklist to ensure all areas of potential concern are considered.

Information is collected on the type of dementia and the functional impact of the illness along with a medical and medication history, tests of vision, executive functioning, reaction times, insight and any family concerns. The results of each area are then fed into an assessment algorithm.

The toolkit identifies the most pertinent question for relatives in 'the granddaughter question': 'Would you feel it was safe if a 5-year-old granddaughter was in the car alone with the person driving?' Relatives who may previously have described the patient as a safe driver often feel that the above situation would be unsafe and this is generally a sensitive indication of an unsafe driver.[28]

The algorithm offers three potential outcomes:

1. The patient may be deemed safe to continue driving and be reassessed in 6 months.
2. The patient may be clearly unsafe and need to stop driving immediately.
3. The patient may lie somewhere in the middle, requiring further assessment.

The toolkit contains resources to support the clinician in telling a patient they need to stop driving, ensuring documentation is completed effectively and helping all patients plan for driving retirement. As the only comprehensive toolkit of its kind, it represents a useful model of an off-road, in-office driving assessment.

The UK

In the UK, research has been more dispersed, although consensus guidelines for clinicians around driving with dementia or MCI were published in 2018, drawing together all the current evidence into clear pathways for appropriate management of all drivers with dementia and MCI.[1]

Psychological batteries developed for neurological conditions such as multiple sclerosis and stroke have been tested on people with dementia and adapted to provide test batteries which can be used to assess driving ability. The two major test batteries of this nature are the Dementia Drivers Screening Assessment (DDSA) developed by Lincoln et al. from the earlier Stroke Drivers Screening Assessment, and the Rookwood Driving Battery (RDB) developed by McKenna et al. for anyone with acquired brain pathology.[29,30]

The RDB was initially proposed in 1998 by McKenna, who noted that traditional psychometric tests used to assess fitness to drive were often IQ-related and bore little relation to the cognitive systems specifically involved in driving behaviour. McKenna aimed to construct a flexible test battery incorporating specific tests for 'each identifiable function underlying movement and analysis of the visual world as they relate to driving' and 'a method of measuring the integrity of cognitive functioning as it relates to driving'.[31]

The RDB was launched in 2004 and comprised a battery of 12 tests.[30] In a comparison with an on-road driving test, the RDB had 92% accuracy in predicting those with brain injury or pathology who would fail the on-road test and a 91% predictive accuracy of those who would pass. The test was much less accurate for those aged 70 years and above, with only 85% accuracy for predicting an on-road fail and 37% for a pass.

The DDSA was published in 2006, following work by Radford in 2001. It looked at nine cognitive assessments covering a range of cognitive domains likely to affect driving ability, such as attention, memory, executive functioning, reasoning and visuospatial skills. When validated against an on-road driving test, no single test was able to differentiate between safe and unsafe drivers, consistent with the findings of Molnar et al.[24] Further analysis identified a combination of six tests which correctly classified 92% of drivers with dementia as safe or unsafe.

Given the variability in driving experience, confidence and translation of in-office testing to on-road performance, both assessment batteries are best used as stratification tools, identifying those who are clearly safe or unsafe to drive; but also identifying a third, indeterminate group who would benefit from an on-road driving assessment to assess their driving ability accurately in real-world scenarios.

Although these two tests may be too long and cumbersome to complete in a 30-minute memory clinic appointment alongside medication reviews and issues raised by the patient and their relatives (both tests take about 30 minutes to administer), they may be manageable in 6-monthly appointments with a clinical psychologist if this resource were available. This is likely to be more acceptable to the patient and more cost-effective than referring every driver with dementia for a regular on-road assessment.

Conclusions

The key points of this chapter are summarized in Box 10.3.

Doctors in the UK should inform drivers with dementia to advise the DVLA of their diagnosis. Not all patients with this condition will follow this advice and if a patient is deemed unsafe to drive but continues to do so, the GMC provides guidance on contacting the DVLA without the patient's consent. It is important to differentiate diagnostic subtypes as specific cognitive deficits more likely to be associated with increased risk. Patients with FTD or DLB

Box 10.3: Key points

- Decisions regarding possession of a driving licence are ultimately made by the DVLA.
- Driving is usually safe for 3 years after the onset of AD.
- The risks are much greater with dementia with Lewy bodies and frontotemporal dementia.
- Early discussion of driving retirement is imperative in helping older people prepare for cessation.
- Older people are more likely to accept a recommendation to stop driving from a doctor or authority figure than from a relative or friend.
- In-office tests offer three outcomes: pass, fail or need for further assessment.
- An on-road driving test is the gold standard assessment, but availability is limited.
- Consensus guidelines for clinicians regarding driving with dementia or mild cognitive impairment are available.

pose the greatest risk. Cognitive assessments, algorithms and pertinent questions are available to categorize patients as safe, unsafe or needing further assessment. The gold standard assessment is an on-road driving test, where this is available. It is advisable to discuss driving cessation as early as possible with all elderly patients to help them prepare for the future.

Acknowledgement

For information, the original paper on which this chapter is based was:

Wilson S, Pinner G. Driving and dementia: a clinician's guide. *Adv Psychiatr Treat* 2013; **19**: 89–96.

References

1. UK Guideline Development Group. *Driving with Dementia or Mild Cognitive Impairment: Consensus Guidelines for Clinicians*, Newcastle University, 2018. Last accessed on 12 September 2019 via: https://research.ncl.ac.uk/driving-and-dementia/consensusguidelinesforclinicians/Final%20Guideline.pdf

2. Holland C. Self-bias in older drivers' judgments of accident likelihood. *Accid Anal Prev* 1993; **25**: 431–441.

3. Johnson J. Older rural adults and the decision to stop driving: the influence of family and friends. *J Community Health Nurs* 1998; **15**: 205–216.

4. Adler G, Rottunda S, Bauer M, et al. Driving cessation and Alzheimer's Dementia: issues confronting patients and family. *Am J Alzheimers Dis Other Demen* 2000; **15**: 212–216.

5. Brown L, Ott B, Papandonatos D, et al. Prediction of on-road driving performance in patients with early Alzheimer's disease. *J Am Geriatr Soc* 2005; **53**: 94–98.

6. Croston J, Meuser T, Berg-Weger M, et al. Driving retirement in older adults with dementia. *Top Geriatr Rehabil* 2009; **25**: 154–162.

7. Trobe J, Waller P, Cook-Flannagan C, et al. Crashes and violations among drivers with Alzheimer disease. *Arch Neurol* 1996; **53**: 411–416.

8. Carr D, Duchek J, Morris J. Characteristics of motor vehicle crashes of drivers with dementia of the Alzheimer type. *J Am Geriatr Soc* 2000; **48**: 18–22.

9. British Psychological Society (BPS). *Fitness to Drive and Cognition: A Document of the Multi-Disciplinary Working Party on Acquired Neuropsychological Deficits and Fitness to Drive* 1999. BPS, 2001. Last accessed on 12th September 2019 via: www.assessmentpsychology.com/fitness_to_drive.pdf

10. Wood J, Worringham C, Kerr G, et al. Quantitative assessment of driving performance in Parkinson's disease. *J Neurol Neurosurg Psychiatry* 2005; **76**: 176–180.

11. Dubinsky R, Stein A, Lyons K. Practice parameter: risk of driving and Alzheimer's disease (an evidence-based review): report of the quality standards subcommittee of the American Academy of Neurology. *Neurology* 2000; **54**: 2205–2211.

12. Hopkins R, Kilik L, Day D, et al. Driving and dementia in Ontario: a quantitative assessment of the problem. *Can J Psychiatry* 2004; **49**: 434–438.

13. Breen D, Breen D, Moore J, et al. Driving and dementia. *Brit Med J* 2007; **334**: 1365–1369.

14. Gilley D, Wilson R, Bennett D, et al. Cessation of driving and unsafe motor vehicle operation by dementia patients. *Arch Intern Med* 1991; **151**: 941–946.

15. Langford J, Methorst R, Hakamies-Blomqvist L. Older drivers do not have a high crash risk – a replication of low mileage bias. *Accid Anal Prev* 2006; **38**: 574–578.

16. Man-Son-Hing M, Marshall S, Molnar F, Wilson K. Systematic review of driving risk and the efficacy of compensatory strategies in persons with dementia. *J Am Geriatr Soc* 2007; **55**: 878–884.

17. Marottoli R, Mendes de Leon C, Glass T, et al. Consequences of driving cessation: decreased out-of-home activity levels. *J Gerontol B Psychol Sci Soc Sci* 2000; **55B**: S334–S340.

18. Foley D, Heimovitz H, Guralnik J, Brock D. Driving life expectancy of persons aged 70 years and older in the United States. *Am J Public Health* 2002; **92**: 1284–1289.

19. Marottoli R, Mendes de Leon C, Glass T, et al. Driving cessation and increased depressive symptoms: prospective evidence from the New Haven EPESE. *J Am Geriatr Soc* 1997; **45**: 202–206.

20. Rosser M. Dementia and driving: European National Guidelines. *Eur J Neurol* 2000; **7**: 745.

21. Driver and Vehicle Licensing Agency. *Assessing Fitness to Drive: A Guide for Medical Professionals.* DVLA, 2019.

22. Naidu A, McKeith I. Driving, dementia and the Driver and Vehicle Licensing Agency: a survey of old age psychiatrists. *Psychiatr Bull* 2006; **30**: 265–268.

23. General Medical Council (GMC). *Confidentiality: Patients' Fitness to Drive and Reporting Concerns to the DVLA or DVA.* GMC, 2019.

24. Molnar F, Patel A, Marshall S, et al. Clinical utility of office-based cognitive predictors of fitness to drive in persons with dementia: a systematic review. *J Am Geriatr Soc* 2006; **54**: 1809–1824.

25. Wiseman E, Souder E. The older driver: a handy tool to assess competence behind the wheel. *Geriatrics* 1996; **51**: 36–45.

26. Man-Son-Hing M, Marshall S, Molnar F, et al. A Canadian research strategy for older drivers: the CanDRIVE Program. *Geriatrics Today: J Can Geriatr Soc* 2004; **7**: 86–92.

27. Champlain Dementia Network, Regional Geriatric Program of Eastern Ontario. *The Driving and Dementia Toolkit for Health Professionals (3rd Edn)*, 2009. Last accessed on 12 September 2019 via: www.rgpeo.com/media/30695/dementia%20toolkit.pdf

28. Molnar F, Byszewski A, Marshall S, Man-Son-Hing M. In-office evaluation of medical fitness to drive: practical approaches for assessing older people. *Can Fam Physician* 2005; **51**: 372–379.

29. Lincoln N, Radford K, Lee E, Reay A. The assessment of fitness to drive in people with dementia. *Int J Geriatr Psychiatry* 2006; **21**: 1044–1051.

30. McKenna P, Jefferies L, Dobson A, Frude N. The use of a cognitive battery to predict who will fail an on-road driving test. *Brit J Clin Psychol* 2004; **43**: 325–336.

31. McKenna P. Fitness to drive: a neuropsychological perspective. *J Ment Health* 1998; **7**: 9–18.

Mini-Mental State Examination for the Detection and Prediction of Dementia in People with and without Mild Cognitive Impairment

Alex J Mitchell

Introduction

Screening for dementia is usually considered important, but only if accuracy of detection is sufficient and treatments are available and effective. In the National Dementia Strategy for England, one of the three main areas promoted was early diagnosis with acknowledgement that much of this role falls to primary care.[1] The majority of dementia and pre-dementia cases in the community and in primary care remain undetected.[2] One in three of those diagnosed remains unaware of their diagnosis.[3] GPs in the UK are encouraged actively to look for people with dementia through annual screening as well as opportunistic testing of older people attending primary care with any significant health concern.[4] The UK government has also encouraged case finding for dementia on acute admission to secondary care services using a dementia CQUIN (Commissioning for Quality and Innovation), which meant that overall, between 80% and 90% of patients aged 75 years and over were screened and assessed.[5] Similarly, the Alzheimer's Foundation of America has run a National Memory Screening Program, and cognitive assessments have formed part of the Medicare Annual Wellness Visit in the United States.[6,7]

Without tools, clinical recognition of dementia is often low especially in cases of those who have mild dementia or mild cognitive impairment (MCI).[8] Rarely do clinicians use standardized criteria, such as those provided by DSM-5, let alone advanced cognitive tests.[9] Most GPs rely on their clinical judgement, occasionally enriched with a basic cognitive screening tool such as the Mini-Mental State Examination (MMSE).[10] It is thought that systematic, routine use of a simple tool in primary care would prove cost-effective.[11] Beyond the detection of early dementia, some hope to identify pre-dementia in the form of MCI, which affects 15% of adults over 75 and progresses to dementia at a rate of about 5% per year, depending on risk factors.[12] That said, there is also a case against routine screening. In particular, inaccurate screening would be problematic and false positives (without a second stage screener) could create anxiety, excessive medical tests, and inappropriate treatment. Additionally, false negatives would give patients and families false reassurance and potentially delay essential treatment or support.

Mini-Mental State Examination

The MMSE was published in 1975 as a relatively simple practical method of grading cognitive impairment.[13] Since then it has become the most commonly used cognitive screener in clinical practice, both for dementia and MCI.[14] While the MMSE may never have been intended as a diagnostic (case-finding) tool, it has been extensively investigated as a diagnostic test of dementia and, to a lesser extent, examined as a diagnostic screen for MCI. Many are attracted by the brevity of the instrument, which typically takes a little over 5 minutes in healthy individuals, and the fact it used to be royalty free (although in 2001 copyright was acquired by Psychological Assessment Resources [www.minimental.com/] so that there is now a fee attached to its use). In clinical practice, the main applications of the MMSE are to help clinicians grade the severity of cognitive change and to help with cognitive screening, either by ruling out those without a cognitive disorder with as few false negatives as possible, or perhaps by pointing towards cases with suspected but unconfirmed dementia.

The MMSE has an internal structure of 20 individual tests covering 11 domains, including: orientation, registration, attention or calculation (serial sevens or spelling), recall, naming, repetition, comprehension (verbal and written), writing, and construction. However, it only tests for recall of three items whereas more modern tools use five or more item recall. Internal consistency appears to be moderate with Cronbach alpha scores reported between 0.6 and 0.9.[15] Test-retest reliability has been examined in several studies, and in those where re-examination took place within 24 hours, reliability by Pearson correlation was usually above 0.85. Using RASCH analysis (named after Georg Rasch), it is possible to grade the completion difficulty of each item on the MMSE. Relatively difficult items are: the recall of three words, citing the correct date, copying the pentagon design, spelling 'world' backwards, and completing serial sevens. Conversely, relatively simple items are: naming the correct country, registering three words, following the command, and naming an object. Acceptability is generally high, but it falls in those with definite or suspected impairment, who may be reluctant to expose perceived deficits. All questions are designed to be asked in the order listed, with omissions scored as errors, giving a maximum score of 30. However, there is some ambiguity in several items, leading to the structured MMSE.[16]

Approximately 250 validation studies have been published using the MMSE as the principal tool, or as a comparator tool, but many are underpowered and/or lack an adequate criterion standard, and hence can give a misleading impression of accuracy. Nevertheless, this extensive evidence base means scores are fairly well understood by health professionals and can be adjusted on the basis of normative population data. For example, Crum et al. tested an extensive group of 18,056 participants in the US Epidemiologic Catchment Area study and presented distributions by age and educational levels.[17] Some groups have provided norms for each item on the MMSE by age group, yet there remains uncertainty regarding optimal cut-off threshold for each condition under study. A cut-off of <24 in persons with at least 8 years of education was recommended as significant by Folstein and colleagues.[8] [13] Some individuals with MCI or early dementia and a background of extensive education may experience a ceiling effect with the MMSE. In other words, the MMSE may lack subtle tests necessary to detect early cognitive changes, particularly regarding recall.

MMSE as a Method to Diagnose Dementia

The MMSE has been extensively investigated as a diagnostic test for current dementia, either on its own or against comparison scales. O'Connor et al. conducted one of the first adequately powered studies of the MMSE, using a cut-off <24 in 586 who received a Cambridge Examination for Mental Disorders of the Elderly (CAMDEX)/Cambridge Cognition Examination (CAMCOG) interview as a gold standard.[18] They found that the sensitivity of the MMSE was 86% and specificity 92%. In 2013, Linn et al. found a pooled sensitivity estimate of 88.3% (95% confidence interval [CI] 81.3–92.9) and a pooled specificity estimate of 86.2% (95%CI 81.8–89.7) but only in a small sample of studies.[19] In 2009, Mitchell undertook the first meta-analysis of the MMSE in dementia; however, sample size was limited and this meta-analysis was updated and revised in 2013 with 45 studies.[20, 21] This included community studies, primary care studies, and, most commonly, studies in specialist settings where the prevalence of dementia is relatively high. The prevalence of each condition in each setting strongly influences the performance of a test. High-prevalence settings favour case-finding with few false positives, but at the expense of false negatives. Low-prevalence settings favour screening with few false negatives but at the expense of frequent false positives. The most recent meta-analysis was published in 2015 and included 108 MMSE studies involving 36,080 subjects (of whom 10,263 had dementia).[22] The most common cut-off values to define participants with dementia were <23 and <24, and the prevalence was 28%. Taking all studies to date (see Table 11.1), the best estimate (using a meta-analytic bivariate random-effects model) is that the MMSE has a sensitivity of 81.3% (CI 80.6–82.1%) and specificity of 89.1% (CI 88.7–89.5%). Positive predictive value (PPV) was calculated as 74.8% (CI 74.0–75.6%) and the negative predictive value (NPV) was 92.3% (CI 92.0–92.6%). The positive clinical utility index was 0.608 (95% CI 0.598–0.618), suggesting that this can be categorized as 'fair' for case-finding; negative clinical utility index was 0.822 (CI 0.819–0.825), suggesting that this can be categorized as 'excellent' for screening. However, performance deteriorates when clinicians use the MMSE to look for dementia in a combined group of healthy people mixed with those with MCI.

A Cochrane review specifically examined the merits of the MMSE in people aged 65 years and over in community and primary care settings.[23] The authors conducted a meta-analysis of 28 studies in the community (44 articles) and six studies in primary care (eight articles). In the community, the pooled accuracy at a cut point of 24 (15 studies) showed a pooled sensitivity of 0.85 (95% CI 0.74–0.92) and a specificity of 0.90 (95% CI 0.82–0.95); at a cut point of 25 (10 studies) its sensitivity was 0.87 (95% CI 0.78–0.93), whereas specificity was 0.82 (95% CI 0.65–0.92). The authors estimated that based on these results, one would expect 85% of people with dementia to be correctly identified with the MMSE, while 15% would be wrongly classified as not having dementia; 90% of those tested would be correctly identified as not having dementia while 10% would be false positives and might be referred for further testing. In other words, although the MMSE can be used as part of a diagnostic evaluation for dementia, it should not be used in isolation to confirm or exclude disease.

Diagnostic Validity in Early Dementia

One critical question is whether the MMSE retains sufficient accuracy when screening for early stages of dementia. People with early dementia are particularly at risk of being overlooked.[24] Provisional evidence from three studies suggests a small reduction in

Table 11.1 Summary table of diagnostic accuracy of the MMSE for cognitive impairment

Purpose of test	Sensitivity	Specificity	PPV	NPV	Overall correct	LR+	LR–	CUI+	CUI–
Dementia vs healthy controls									
Detection of dementia	81.3% (80.6–82.1%)	89.1% (88.7–89.5%)	74.8% (74.0–75.6%)	92.3% (92.0–92.6%)	86.9% (86.5–87.2%)	7.45 (7.19–7.73)	0.21 (0.20–0.22)	0.608 'fair' (0.598–0.618)	0.822 'excellent' (0.819–0.825)
Dementia vs mixed MCI/ healthy									
Detection of dementia	71.6% (69.8–73.4%)	93.5% (92.8–94.2%)	85.1% (83.5–86.7%)	86.4% (85.4–87.3%)	86.0 (85.2–86.8)	11.01 (9.863–12.33)	0.30 (0.28–0.32)	0.609 'fair' (0.588–0.631)	0.808 'good' (0.800–0.815)
Mild cognitive impairment vs healthy controls									
Detection of MCI vs HC	59.7% (58.6–60.7%)	80.2% (79.4–81.0%)	72.1% (71.1–73.2%)	69.9% (69.0–70.7%)	70.7% (70.1–71.4%)	3.02 (2.89–3.15)	0.50 (0.49–0.52)	0.431% 'poor' (0.418–0.444)	0.561 'fair' (0.553–0.568)

HC = healthy controls; MCI = mild cognitive impairment; PPV = positive predictive value; NPV = negative predictive value; LR+ (likelihood ratio+) = sensitivity/(1 – specificity); LR– (likelihood ratio–) = (1 – sensitivity)/specificity; CUI+ (Clinical Utility Index +) = sensitivity × PPV; Clinical Utility Index – (Clinical Utility Index –) = specificity × NPV.

accuracy when attempting to detect those with mild dementia. For example, in a specialist hospital or memory clinic, Heinik et al. found that the area under the receiver operating characteristic (ROC) curve was 0.96 for all dementias, but 0.89 for very mild dementia;[25] similarly, Meulen and colleagues found that the area under the ROC curve was 0.95 for all dementias, but only 0.87 for mild dementia.[26] However, it should be noted that a cut-off threshold higher than ≤23 is recommended when looking for mild dementia. Yoshida et al. found a 95% sensitivity and an 83% specificity looking for mild dementia in a Japanese memory clinic at a threshold of ≤28, which would give 'good' clinical utility for screening (clinical utility index + = 0.789) and case-finding (clinical utility index – = 0.786).[27] At a lower threshold of ≤25, sensitivity fell to 76% but specificity increased to 97%, which would also have 'good' clinical utility for screening (clinical utility index + = 0.800) and case-finding (clinical utility index – = 0.727). In a sub-analysis of 88 people with mild Alzheimer's scoring >20 on the MMSE, Kalbe and colleagues found that the MMSE had a sensitivity of 92% and a specificity of 86% (PPV 85.2%, NPV 92.2%), which again would imply 'good' clinical utility for screening (clinical utility index + = 0.781) and case-finding (clinical utility index – = 0.796).[28] Regarding diagnosis of mild dementia in primary care, Kilada and colleagues found adjustment of the MMSE cut-off to ≤27 was required. Grober et al. examined the value of MMSE in 317 primary care attendees with mild dementia (Clinical Dementia Rating [CDR] of 1.0 and 0.5 but without MCI). In this study, at a cut-off of ≤23 sensitivity was 53% and specificity 90% (PPV 52.7%, NPV 90.1), but at a cut-off of ≤26 sensitivity was 73% and specificity 73% (PPV 36.0%, NPV 92.7%), suggesting only 'fair' clinical utility.[29]

Diagnostic Accuracy in the Detection of MCI

MCI is not the only pre-dementia condition, but it is the most studied. In 2015, a meta-analysis found 21 qualifying studies with a sensitivity estimate of 0.62 (95% Cl, 0.52–0.71) and specificity of 0.87 (95% Cl, 0.80–0.92).[15] Mitchell re-examined this data in 2016 and found 40 relevant studies.[30] In 2018, the most recent meta-analysis expanded this to 46 qualifying studies.[31] Most used less robust cross-sectional definitions of MCI, rather than longitudinal. The majority used the Mayo clinic criteria suggested by Petersen and colleagues,[32] and recruited from memory clinics or secondary care, with only a handful recruited directly from the community. Samples were not matched but recruited from convenience samples. Thus, the mean age of those with MCI was 73.2 years and healthy controls 71.0 years. The proportion of females in MCI studies was 44% and in controls 46.9%. Regarding education, the mean number of years of education in people with MCI was 9.79 versus 9.64 in controls. Perhaps the major question regards cut-off thresholds. In terms of cut-off scores, 12 studies examined <29, 9 studies <28, 17 studies <27, and 9 studies <26. After weighting, Mitchell found that the meta-analytic sensitivity was 59.7% (58.6–60.7%) and specificity was 80.2% (79.4–81.0%). PPV was 72.1% (71.1–73.2%) and NPV 69.9% (69.0–70.7%).[30] This data is summarized in Table 11.1. Breton et al. found slightly lower accuracy rates with a sensitivity of 66.4% (95% CI 60.5–71.8%) and specificity of 73.5% (95% CI 68.6–77.8%).[31] The positive clinical utility index was 0.431%, suggesting that this can be categorized as 'poor' for case-finding MCI (95% CI 0.418–0.444) and negative clinical utility index was 0.561 (95% CI 0.553–0.568), suggesting that this can be categorized as 'fair' for screening (ruling out) those without MCI.

Prediction of Future Dementia in Those with MCI

Given the limitations of the MMSE diagnostically, it would be surprising but not impossible that the MMSE might be a valuable risk prediction tool. A Cochrane review from Arevalo-Rodriguez and colleagues examined whether the MMSE can be used to predict (rather than diagnose) dementia.[33] They included 11 studies comprising 1,569 people with MCI who were followed for conversion to dementia ($n = 4$), AD ($n = 8$), or VaD ($n = 1$). Arevalo-Rodriguez established the diagnosis of MCI not just using conventional Petersen and revised Petersen criteria, but also using Matthews 2008 criteria, and using the CDR scale score of 0.5, criteria which are fairly broad. It should be noted that using the QUANDAS2 appraisal tool,[34] all 11 studies had a high risk of bias in at least one domain. Looking in more detail, most studies came from samples of older people in memory clinics. Various thresholds were used to define a positive MMSE (≤ 21, ≤ 26, ≤ 28, ≤ 29), and follow-up times ranged from 15 months to seven years; over this time 36% on average developed dementia.

Results suggested that the accuracy of a baseline MMSE showed a wide range of sensitivities (23–76%) and specificities (40–94%). Overall, the authors found that at the median specificity of 88%, the sensitivity was only 40% for prediction of dementia and 54% for prediction of AD.[33] They calculated that in a hypothetical cohort of 100 MCI patients with a 36% incidence of dementia, the number of missed cases (false negatives) would be 18 patients, while eight MCI patients would be overdiagnosed (false positives). Further modelling of the accuracy can be generated from a pre-test/post-test Baysian graph, calculated in a commentary by Mitchell.[35] This showed that the predictive accuracy of using the MMSE to spot later dementia (or AD) at a prevalence of 36%, would be 45% for dementia and 52% for AD when the test is positive (PPV); and 86% for dementia and 89% for AD when the test is negative (NPV).

Conclusion and Implementation

This is an up-to-date review of the evidence concerning the application of the MMSE as a diagnostic and predictive test for dementia and/or MCI. It is worth acknowledging that the MMSE has a number of limitations.[36] It has a floor effect (imprecise measurement in the very severe range) which is notable in advanced dementia patients with little formal education and in those with severe language problems. There is also a ceiling effect, meaning it may well not perform well in people with very mild dementia or indeed MCI. This is thought to relate to its relatively crude testing of recall based solely on three objects. This problem is likely to be amplified when testing highly educated individuals. Most cognitive tests are influenced by age, education, and ethnicity, and the MMSE is no exception.[37] Twelve per cent of the variance in MMSE scores can be attributed to age and education alone.[38] Tables of adjustment by age and education have been published but are often overlooked by busy clinicians.[39] Another important limitation is its length, particularly when its intended use is in primary care. While it can be completed and scored in about 5 minutes in unimpaired healthy individuals, it often takes 15 minutes or more in patients with dementia.[40]

When discussing the accuracy of the MMSE in helping establish a diagnosis, it should be remembered that the tool can be used to reassure those without cognitive impairment (that is a screening role), or as a case-finding tool to confirm those with cognitive impairment. The MMSE performs differently in each capacity and depending on the underlying prevalence. Overall, results from 108 studies suggest it performs best when helping detect dementia in a pool of otherwise healthy cognitively unimpaired individuals. Here, clinical utility index indicates it can be considered 'fair' (0.608) for case-finding and 'excellent'

(0.822) for screening. Performance was slightly weaker in looking specifically for early dementia, but the MMSE still achieved a 'good' rating on the clinical utility index. For MCI, however, the MMSE had a poor positive clinical utility index (0.431) for case-finding and the negative clinical utility index was only 'fair' (0.561) for screening, illustrating limited usefulness when looking for MCI. In most memory clinics people are not simply divided into dementia or healthy, therefore the comparison of dementia versus healthy combined with MCI is needed. In the detection of dementia versus healthy controls combined with MCI the clinical utility is no longer 'good' but 'fair' for case-finding (CUI+ 0.609), but a 'good' rating is preserved for screening (CUI – 0.808). However, an adjustment of cut-off threshold to ≤26 is necessary. Thus, in specialist settings the MMSE is likely to be useful for initial reassurance in those who score 27 or above. However, there is a complication. In 2013, the American Psychiatric Association introduced the Fifth Edition of the *Diagnostic and Statistical Manual of Mental Disorders* (DSM-5). With it came a new classification of major cognitive disorder (instead of dementia) and minor cognitive disorders (instead of MCI and pre-dementia). Only one study to date has examined the MMSE in relation to these categories.[41]

The final decision about whether to use the MMSE as a diagnostic tool will depend on the consequences of false positives and false negatives and the acceptability of the tool in practice. The following examples are illustrative of screening yield. In the case of the MMSE for dementia versus healthy controls, out of 100 people tested, the MMSE would correctly identify 23 with dementia missing 5; and it would correctly reassure 64 with 8 false positives (assumptions: sensitivity 81.3%, specificity 89.1%, prevalence 28.4%) (see Figure 11.1). In

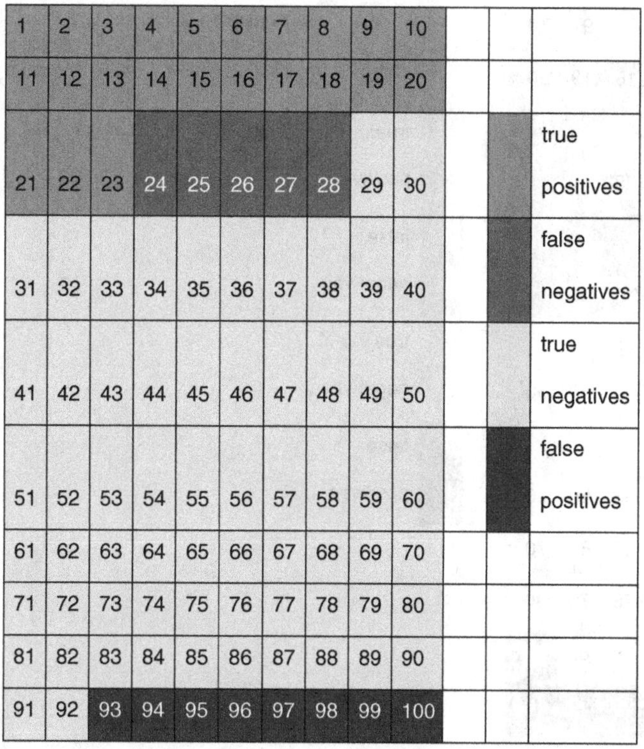

Figure 11.1 Yield of MMSE screening for dementia in 100 typical elderly primary care attendees

the case of the MMSE for MCI versus healthy controls, out of 100 patients tested, the MMSE would correctly identify 28 with MCI missing 18; and it would correctly reassure 43 with 11 false positives (assumptions: sensitivity 59.7%, specificity 80.2%, prevalence 46.2%) (see Figure 11.2). If those with false negatives and positives received further evaluation then the adverse consequences could be minimized; however, if those with false negatives received no follow-up, and those with false positives received an erroneous diagnosis, then the consequences could be serious. Certainly, taking evidence to date the MMSE does not seem a good choice for helping clinicians specifically detect MCI, especially an given other tool, the Montreal Cognitive Assessment (MoCA), which is both accurate and freely available in 35 languages.[29]

Many would argue that data on the accuracy of a tool does not prove that it is effective in clinical practice. Few studies have actually evaluated whether the MMSE (or indeed any cognitive tool) improves outcomes when implemented in a clinical setting such as primary care. In one study, after 3,340 patients were screened, 434 scored positive, but only 227 would agree to a formal diagnostic assessment, and 47% were diagnosed with dementia; 33% had cognitive impairment-no dementia (CIND), and 20% were considered to have no cognitive deficit.[42] A non-randomized study by Van Hout and colleagues found GPs opted to use the MMSE in only 18 out of 93 cases, and use of the MMSE was not associated with better diagnostic accuracy.[43] However, in a 24-month, cluster-randomized study, Fowler et al. found those who received cognitive test results were more likely to order diagnostic tests and discuss memory problems with patients, and patients were more likely

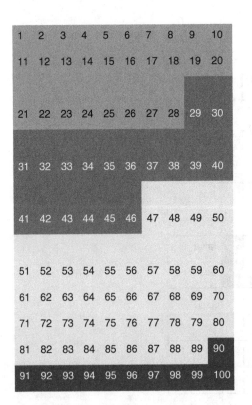

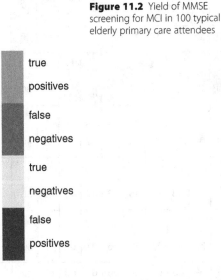

Figure 11.2 Yield of MMSE screening for MCI in 100 typical elderly primary care attendees

to be taking cognitive-enhancing medication at follow-up.[44] Overall, this lack of evidence from implementation studies has led some guidelines to advise against routine (and/or population based) screening for cognitive impairment in asymptomatic individuals until further evidence is forthcoming.[45]

Regarding the question of the prediction of later dementia, evidence suggests that when the MMSE is used alone it is not a good tool for prediction of future decline in those with MCI. It has a limited role in reassuring those scoring above threshold that a decline to dementia is unlikely. However, even here there is a substantial error rate because about 14% of those with MCI did decline, even with an initially high (that is near normal) MMSE score. Remember, this is in a cohort where 36% declined over approximately a mean of 3–4 years and therefore a high initial MMSE score cuts the projected risk of decline by about 22% of 36% (or a relative risk reduction of 0.61). What would be the effect in a primary care setting when the risk of dementia and hence incidence of dementia is substantially lower? Assuming only 10% declined to dementia, an above-threshold score on the MMSE would reduce the risk of decline from 10% to 3%. A positive MMSE score would suggest a future risk increase from 10% to 14%, which is far from providing useful clarity. Overall, results are not encouraging regarding use of the MMSE in a predictive capacity, and therefore other methods should be sought.

The MMSE has gained tremendous popularity as a relatively quick 'bedside' cognitive test, but its diagnostic accuracy has been hitherto unclear. The best evidence available to date suggests it is not an ideal tool for case-finding dementia and it is frankly poor at case-finding MCI. It is also not suitable as a predictive tool which might indicate future decline. However, it can have a role as an initial first step screener for dementia and/or MCI. In fact, for a perhaps rarefied group of suspected dementia compared with purely healthy controls it has excellent accuracy, but this falls to 'good' if the population is mixed into a more realistic healthy control and MCI (i.e. healthy control and pre-dementia) cohort. It should be remembered that there is no perfect single tool for case-finding and/or screening especially for mild cases. Here the MMSE performs relatively poorly compared with more modern tools like the Addenbrooke's Cognitive Examination III and the MoCA.[46] Finally, no tool is able to clarify the cause of cognitive impairment or the type of dementia and as such none is a replacement for expert clinical assessment and investigation.

Acknowledgement

For information, the original paper on which this chapter is based was:

Mitchell A. Can the MMSE help clinicians predict progression from mild cognitive impairment to dementia?: commentary on. . . Cochrane Corner. *Adv Psychiatr Treat* 2015; **6**: 363–6.

References

1. Department of Health. *Living Well with Dementia: A National Dementia Strategy.* DoH, 2009.

2. Lang L, Clifford A, Wei L, et al. Prevalence and determinants of undetected dementia in the community: a systematic literature review and a meta-analysis. *BMJ Open* 2017; **7**: e011146.

3. Amjad H, Roth DL, Sheehan OC, et al. Underdiagnosis of dementia: an observational study of patterns in diagnosis and awareness in US older adults. *J Gen Intern Med* 2018; **33**: 1131–8.

4. Department of Health. General medical services – contractual changes 2013–2014

[Letter to chairman of BMA General Practitioners Committee]. DoH, 6th December 2012. www.wp.dh.gov.uk/publications/files/2012/12/GMS-Contract-letter.pdf (last accessed 30 November 2019).

5. www.england.nhs.uk/statistics/statistical-work-areas/dementia/dementia-assessment-and-referral-2018-19/ (last accessed 30 November 2019).

6. Bayley PJ, Kong JY, Mendiondo M, et al. Findings from the national memory screening day program. *J Am Geriatr Soc* 2015; **63**: 309–14.

7. Cordell CB, Borson S, Boustani M, et al. Alzheimer's Association recommendations for operationalizing the detection of cognitive impairment during the Medicare Annual Wellness Visit in a primary care setting. *Alzheimer's & Dementia* 2013; **9**: 141–50.

8. Mitchell, AJ, Meader N, Pentzek . Clinical recognition of dementia and cognitive impairment in primary care: a meta-analysis of physician accuracy. *Acta Psychiatr Scand* 2011; **124**: 165–83.

9. Iracleous P, Nie JX, Tracy CS, et al. Primary care physicians' attitudes towards cognitive screening: findings from a national postal survey. *Int J Geriatr Psychiatry* 2010; **25**: 23–9.

10. Brodaty H, Howarth GC, Mant A, Kurrle SE. General practice and dementia. A national survey of Australian GPs. *Med J Aust* 1994; **160**: 10–14.

11. Tong T, Thokala P, McMillan B, Ghosh R, Brazier J. Cost effectiveness of using cognitive screening tests for detecting dementia and mild cognitive impairment in primary care. *Int J Geriatr Psychiatry* 2017; **32**: 1392–1400.

12. Mitchell AJ, Shiri-Feshki M. Rate of progression of mild cognitive impairment to dementia–meta-analysis of 41 robust inception cohort studies. *Acta Psychiatr Scand* 2009; **119**: 252–65.

13. Folstein MF, Folstein SE, McHugh PR. 'Mini-mental state'. A practical method for grading the cognitive state of patients for the clinician. *J Psychiatr Res* 1975; **12**: 189–98.

14. Christa Maree Stephan B, Minett T, Pagett E, et al. Diagnosing mild cognitive impairment (MCI) in clinical trials: a systematic review. *BMJ Open* 2013; **3**(2). http://dx.doi.org/10.1136/bmjopen-2012-001909 (last Accessed 5 November 2019).

15. Toglia J, Fitzgerald KA, O'Dell MW, Mastrogiovanni AR, Lin CD. The Mini-Mental State Examination and Montreal Cognitive Assessment in persons with mild subacute stroke: relationship to functional outcome. *Arch Phys Med Rehabil* 2011; **92**: 792–8.

16. Molloy DW, Alemayehu E, Roberts R. Reliability of a standardized mini-mental-state-examination compared with the traditional mini-mental-state-examination. *Am J Psychiatry* 1991; **148**: 102–5.

17. Crum RM, Anthony JC, Bassett SS, Folstein MF. Population-based norms for the Mini-Mental State Examination by age and educational level. *JAMA* 1993; **269**: 2386–91.

18. O'Connor DW, Pollitt PA, Hyde JB, et al. The reliability and validity of the Mini-Mental State in a British community survey. *J Psychiatr Res* 1989; **23**: 87–96.

19. Lin JS. O'Connor E. Rossom RC, et al. *Screening for Cognitive Impairment in Older Adults: An Evidence Update for the U.S. Preventative Services Task Force. Evidence Synthesis Number 107*. AHRQ Publication No. 14–05198-EF-1. Agency for Healthcare Research and Quality, 2013.

20. Mitchell AJ. A meta-analysis of the accuracy of the mini-mental state examination in the detection of dementia and mild cognitive impairment. *J Psychiatr Res* 2009; **43**: 411–31.

21. Mitchell AJ. The Mini-Mental State Examination (MMSE): an update on its diagnostic validity for cognitive disorders. In *Cognitive Screening Instruments: A Practical Approach* (ed. AJ Larner): 15–46. Springer, 2013.

22. Tsoi KK, Chan JY, Hirai HW, Wong SY, Kwok TC. Cognitive tests to detect dementia: a systematic review and meta-analysis. *JAMA Intern Med* 2015; **175**: 1450–8.

23. Creavin ST, Wisniewski S, Noel-Storr AH, et al. Mini-Mental State Examination (MMSE) for the detection of dementia in clinically unevaluated people aged 65 and over in community and primary care populations. *Cochrane Database Syst Rev* 2016; **1**: CD011145.

24. Mitchell AJ, Meader N, Pentzek M. Clinical recognition of dementia and cognitive impairment in primary care: a meta-analysis of physician accuracy. *Acta Psychiatr Scand* 2011; **124**: 165–83.

25. Heinik J, Solomesh I, Bleich A, et al. Are the clock-drawing test and the MMSE combined interchangeable with CAMCOG as a dementia evaluation instrument in a specialized outpatient setting? *J Geriatr Psychiatry Neurol* 2003; **16**: 74–9.

26. Meulen EFJ, Schmand B, van Campen JP, et al. The seven minute screen: a neurocognitive screening test highly sensitive to various types of dementia. *J Neurol Neurosurg Psychiatry* 2004; **75**: 700–5.

27. Yoshida H, Terada S, Honda H, et al. Validation of Addenbrooke's cognitive examination for detecting early dementia in a Japanese population. *Psychiatry Res* 2011; **185**: 211–4.

28. Kalbe E, Kessler J, Calabrese P, et al. DemTect: a new, sensitive cognitive screening test to support the diagnosis of mild cognitive impairment and early dementia. *Int J Geriatr Psychiatry* 2004; **19**: 136–43.

29. Grober E, Hall C, Lipton RB, Teresi JA. Primary care screen for early dementia. *J Am Geriatr Soc* 2008; **56**: 206–13.

30. Mitchell A.J. The Mini-Mental State Examination (MMSE): update on its diagnostic accuracy and clinical utility for cognitive disorders. In: *Cognitive Screening Instruments* (ed. AJ Larner): 37–48. Springer, 2017.

31. Breton A, Casey D, Arnaoutoglou NA. Cognitive tests for the detection of mild cognitive impairment (MCI), the prodromal stage of dementia: meta-analysis of diagnostic accuracy studies. *Int J Geriatr Psychiatry* 2019; **34**: 233–42.

32. Petersen RC. Clinical practice. Mild cognitive impairment. *N Engl J Med* 2011; **364**: 2227–34.

33. Arevalo-Rodriguez I, Smailagic N, Roqué I. Mini-Mental State Examination (MMSE) for the detection of Alzheimer's disease and other dementias in people with mild cognitive impairment (MCI). *Cochrane Database Syst Rev* 2015; **3**: CD010783. DOI:10.1002/14651858.CD010783.pub2.

34. Whiting PF, Rutjes AW, Westwood ME, et al. QUADAS-2: a revised tool for the quality assessment of diagnostic accuracy studies. *Ann Intern Med* 2011; **155**: 529–36.

35. Mitchell AJ. Can the MMSE help clinicians predict progression from mild cognitive impairment to dementia? Commentary On. . . Cochrane Corner. *BJPsych Adv* 2015; **21**: 363–66.

36. Diniz BS, Yassuda MS, Nunes PV, Radanovic M, Forlenza OV. Mini-mental State Examination performance in mild cognitive impairment subtypes. *Int Psychogeriatr* 2007; **19**: 647–56.

37. Schultz-Larsen K, Kreiner S, Lomholt RK. Mini-Mental Status Examination: mixed Rasch model item analysis derived two different cognitive dimensions of the MMSE. *J Clin Epidemiol* 2007; **60**: 268–79.

38. Bravo G, Hébert R. Age- and education-specific reference values for the Mini-Mental and Modified Mini-Mental State Examinations derived from a non-demented elderly population. *Int J Geriatr Psychiatry* 1997; **12**: 1008–18.

39. Kahle-Wrobleski K, Corrada MM, Li B, Kawas CH. Sensitivity and specificity of the Mini-Mental State Examination for identifying dementia in the oldest-old: the 90+ Study. *J Am Geriatr Soc* 2007; **55**: 284–9.

40. Meulen EFJ, Schmand B, van Campen JP, et al. The seven minute screen: a neurocognitive screening test highly sensitive to various types of dementia. *J Neurol Neurosurg Psychiatry* 2004; **75**: 700–5.

41. Estrada-Orozco K. Diagnostic performance of minimental against DSM-5 in cognitive disorder. Experience of

a cohort in Colombia. *Rev Ecuat Neurol* 2018; **27** n.3. http://revecuatneurol.com/wp-content/uploads/2019/04/2631-2581-rneuro-27-03-00025.pdf (last accessed 6 November 2019).

42. Boustani M1, Callahan CM, Unverzagt FW, et al. Implementing a screening and diagnosis program for dementia in primary care. *J Gen Intern Med* 2005; **20**: 572–7.

43. Van Hout H, Teunisse S, Derix M, et al. CAMDEX, can it be more efficient? Observational study on the contribution of four screening measures to the diagnosis of dementia by a memory clinic team. *Int J Geriatr Psychiatry* 2001; **16**: 64–9.

44. Fowler NR, Morrow L, Chiappetta L, et al. Cognitive testing in older primary care patients: a cluster-randomized trial. *Alzheimers Dement* 2015; **1**: 349–57.

45. Pittam G, Allaby M. *Screening for Dementia: Can Screening Bring Benefits to Those with Unrecognised Dementia, Their Carers and Society? An Appraisal against UKNSC Criteria. A Report for the UK National Screening Committee.* Solutions for Public Health (SPH), 2015.

46. Wang BR, Zheng HF, Xu C. Comparative diagnostic accuracy of ACE-III and MoCA for detecting mild cognitive impairment. *Neuropsychiatr Dis Treat* 2019; **15**: 2647–53.

Biomarkers and the Diagnosis of Preclinical Alzheimer's Disease

Philippa Lilford and Julian C Hughes

Introduction

More than 47 million people are living with dementia worldwide, and this number is predicted to increase to 131 million by 2050. Not only can dementia be a devastating condition, it carries a large economic burden with a worldwide cost estimated at US$818 billion.[1] With no cure and an ageing population, the increasing prevalence is a worry.

Biomarkers are naturally occurring markers of the underlying pathological process of a particular disease. Numerous biomarkers to detect Alzheimer's disease (AD) have been developed over the past decade. These have helped to develop the theory that AD is a continuum, which starts with the accumulation of Alzheimer's pathology years before the emergence of clinical symptoms. The continuum begins with a preclinical phase (Box 12.1), in which there are pathological changes of AD (which can be detected by biomarkers),

---

Box 12.1 Glossary of terms

Mild cognitive impairment (MCI)

Variously defined, but includes subjective memory symptoms or cognitive symptoms or both, objective memory impairment or cognitive impairment or both, and generally unaffected activities of daily living; affected people do not meet currently accepted diagnostic criteria for dementia or AD.

Amnestic mild cognitive impairment (aMCI)

A more specific term describing a subtype of MCI, in which there are subjective memory symptoms and objective memory impairment; other cognitive domains and activities of daily living are generally unaffected; affected people do not meet currently accepted diagnostic criteria for dementia or AD.

Preclinical Alzheimer's disease

The long asymptomatic period between the first brain lesions and the first appearance of symptoms and signs which concern normal individuals who later fulfil diagnostic criteria for AD.

Prodromal Alzheimer's disease

The symptomatic pre-dementia phase of AD, generally included in the MCI category; this phase is characterized by symptoms not severe enough to meet currently accepted diagnostic criteria for AD.

Dubois B, Feldman H, Jacova C, et al. Research criteria for the diagnosis of Alzheimer's disease: revising the NINCDSADRDA criteria. Lancet Neurol 2007; 6: 734–46.

but no symptoms of dementia. This stage may pre-date AD by decades.[2] It is suggested that this progresses to a prodromal phase of mild symptoms that do not affect daily living. The final stage is established Alzheimer's dementia. Moving through these stages is not inevitable, and biomarkers have been developed to help predict who will show progression along the continuum.[3]

Preclinical AD was initially a hypothetical model, but with the development of biomarkers, the in vivo pathological process can now be detected. The pathological hallmarks of AD are amyloid plaques in the brain and hyperphosphorylated tau fibrillary tangles. Biomarkers of the disease therefore reflect the presumed underlying pathological processes.[4]

The detection of a preclinical phase of AD is considered important for several reasons. First, it may contribute to our understanding of the pathogenesis of the disease itself. Second, this is the stage at which potential future treatments will be crucial, since it will allow disease-modifying drugs to be started before the onset of irreversible neurodegeneration.[5]

A working group of the Research Institute of the Alzheimer's Association and the National Institute on Aging has suggested that useful biomarkers in AD would detect the underlying neuropathology of the disease with a sensitivity of >80% (this would be the true-positive rate) and a specificity of >80% (this would be the true-negative rate and would distinguish AD from other types of dementia).[6] In addition, the test should be affordable, reliable, and non-invasive.[7]

Box 12.1 helps to clarify the terminology used in this field. It will be noted, however, that the terms are not used exclusively: prodromal AD seems to be a subset of MCI and difficult to distinguish from amnestic MCI (aMCI). It is probably true that aMCI is better characterized than prodromal AD, having been investigated as an entity for longer, albeit biomarkers might make these categorizations more precise. Of course, although aMCI is thought to be the type of MCI that is most likely to progress to AD, there is no commitment to this in the name, whereas there is a commitment that prodromal AD is the precursor of AD. If this is not always the case, then 'prodromal Alzheimer's disease' is a misnomer and one that has the potential to cause harm. As we shall suggest towards the end of this chapter, on this ground it would be unethical to label patients in this way if there is uncertainty.

The Pathophysiology of Alzheimer's Disease

The underlying pathophysiology of AD is important in understanding why particular biomarkers have been developed and is depicted in Figure 12.1. AD involves abnormal functioning of amyloid precursor protein, which leads to an excess of amyloid-β in the cortex. This excess of amyloid-β is thought to lead to faulty accumulation of tau proteins, which in turn leads to synaptic dysfunction and neuronal death.[2] The pathological hallmarks of AD are amyloid-β plaques and neurofibrillary tangles of hyperphosphorylated tau. Compared to amyloid-β plaque formation, hyperphosphorylated tau and neurofibrillary tangles are more closely correlated with neurodegeneration and clinical symptoms.[8]

The difference between genetic profiles, other risk factors for dementia, and cognitive reserve may explain the variation in lag time between the development of Alzheimer's pathology and dementia itself. Cognitive reserve is given as one explanation of why there is such individual variability in the time taken between developing Alzheimer's pathology and

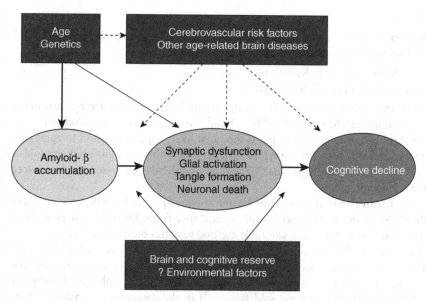

Figure 12.1 A hypothetical model of the pathophysiological cascade in Alzheimer's disease.
Sperling RA, Aisen PS, Beckett LA, et al. Toward defining the preclinical stages of Alzheimer's disease: recommendations from the National Institute on Aging–Alzheimer's Association workgroups on diagnostic guidelines for Alzheimer's disease. *Alzheimers Dement* 2011; 7: 280–92.

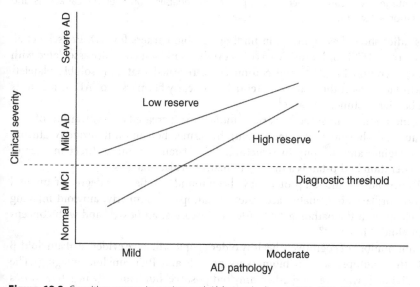

Figure 12.2 Cognitive reserve in ageing and Alzheimer's disease (AD). With high cognitive reserve, more AD pathology can be tolerated before symptoms develop
Stern Y. Cognitive reserve in ageing and Alzheimer's disease. *Lancet Neurol* 2012; 11: 1006–12.

clinical symptoms (Figure 12.2). The greater your cognitive reserve, the more insult you can endure before displaying cognitive symptoms. Cognitive reserve is an active process which can be strengthened by, for example, education and mental activity.[9]

Biomarkers

The main biomarkers of AD can be divided by two major pathological processes: amyloid-β deposition and neurodegeneration. Hence, main biomarkers focus on:

- measures of brain amyloid-β deposition;
- measures of markers of neurodegeneration.

The two key methods currently of detecting amyloid-β deposition are by measuring amyloid-β levels in the cerebrospinal fluid (CSF) and through positron emission tomography (PET) amyloid imaging.[5] Amyloid-β_{42} is the most likely type of amyloid to aggregate and is the most commonly measured amyloid variant. Where there is significant amyloid-β accumulation, levels of amyloid-β_{42} in the CSF are low and there is increased amyloid tracer retention on PET imaging.[10]

Plasma amyloid can also be detected, but plasma amyloid-β_{42} has hitherto been used less frequently than CSF owing to its lower sensitivity and specificity. Recently, however, there have been further advances in finding a suitable method to detect biomarkers in the blood.[11] Acquiring blood, unlike CSF, requires a much less invasive procedure and, unlike PET scanning, is less costly. The researchers, by using immunoprecipitation and mass spectrometry, were able to achieve roughly 90% accuracy (using ^{11}C-labelled Pittsburgh Compound B ([^{11}C]PiB) PET as their gold standard) in the detection of amyloid-β biomarkers. They concluded:

These results demonstrate the potential clinical utility of plasma biomarkers in predicting brain amyloid-β burden at an individual level. These plasma biomarkers also have cost-benefit and scalability advantages over current techniques, potentially enabling broader clinical access and efficient population screening.[11]

Two recent studies show developments in finding new biomarkers for AD. Preische et al. showed that increased CSF and serum levels of neurofilament light chain are associated with early neurodegeneration in AD;[12] and Nation et al. revealed that CSF soluble platelet-derived growth factor receptor β shows potential as an early biomarker of AD as it detects blood–brain barrier dysfunction early.[13]

Neurodegeneration is measured by various indicators: increased concentrations of CSF total tau (t-tau) and phosphorylated tau (p-tau), hypermetabolism on fluorodeoxyglucose (FDG) PET imaging, and atrophy in structural MRI: t-tau is a more direct marker of neuronal degeneration and p-tau is a marker of neurofibrillary tangles.[3]

Both CSF amyloid-β_{42} and tau protein have been found to reflect the degree of amyloid load and neurofibrillary abnormality accurately at autopsy.[14] Similarly, amyloid imaging strongly correlates with the pathological burden of disease at autopsy,[15] and with concentrations of amyloid-β in CSF.[16]

A significant number of cognitively healthy older people will have evidence of amyloid-β deposition both at autopsy and in biomarkers of CSF and PET amyloid imaging. The number of individuals who are biomarker 'amyloid positive' but 'clinically negative' varies from 20% to 40%,[10] which is similar to autopsy findings.[17] One theory is that if 'amyloid-positive' individuals lived longer they would eventually develop symptoms of AD.

Jack et al. have proposed a model to represent the progression of Alzheimer's pathology (Figure 12.3).[2] In this model, amyloid-β deposition occurs first, years before the onset of clinical symptoms. The duration of this phase may vary, depending on the individual's cognitive reserve and risk factors for AD. Next, tau-mediated neurodegeneration begins,

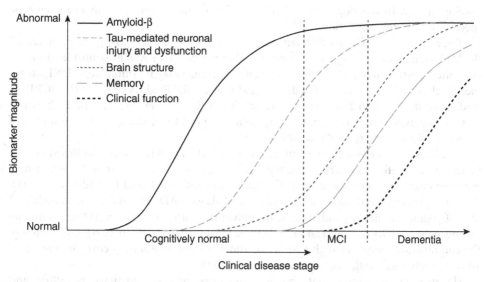

Figure 12.3 Accumulation of markers of disease over time. In this hypothetical model, amyloid-β markers are the first to become abnormal, followed by markers of neurodegeneration, followed by clinical symptoms. MCI, mild cognitive impairment

Jack CR Jr, Knopman DS, Jagust WJ, et al. Hypothetical model of dynamic biomarkers of the Alzheimer's pathological cascade. *Lancet Neurol* 2010; 9: 119–28.

which is evident from changes on structural imaging. Finally, there is progression to cognitive impairment and clinical symptoms become evident. Important to the biomarker model is that Aβ accumulation alone is not sufficient to cause dementia.[2]

Ocular biomarkers are less well-known biomarkers of AD. Ocular biomarkers have been proposed for several reasons. First, individuals with AD often present with visual deterioration, and this appears to predate cognitive changes. Second, the retina is easily visualized and ocular biomarkers do not require invasive tests such as lumbar puncture. There are many proposed ocular biomarkers, which we shall not discuss exhaustively here. For instance, micro-ribonucleic acid (RNA) can be found in tear fluid and is implicated in the regulation of amyloid. Other important approaches include detecting retinal amyloid-β accumulation, or an assessment of functional and clinical changes within the visual system.[18] Amyloid-β detection in the retina has been performed with or without contrast-enhanced imaging. Further work is required to determine whether amyloid accumulation detected in the retina is reflective of brain deposition and, indeed, predictive of future cognitive impairment. Functional changes to the visual system include changes in neuronal responses, such as reduced visually evoked potentials over the occipital cortex, and interrupted neurotransmission between photoreceptors in the retina. Further ocular biomarkers include 'fixation and movement errors', where there is failure to fixate or follow a target, and reduced eye movements.[18]

Do CSF Biomarkers Accurately Predict Who Will Develop Alzheimer's Dementia?

Using biomarkers to help predict who will develop dementia already has a significant history, particularly in determining which individuals with MCI are most at risk of developing AD. In this population, there is evidence that biomarkers enhance diagnostic specificity and prognostication.[19, 20-25]

The combination of high CSF t-tau and p-tau with low CSF amyloid-β_{42} has been termed the 'Alzheimer's disease signature'[7] and is highly predictive of AD, as confirmed in three large multicentre studies: the Alzheimer's Disease Neuroimaging Initiative (ADNI) study, the Development of Screening Guidelines and Criteria for Predementia AD (DESCRIPA) study, and the Swedish Brain Power project. The CSF AD signature has been shown to increase diagnostic accuracy significantly even at a prodromal stage, with a sensitivity of 90–95% and a specificity of about 90% for AD.[26, 27]

De Meyer et al. studied participants from the ADNI.[7] The ADNI was established in 2004 to determine whether biomarkers could predict progression from MCI to AD. Their sample included cognitively normal individuals, individuals with MCI, and individuals with AD. The AD signature was detected in 90% of individuals with AD, 72% of those with MCI, and 36% of cognitively healthy individuals. In individuals with MCI and an AD signature, the diagnostic sensitivity of progression to AD was 90%, with a specificity of 64%. In addition, the combination simply of high CSF p-tau and low CSF amyloid-β_{42} correctly identified 100% of individuals with MCI who progressed to AD.

Hansson et al. found that the AD signature had a sensitivity of >90% and specificity of >85% for individuals with MCI who subsequently developed AD. [21] Similarly, Van Rossum et al. found that the combination of CSF amyloid-β_{42} with either p-tau or t-tau was highly predictive of the development of AD from MCI, with an odds ratio of 18.1 (95% confidence interval [CI] 9.6–32.4).[28]

Most of this evidence relates to individuals who already have MCI. If pathological changes really do start decades before the onset of clinical symptoms, is it possible to tell at this very early stage who will develop AD in their later years? There have not been enough longitudinal studies to answer this conclusively, although some studies have found that amyloid-β positivity confers an increased risk of progression to AD; [25, 29, 30-34] and two found that plasma biomarkers and imaging (MRI and FDG PET) can predict cognitively normal individuals who are at risk of cognitive decline.[35, 36] Fagan et al. found that non-cognitively impaired individuals with the AD signature progress to symptomatic cognitive impairment more quickly than do the remainder of the cohort.[29]

Are CSF Biomarkers Useful in People Who Already Have Alzheimer's Disease?

A marked reduction in CSF amyloid-β_{42} has consistently been noted in patients at different stages of AD. On the one hand, an isolated low amyloid-β_{42} is not sufficiently specific for a diagnosis. Non-AD dementias, such as Lewy body disease and vascular dementia, are also associated with low CSF amyloid-β_{42}.[3] CSF p-tau appears to be the most specific CSF biomarker, distinguishing AD from non-Alzheimer's dementias.[37] On the other hand, combinations of CSF biomarkers appear to enhance the sensitivity of an AD diagnosis, but there is no consensus as to which specific combination has the greatest accuracy.[3] CSF biomarkers may also have a role in predicting the course of AD. Snider et al. found that individuals with AD and the CSF AD signature progressed more rapidly than those without.[26] Markers of amyloid load tend to remain constant throughout the course of AD, whereas t-tau and p-tau rise as AD progresses.[7]

Neuroimaging

Studies investigating the value of FDG PET (Box 12.2) in diagnosing prodromal AD are few and have short follow-up periods. Metabolic reductions in the medial, temporal, and parietal cortices, as well as the anterior and posterior cingulate, detected prodromal AD with an accuracy of 75–84%.[38] Differences between MCI and AD have been consistently found on FDG PET.[39]

There are PET techniques that provide in vivo detection of amyloid and, potentially, of neurofibrillary tangles. Imaging using [^{11}C]PiB (N-methyl-[^{11}C]2-(4'-methyl aminophe-nyl)-6-hydroxybenzothiazole) and [^{18}F]FDDNP (2-(1-{6-[(2-[^{18}F]fluoroethyl)(methyl) amino]-2-naphthyl}ethylidene)malononitrile) have detected enhanced radio-ligand reten-tion patterns in patients with AD compared with controls; and positive [^{11}C]PiB patterns are correlated with low CSF amyloid-β_{42}.[38] There is evidence of enhanced [^{11}C]PiB reten-tion in cognitively normal people and in those with MCI.[38] Longitudinal follow-up is required to determine whether these are people with a preclinical or prodromal dementia.

Diagnostic Criteria

In 1984, a workgroup from the National Institute of Neurological and Communicative Disorders and Stroke and the Alzheimer's Disease and Related Disorders Association (NINCDS–ADRDA) published criteria for the diagnosis of AD.[40] These criteria allowed only a 'probable' diagnosis of AD to be reached while the person was alive: a definitive diagnosis could be made only if Alzheimer's pathology was found at autopsy. Furthermore, the (probable) diagnosis required the presence of significant disability and impact on daily living, thus excluding MCI (which was not recognized as such at the time). The specificity of these diagnostic criteria, in terms of distinguishing AD from other types of dementia, was low.[3]

In 2011, the National Institute on Aging and the Alzheimer's Association (NIA–AA) published guidelines revising the 1984 diagnostic criteria.[41] All-cause dementia continues to be diagnosed by history and neuropsychological testing, with impairment in function required for a diagnosis to be made. This is then further subdivided into 'probable' or 'possible' AD, and biomarkers may be used as supportive information to help guide a diagnosis and to help distinguish AD from other forms of dementia. There is also a shift away from concentrating only on memory problems as the clinical phenotype of AD towards including impairments of other cognitive domains, such as language.[3]

Furthermore, the NIA–AA guidelines of 2011 recognize the spectrum of AD, such as preclinical AD and MCI, and the use of CSF and imaging biomarkers in identifying these states. Dubois and Albert describe prodromal MCI as a heterogeneous state that may or may

---

Box 12.2 FDG PET

Fludeoxyglucose (FDG) is an analogue of glucose and is used as a radiotracer in positron emission tomography (PET) imaging. FDG is taken up by cells and as a result acts as a marker of tissue metabolism. In Alzheimer's disease there are patterns of hypometabolism that are detected by poor FDG uptake. Different forms of dementia show distinct patterns of hypometabolism, which can aid diagnosis.

not lead to dementia of multiple different aetiologies.[42] They describe prodromal AD as 'MCI of the Alzheimer type' and advocate the use of CSF and imaging biomarkers to help make this distinction. For preclinical AD, however, the NIA–AA guidelines only apply in a research setting.[43] Research criteria for diagnosing preclinical states of AD developed by the International Working Group (the IWG-2 criteria) require the individual to be asymptomatic, have a marker of AD pathology, or have an AD autosomal dominant mutation on chromosome 1, 14 or 21.[3] This is describing an at-risk state where progression to AD is not inevitable.

Limitations in the Use of Biomarkers

Biomarker results are often taken from highly selected populations, so that the predictability of the results is likely to be exaggerated.[4] A major limitation is that participants in these studies are generally volunteers and one wonders who volunteers for invasive trials such as these. They may be individuals with concerns about their cognitive performance or with a family history of dementia. This is supported by the higher rates of apolipoprotein E (ApoE) ε4 carriers detected in many of these cohorts.[10] This would lead to an overly high prediction of biomarkers in the general population.

Lumbar punctures are not without risk and there is no standardized analytic technique or reference range for CSF biomarkers. [4] CSF biomarkers show 20–30% inter-laboratory and inter-assay variability.[5] The Alzheimer's Association has funded the Alzheimer's Association QC (Quality Control) Program for CSF Biomarkers to try to reduce this variability by using reference laboratories to compare samples.[44]

Ethical Implications

With this new concept of preclinical dementia comes numerous ethical implications. Finding out that a cognitively healthy individual has Alzheimer's pathology leaves the researcher with a difficult question regarding an unknown risk that the participant will develop an incredibly debilitating disease. With such a significant number (20–40%) of cognitively normal individuals with evidence of amyloid-β plaques, more information is needed on the sensitivity of such a test so that the implication of this result can be communicated to participants. Currently, establishing preclinical dementia has no clinical utility and an unknown prognosis, therefore provides unsettling and uncertain information for the patient.[45]

Hughes et al. carried out a scoping review of the literature to explore some of the issues that arise following detection of preclinical dementia and identified four main themes: stigma, ethical questions, psychological burden, and language or terminology.[46]

First, individuals with preclinical dementia may face stigma, including difficulties at work and insurance implications. In addition, social stigma can lead to isolation and cause the individual to form negative self-perceptions.[46]

Second, the idea of non-maleficence has recurred in the literature. Harm may be done by telling someone about biomarker positivity, particularly if, as is currently the case, there are no effective treatments for AD. However, the Risk Evaluation and Education for Alzheimer's Disease (REVEAL) project reported that participants were no more likely to develop depression, anxiety, or distress on being told their *APoE* genotype in addition to general risk factors for AD (such as family history, age, and gender) than those who were told the general risk factors alone.[47] In terms of beneficence, individuals with a positive amyloid profile can alter their lifestyle choices to reduce their risk of dementia in the future or have time to make advance care planning decisions.

Third, there are psychological burdens associated with these studies, including anxiety about the test results. Psychoeducation to help participants and their families understand and reflect on the results may help.

The final theme in the literature is the importance of language. How things are communicated will shape how the person understands the meaning of results that may be ambiguous. Indeed, language itself can cause harm. A question can be raised, given the level of uncertainty, about whether the label of 'preclinical AD' should ever be used, except perhaps in the context of research. The situation described by 'preclinical AD' can also be called 'non-dementia AD'. It could be said that those affected are not ill, but have a disease. This is not uncommon in medicine: for example, many people may have cancer but no symptoms. It is more problematic when people have the putative pathology, but never go on to have symptoms. So, for example, many normal older people will have amyloid in their brains and it seems odd on this account alone to describe them as diseased. The worry here is a broad one about the medicalization of ageing.[48]

Conclusions

At present, CSF biomarkers are not radically altering the diagnostic pathway for AD. The core criteria for diagnosing AD remain a gradual, progressive, cognitive impairment that is documented on objective testing. History and examination, therefore, remain the crucial elements of diagnosis, which can be supported by the use of in vivo markers of AD pathology. CSF and imaging biomarkers are providing more information, which will need to be applied in light of the individual presentation, and diagnostic criteria may continue to change as we learn more about their diagnostic accuracy.[3] In MCI and in established dementia, biomarkers do appear to provide useful diagnostic and prognostic information.

According to the working group for the Alzheimer's Association and the National Institute on Aging, the CSF AD signature is coming close to fulfilling the desirable features of a useful biomarker.[6, 7] What about using AD biomarkers as a screening tool (Box 12.3)? According to Wilson's criteria for screening,[49] AD is an important health problem with a recognizable pathophysiological process. There is an early symptomatic stage (prodromal AD) and there are tests which are (arguably) easy and acceptable to perform. The tests, however, are not definitely sensitive or specific enough and there currently is not an effective treatment for AD. A sensible consensus, therefore, would be that these biomarkers are not appropriate for screening the general population and should be reserved for detecting preclinical dementia in research settings only.

Acknowledgement

For information, the original paper on which this chapter is based was:

Lilford P, Hughes JC. Biomarkers and the diagnosis of preclinical dementia. *Adv Psychiatr Treat* 2018; **24**: 422–30.

Box 12.3 Further questions

Should we be using CSF biomarkers in routine clinical practice?

This is a controversial question and the answer varies between different countries. In Scandinavia, CSF biomarkers are part of a routine work-up to diagnose Alzheimer's disease (AD).

How invasive and safe are lumbar punctures?

The threshold varies between individuals. They are certainly more invasive than blood tests and they are associated with adverse effects, including pain, infection, and headaches. Serious side effects, however, are very rare.[6]

How would using CSF biomarkers work practically?

In the UK, patients with memory impairment are not necessarily reviewed by a neurologist. Psychiatrists are not trained to perform lumbar punctures so they would have to refer to a neurological (or other appropriate) team; this service design will require thought and may depend on local services and relationships.

What to do with the results?

In MCI, there is evidence that CSF biomarkers help to determine who will develop full-blown AD. Similarly, in established AD, CSF biomarkers may help in estimating the rate of progression or provide supportive evidence for a diagnosis to be made. However, in those who are cognitively normal, it will be more difficult to interpret the results. The results of studies to date are likely to be overly optimistic, as the participants may have volunteered because of concerns regarding their memory or a positive family history of AD. More longitudinal studies are required further to clarify sensitivities and specificities to establish whether these biomarkers will be useful in the cognitively normal.

References

1. Prince M, Comas-Herrera A, Knapp M, Guerchet M, Karagiannidou M. *World Alzheimer Report 2016: Improving Healthcare for People Living with Dementia. Coverage, Quality and Costs Now and in the Future.* Alzheimer's Disease International, 2016.

2. Jack CR Jr, Knopman DS, Jagust WJ, et al. Hypothetical model of dynamic biomarkers of the Alzheimer's pathological cascade. *Lancet Neurol* 2010; **9**: 119–28.

3. Dubois B, Feldman HH, Jacova C, et al. Advancing research diagnostic criteria for Alzheimer's disease: the IWG-2 criteria. *Lancet Neurol* 2014; **13**: 614–29.

4. Livingston G, Sommerlad A, Orgeta V, et al. Dementia prevention, intervention, and care. *Lancet* 2017; **390**: 2673–734.

5. Berti V, Polio C, Lombardi G, Ferrari C, Sorbi S, Pupi A. Rethinking on the concept of biomarkers in preclinical Alzheimer's disease. *Neurol Sci* 2016; **37**: 663–72.

6. Herskovits Z, Growden J. Sharpen that needle. *Arch Neurol* 2010; **67**: 918–20.

7. De Meyer G, Shapiro F, Vanderstichele H, et al. Diagnosis-independent Alzheimer disease biomarker signature in cognitively normal elderly people. *Arch Neurol* 2010; **67**: 949–56.

8. Bennett DA, Schneider JA, Wilson RS, et al. Neurofibrillary tangles mediate the association of amyloid load with clinic Alzheimer disease and level of cognitive function. *Arch Neurol* 2004; **61**: 378–84.

9. Stern Y. Cognitive reserve in ageing and Alzheimer's disease. *Lancet Neurol* 2012; **11**: 1006–12.

10. Sperling RA, Aisen PS, Beckett LA, et al. Toward defining the preclinical stages of

Alzheimer's disease: recommendations from the National Institute on Aging–Alzheimer's Association workgroups on diagnostic guidelines for Alzheimer's disease. *Alzheimers Dement* 2011; **7**: 280–92.

11. Nakamura A, Kaneko N, Villemagne VL, et al. High performance plasma amyloid-β biomarkers for Alzheimer's disease. *Nature* 2018; **554**: 249–54.

12. Preische O, Schultz S, et al. Serum neurofilament dynamics predicts neurodegeneration and clinical progression in presymptomatic Alzheimer's disease. *Nat Med* 2019; **25**: 277–282.

13. Nation D, Sweeney M, Montagne A, et al. Blood-brain barrier breakdown is an early biomarker of human cognitive dysfunction. *Nat Med* 2019; **25**: 270–276.

14. Tapiola T, Alafuzoff I, Herukka SK, et al. Cerebrospinal fluid β-amyloid 42 and tau proteins as biomarkers of Alzheimer-type pathologic changes in the brain. *Arch Neurol* 2009; **66**: 382–89.

15. Bacskai B, Frosch J, Freeman M, et al. Molecular imaging with Pittsburgh Compound B confirmed at autopsy: a case report. *Arch Neurol* 2007; **64**: 431–4.

16. Fagan A, Mintum M, Mach R, et al. Inverse relation between in vivo amyloid imaging load and cerebrospinal fluid Aβ42 in humans. *Ann Neurol* 2006; **59**: 512–9.

17. Morris JC, Storandt M, McKeel DW Jr, et al. Cerebral amyloid deposition and diffuse plaques in 'normal' aging: evidence for presymptomatic and very mild Alzheimer's disease. *Neurology* 1996; **46**: 707–19.

18. Lim J, Li Q, He Z, et al. The eye as a biomarker for Alzheimer's disease. *Front Neurosci* 2016; **10**: 536.

19. Hardy, J, Selkoe, DJ The amyloid hypothesis of Alzheimer's disease: progress and problems on the road to therapeutics. *Science* 2002; **297**: 353–6.

20. Klein WL, Stine WB Jr, Teplow DB Small assemblies of unmodified amyloid beta protein are the proximate neurotoxin in Alzheimer's disease. *Neurobiol Aging* 2004; **25**: 569–80.

21. Hansson O, Zetterberg H, Buchhave P, et al. Association between CSF biomarkers and incipient Alzheimer's disease in patients with mild cognitive impairment: a follow-up study. *Lancet Neurol* 2006; **5**: 228–34.

22. Parnetti L, Lanari A, Silvestrelli G, Saggese E, Reboldi P. Diagnosing prodromal Alzheimer's disease: role of CSF biochemical markers. *Mech Ageing Dev* 2006; **127**: 129–32.

23. Mattsson N, Zetterberg H, Hansson O, et al. CSF biomarkers and incipient Alzheimer disease in patients with mild cognitive impairment. *JAMA* 2009; **302**: 385–93.

24. Visser PJ, Verhey F, Knol D, et al. Prevalence and prognostic value of CSF markers of Alzheimer's disease pathology in patients with subjective cognitive impairment or mild cognitive impairment in the DESCRIPA study: a prospective cohort study. *Lancet Neurol* 2009; **8**: 619–27.

25. Chetelat G, Villemagne VL, Pike K, et al. Independent contribution of temporal beta-amyloid deposition to memory decline in the pre-dementia phase of Alzheimer's disease. *Brain* 2011; **134**: 798–807.

26. Snider BJ, Fagan AM, Roe C, et al. Cerebrospinal fluid biomarkers and rate of cognitive decline in very mild dementia of the Alzheimer type. *Arch Neurol* 2009; **66**: 638–45.

27. De Souza, LC, Lamari, F, Belliard, S, et al. Cerebrospinal fluid biomarkers in the differential diagnosis of Alzheimer's disease from other cortical dementias. *J Neurol Neurosurg Psychiatry* 2011; **82**: 240–6.

28. Van Rossum IA, Vos S, Handels R, et al. Biomarkers as predictors for conversion from mild cognitive impairment to Alzheimer-type dementia: implications for trial design. *J Alzheimers Dis* 2010; **20**: 881–91.

29. Fagan AM, Roe CM, Xiong C, et al. Cerebrospinal fluid tau/β-amyloid42 ratio as a prediction of cognitive decline in nondemented older adults. *Arch Neurol* 2007; **64**: 343–9.

30. Li G, Sokal I, Quinn JF, et al. CSF tau/Abeta42 ratio for increased risk of mild cognitive impairment: a follow-up study. *Neurology* 2007; **69**: 631–9.

31. Villemagne VL, Pike KE, Darby D, et al. Aß deposits in older non-demented individuals with cognitive decline are indicative of preclinical Alzheimer's disease. *Neuropsychologia* 2008; **46**: 1688–97.

32. Morris JC, Roe CM, Grant EA, et al. Pittsburgh Compound B imaging and prediction of progression from cognitive normality to symptomatic Alzheimer disease. *Arch Neurol* 2009; **66**: 1469–75.

33. Storandt M, Mintun MA, Head D, et al. Cognitive decline and brain volume loss as signatures of cerebral amyloid-beta peptide deposition identified with Pittsburgh compound B: cognitive decline associated with Abeta deposition. *Arch Neurol* 2009; **66**: 1476–81.

34. Resnick SM, Sojkova J, Zhou Y, et al. Longitudinal cognitive decline is associated with fibrillar amyloid-beta measured by [11C]PiB. *Neurology* 2010; **74**: 807–15.

35. Vemuri P, Wiste HJ, Weigand SD, et al. MRI and CSF biomarkers in normal, MCI, and AD subjects: predicting future clinical change. *Neurology* 2009; **73**: 294–301.

36. Yaffe K, Weston A, Graff-Radford NR, et al. Association of plasma beta-amyloid level and cognitive reserve with subsequent cognitive decline. *JAMA* 2011; **305**: 261–6.

37. Koopman K, Le Bastard N, Martin JJ, et al. Improved discrimination of autopsy-confirmed Alzheimer's disease from non-AD dementias using CSF P-tau. *Neurochem Int* 2009; **55**: 214–8.

38. Dubois B, Feldman H, Jacova C, et al. Research criteria for the diagnosis of Alzheimer's disease: revising the NINCDS-ADRDA criteria. *Lancet Neurol* 2007; **6**: 734–46.

39. Shivamurthy V, Tahari A, Marcus C, et al. Brain FDG PET and the diagnosis of dementia. *Nucl Med Mol Imaging* 2015; **204**: 76–85.

40. McKhann G, Drachman D, Folstein M, et al. Clinical diagnosis of Alzheimer's disease: report of the NINCDS-ADRDA Work Group under the auspices of Department of Health and Human Services Task Force on Alzheimer's Disease. *Neurology* 1984; **34**: 939–44.

41. Jack CR Jr, Albert MS, Knopman DS, et al. Introduction to the recommendations from the National Institute on Aging–Alzheimer's Association workgroups on diagnostic guidelines for Alzheimer's disease. *Alzheimers Dement* 2011; **7**: 257–62.

42. Dubois B, Albert ML. Amnestic MCI or prodromal Alzheimer's disease? *Lancet Neurol* 2004; **3**: 246–8.

43. Watkin A, Sikdar S, Majurndar B, et al. New diagnostic concepts in Alzheimer's disease. *BJPsych Adv* 2013; **19**: 242–9.

44. Mattsson N, Andreasson U, Persson S, et al. CSF biomarker variability in the Alzheimer's Association quality control program. *Alzheimers Dement* 2013; **9**: 251–61.

45. Harkins K, Sankar P, Sperling R, et al. Development of a process to disclose amyloid imaging results to cognitively normal older adult research participants. *Alzheimers Res Ther* 2015; **7**: 26.

46. Hughes JC, Ingram TA, Jarvis A, Denton E, Lampshire Z, Wernham C. Consent for the diagnosis of preclinical dementia states: a review. *Maturitas* 2017; **98**: 30–4.

47. Green R, Roberts J, Cupples L, et al. Disclosure of APOE genotype for risk of Alzheimer's disease. *N Engl J Med* 2009; **361**: 245–54.

48. Estes CL, Binney EA. The biomedicalization of aging: dangers and dilemmas. *Gerontologist* 1989; **29**: 587–96.

49. Wilson JMG, Jungner G. *Principles and Practice of Screening for Disease* (Public Health Papers 34). World Health Organization, 1968.

Chapter 13

To Scan or Not to Scan

Neuroimaging in Mild Cognitive Impairment and Dementia

Victoria Sullivan, Biswadeep Majumdar, Anna Richman, and Sobhan Vinjamuri

Introduction

There is currently a huge variation in clinical practice as to whether patients being assessed for dementia undergo neuroimaging. With an ageing population it is likely that there will be greater pressures on psychogeriatric services, so accurate assessment, diagnosis, and prompt treatment will be required. This chapter will examine the evidence for the use of different neuroimaging techniques in the diagnosis of mild cognitive impairment (MCI) and dementia.

The UK has an ageing population. In the 25 years to 2016, the number of UK residents aged 65 years and over rose from 9.1 million (15.8% of the population) to 11.8 million (18% of the population). By 2066, there are predicted to be a further 8.6 million UK residents aged 65 years and over.[1] The total number of those 65 years and over will then be 20.4 million or 26% of the total population. The fastest increase will be seen in those 85 years and over.[1] In mid-2016, there were 1.6 million people aged 85 years and over (2% of the total population); by 2066 there will be 5.1 million people aged 85 years and over (7% of the total UK population). Meanwhile, the population aged 16–64 years is projected to increase by only 5% by 2066.[1] Dementia is one of the most common conditions in the elderly and it is estimated that in 2013, approximately 815,000 people were affected in the UK.[2] This number is expected to double over the next 30 years, which will increase financial pressures on clinical budgets, so there is a significant emphasis on early assessment, diagnosis, and prompt initiation of treatment.

NICE recommends an initial approach to improving the rate of diagnosis of dementia.[3] A significant number (up to 32%) of people living with dementia may not have a formal diagnosis of dementia. It suggests that the diagnosis of dementia should be timely, personalized, and accurate, and that it is vital to rule out reversible causes of cognitive decline, and to distinguish dementia from delirium. Referral to a specialist dementia diagnostic service is then recommended if reversible causes of cognitive decline have been excluded and dementia is still suspected. The role of structural imaging, such as computed tomography (CT) and magnetic resonance imaging (MRI), is to rule out reversible causes of cognitive decline, such as normal pressure hydrocephalus, subdural haemorrhage, and brain tumour; and to assist with subtype diagnosis, unless dementia is well established and the subtype diagnosis is clear.

Further imaging tests are only recommended if those would help to diagnose a dementia subtype and knowing more about the dementia subtype would change management. In the setting of an uncertain diagnosis of Alzheimer's disease (AD) or frontotemporal dementia

(FTD) and high clinical suspicion, positron emission tomography (PET) using the tracer fluorine-18 (F-18) fluorodeoxyglucose (FDG), therefore known as ^{18}F-FDG PET, or perfusion single-photon emission computed tomography (SPECT) are to be considered, along with cerebrospinal fluid (CSF) for tau or amyloid proteins for AD. If dementia with Lewy bodies (DLB) is suspected, but the diagnosis is uncertain,^{123} I-FP-CIT SPECT scanning is recommended. The full name for the compound is ioflupane (^{123}I)-N-omega-fluoropropyl-2beta-carbomethoxy-3beta-(4-iodophenyl)nortropane. More simply, the scan is known as a DaTSCAN. Table 13.1 outlines the basic details of CT, MRI, SPECT, and PET in terms of indications, benefits, risks, adverse effects, costs, and tolerability in the elderly.

There has been a greater clinical emphasis on functional neuroimaging, such as technetium-99m hexamethyl propylene amine oxime (Tc-99m HMPAO) SPECT PET scanning with 18F FDG and DaTSCANs. Single-photon emission CT uses radio-labelled tracers such as Tc-99m HMPAO to measure cerebral perfusion to show areas where blood flow is reduced. This procedure takes about 30 minutes to perform and can help in the differential diagnosis of dementia. DaTSCANs use a tracer that binds to the presynaptic dopamine transporter and is useful in the investigation of DLB and Parkinson's disease (PD), in which there is decreased uptake in the transporters of the tracer ^{123}I ioflupane.

Alzheimer's Disease

In the clinical diagnosis of AD, NICE recommends that clinicians use the updated version of the NINCDS–ADRDA diagnostic criteria, sometimes known as the McKhann criteria.[4] The McKhann criteria have a sensitivity of 81% (i.e. will correctly detect patients who have AD); however, they only have a specificity of 70%, as patients with other forms of dementia often fulfil the criteria.[5] The updated criteria were published in 2011 and are shown in Box 13.1.[6] The criteria also cover possible AD dementia and probable or possible AD dementia with evidence of the AD pathophysiological process (these are not shown in Box 13.1).

Computed Tomography

CT is a well-established, widely available, quick, and relatively inexpensive tool. However, it is associated with radiation exposure, which can limit the use of serial scanning. It is most commonly used to exclude potentially reversible causes of cognitive impairment, but it can have some diagnostic value in AD. Normal ageing (without cognitive impairment) is associated with general brain atrophy. Therefore, neuroimaging studies of brain volume show very little discrimination between normal ageing, cognitive impairment, and dementia.[7] However, there are several studies that show atrophy of specific brain regions on CT and MRI: notably, the hippocampus and entorhinal cortices in the medial temporal lobes are associated with cognitive impairment in AD.[8] The sensitivity and specificity of using CT alone in detecting medial temporal lobe atrophy are 94% and 93%, respectively.[9]

Magnetic Resonance Imaging

MRI is becoming more widely used as a diagnostic tool in the investigation of dementia. Studies have shown that patients with AD have a greater reduction in the volume of entorhinal cortices (37%) and hippocampus (27%) compared with normal elderly adults and patients with MCI (combined data: entorhinal cortices 11%, hippocampus 13%), and

Table 13.1 Comparison of neuroimaging techniques used in dementia

	CT	MRI	SPECT	PET
Scan details	X-rays producing cross-sectional images	Magnetic field alters the axes of spinning protons, which is detected by scanner	Uses a gamma camera to detect gamma-emitting radioisotopes. Can involve a CT scan at same time	Uses a gamma camera to detect a positron-emitting radioisotope. CT scan can be performed during same session
Benefits	Quick, painless, quiet, readily available, well-established	Non-invasive, painless, no exposure to ionising radiation, post-scan modification of images	Allows assessment of blood flow to brain. Relatively quick (about 15 minutes)	Allows assessment of biological activity such as glucose activity. Non-invasive
Cost	Least expensive	Slightly more expensive than CT	Relatively inexpensive compared with PET	Most expensive, particularly if CT used in combination
Invasiveness	Standard CT non-invasive. Contrast media can cause allergic reactions	Standard MRI non-invasive. Contrast media can cause allergic reactions	Intravenous injection, with rare possibility of allergy	Potential allergies to radioisotopes (these are short-lived isotopes)
Risks	Radiation exposure Radiologist experience in interpretation	Contraindicated with some metal implants	Radiation exposure. Allergic reaction to radioisotope	Exposure to ionising radiation – substantial if concomitant CT
Tolerability in elderly patients	Generally well tolerated	Can be less well tolerated, as longer to perform, claustrophobic, and noisy	Can be less well tolerated because of the invasiveness and claustrophobia	Generally well tolerated

Box 13.1 The revised McKhann criteria for probable Alzheimer's disease

Core clinical criteria for dementia

Cognitive or behavioural (neuropsychiatric) symptoms that:

1 interfere with the ability to function at work or at usual activities;
2 represent a decline from previous levels of functioning and performing; and
3 are not explained by delirium or major psychiatric disorder.
4 Cognitive impairment is detected and diagnosed through a combination of

   (i) history-taking from the patient and a knowledgeable informant, and
   (ii) an objective cognitive assessment.

5. The cognitive or behavioural impairment involves a minimum of two of the following domains:

   a. Impaired ability to acquire and remember new information
   b. Impaired reasoning and handling of complex tasks, poor judgement
   c. Impaired visuospatial abilities
   d. Impaired language functions (speaking, reading, writing)
   e. Changes in personality, behaviour, or comportment

Probable AD dementia

1. Meets core clinical criteria for dementia and has the following characteristics:

   A. Insidious onset
   B. Clear-cut history of worsening of cognition by report or observation
   C. The initial and most prominent cognitive deficits are evident on history and examination in one of the following categories:

      a. Amnestic presentation
      b. Non-amnestic presentations

   D. The diagnosis of probable AD dementia should *not* be applied when there is evidence of

      (a) substantial concomitant cerebrovascular disease;
      (b) core features of dementia with Lewy bodies other than dementia itself;
      (c) prominent features of behavioural variant FTD;
      (d) prominent features of semantic variant primary progressive aphasia or nonfluent/ agrammatic variant primary progressive aphasia; or
      (e) evidence for another concurrent, active neurological disease, or a non-neurological medical comorbidity, or use of medication that could have a substantial effect on cognition.

McKhann GM, Knopmanc DS, Howard Chertkow H, et al. The diagnosis of dementia due to Alzheimer's disease: Recommendations from the National Institute on Aging Alzheimer's Association workgroups on diagnostic guidelines for Alzheimer's disease. *Alzheimers Dement* 2011; 7: 263–9. DOI:10.1016/j.jalz.2011.03.005

that these findings correlate well with neuropsychological testing.[10] Although these changes are seen in up to two-thirds of cases of AD, they are often absent on CT scans of patients with clinical diagnoses of the disease and are seen in about 5–10% of normal elderly individuals.[9] In patients over 80 years old, these changes are much less specific, and it may be more difficult to differentiate between normal ageing and AD.[9]

Serial MRI has been used to assess the progression of changes in MRI findings; however, this has tended to be in clinical trial settings, with very little diagnostic applicability. In AD, brain atrophy progresses at a rate of about 2% per year, in contrast to 0.1–0.5% per year in controls who are cognitively intact,[9] but it remains to be seen whether this could be used diagnostically. Some studies suggest that serial MRI, in combination with other markers such as CSF biomarkers and pattern classification, may be useful in differentiating patients with MCI from patients with AD by assessing the rate of neurodegeneration.[10]

Functional Neuroimaging

Functional neuroimaging – SPECT, PET, proton or ¹hydrogen magnetic resonance spectroscopy (1H-MRS), and magnetic resonance volumetry (MRV) – can be as effective as postmortem pathological examination in differentiating elderly patients with normal cognition from patients with AD .[11]

Single-Photon Emission Computed Tomography

SPECT findings in AD centre on the detection of hypoperfusion of the temporal and parietal brain regions (Figure 13.1).[11]

A comparison of clinical diagnosis, SPECT findings, and post-mortem examination showed that SPECT increased the diagnostic certainty in patients who were clinically diagnosed with AD from 84% to 92%.[12] This study found that a negative SPECT in these patients reduced the diagnostic certainty to 70%.

Positron Emission Tomography

PET imaging uses PiB to detect amyloid deposition in AD, which can be seen early in the disease process. As the disease progresses, amyloid deposits are less of a burden than neurodegeneration,[13] so PET imaging may be more useful in detecting cases of AD in the early stages. Pittsburgh Compound-B PET imaging is sensitive in detecting deposition of amyloid in AD, but it is less specific, as 10–30% of cognitively intact elderly people have PiB-PET-detected amyloid deposition.[13]

The evidence has gradually built that $^{(18)}$F-FDG PET is significantly superior to perfusion (HMPAO) SPECT in the differential diagnosis of degenerative dementia.[14] Moreover,

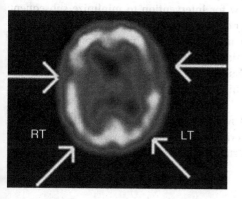

Figure 13.1 Tc-99m HMPAO single-photon emission computed tomography findings in a patient with clinical dementia. The scan shows reduced perfusion in the left frontotemporal, right temporal, left parietal, and right parietal lobes. These findings suggest Alzheimer's disease

patients seemed no more stressed by the process of undergoing PET or SPECT than they did by a home visit from a researcher and they showed no preference for one type of scan over the other, although carers seemed slightly to prefer SPECT, presumably because they were able to remain with the patient through the procedure.[15] [(18)]F-fluorodeoxyglucose ([(18)]FDG) PET detects glucose metabolism, and studies suggest that bilateral hypometabolism of the corpus callosum, temporoparietal, and frontal association areas may be associated with AD.[16] Investigations using FDG PET can detect hypometabolism up to 1 year before subjective complaints of memory impairment in patients who later develop AD.[16]

Future Imaging Techniques

Future imaging techniques may centre on the use of more detailed MRI such as functional MRI (fMRI), spin-labelled MRI, magnetic resonance microscopy, and magnetization transfer MRI. fMRI measures cerebral blood flow in relation to functional activity in the brain and early studies show that inferior prefrontal and left temporal activation is associated with better scoring on cognitive testing.[9] However, fMRI is still in the early stages of trial for this use and is not a routine investigation. Advances in radioligands and tracers used in SPECT and PET scanning, such as monoclonal antibodies to β-amyloid and flumazenil, are likely to allow for further development in diagnostic validity. The development of new biomarkers increases the possibility of greater understanding of pathophysiological changes. In recent years this has included, for instance, the development of ligands that allow tau deposition to be visualized in the brain using PET scanning.[17]

The complicating factor is that amyloid is found in the brains of normal older people. None the less, amyloid-PET scans are already proving useful. In one study, the progression from amnestic mild cognitive impairment (aMCI) to probable AD was 2.5 times more likely within three years if the person's PET scan was β-amyloid-positive in comparison with those whose scans were negative.[18] When additional biomarkers (see Chapter 12), namely hippocampal volume loss and cognitive status, were added to the result of the amyloid-PET scan, the risk of progression increased to 8.5 times the risk in amyloid-negative participants. Meanwhile, there is evidence emerging that amyloid-positivity on a PET scan is helpful in changing the management of patients where the diagnosis is challenging. [19]

Vascular Dementia

To some extent vascular dementia (VaD) may be preventable, as early detection of potentially modifiable vascular risk factors can allow for intervention to minimize subsequent cardiac and cerebrovascular disease (for further discussion of VaD, see also Chapter 2). For the clinical diagnosis of VaD, NICE recommends the National Institute of Neurological Disorders and Stroke and Association Internationale pour le Recherche et l'Enseignement en Neurosciences (NINDS–AIREN) criteria (Box 13.2),[3] which are widely used across the globe.[20] However, although the criteria have a high specificity at 0.80, they have a relatively low sensitivity at 0.58 in diagnosing VaD.[21]

Importantly, O'Brien demonstrated that it was not possible to differentiate those with and without dementia using the diagnostic criteria and imaging results alone in older patients who had had a stroke.[9] Therefore, structural neuroimaging can only be used to support a clinical diagnosis.

Box 13.2 Summary of the NINDS–AIREN criteria for the diagnosis of vascular dementia

- Dementia:
  Memory impairment
  Deficits in two other cognitive domains
- Neurological signs of cerebrovascular disease[a] on neuroimaging:
  Multiple large vessel infarcts/single strategically placed infarct
  Multiple basal ganglia and white matter lacunes
  Bilateral thalamic lesions or extensive periventricular white matter lesions
- A relationship between the first two disorders: onset of dementia within 3 months of a stroke or stepwise deterioration of cognitive deficits
- Clinical features consistent with VaD:
  Early gait disturbance
  Frequent and unprovoked falls
  Urinary symptoms not explained by urological disease
  Pseudobulbar palsy
  Personality change, apathy, and abulia

[a]The NINDS–AIREN criteria propose that up to 25% of white matter needs to be affected.

Based on Román GC, Tatemichi, TK, Erkinjuntti, T et al. Vascular dementia: diagnostic criteria for research studies. Report of the NINDS-AIREN International Workshop. *Neurology* 1993; 43: 250–60.

Periventricular White Matter Lesions

Periventricular white matter lesions are an important component of the diagnostic criteria for VaD (Box 13.2). However, these lesions are present in other forms of dementia, depression, and even in normal ageing. It is felt that bilateral or left-sided white matter lesions may be important predictors of dementia and cognitive impairment.[8] Structural neuroimaging (CT/MRI) provides information about the volume, location, and severity of vascular lesions and is an important tool for excluding other causes of cognitive impairment. MRI is more sensitive than CT in detecting ischaemic lesions.[9] It has been suggested that the presence of periventricular white matter changes can help differentiate VaD from AD, as both conditions are associated with cortical atrophy and ventricular enlargement on imaging.[8]

Functional Neuroimaging

Technetium-99m HMPAO SPECT findings in VaD reveal considerably reduced cerebral blood flow to certain brain areas compared with Alzheimer's dementia; a typical SPECT scan is shown in Figure 13.2. These brain regions include frontal lobes and the basal ganglia. Other studies have demonstrated reduced cerebral blood flow in bilateral thalami, anterior cingulate gyri, superior temporal gyri, caudate, and the left parahippocampal gyrus in patients with VaD compared with controls.[22] However, SPECT is not routinely recommended in the investigation of dementia owing to a lower diagnostic accuracy than that of clinical guidelines; sensitivity is reported to be as low as 43%.[22]

PET imaging in VaD shows hypometabolism of cortical and subcortical brain areas. One PET study of patients with AD and VaD found deficits in metabolism in thalamus, caudate, and frontal lobe which were strongly associated with VaD.[23]

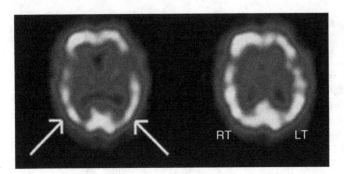

Figure 13.2 Tc-99m HMPAO single-photon emission computed tomography findings in a patient with cognitive impairment. The scan shows patchy perfusion defects in temporal and parietal lobes bilaterally, with reduction in perfusion to the occipital lobes (right > left). These findings are in keeping with vascular dementia

Dementia with Lewy Bodies

DLB shares clinical symptoms with AD and PD (Box 13.3).

It can be distinguished from PD in that the cognitive symptoms and parkinsonian symptoms are relative and appear within 1 year of each other. PD can be diagnosed if cognitive symptoms appear more than 1 year after the onset of motor symptoms. DLB has pathological changes which can separate it from AD: the presence of Lewy bodies (which are neuronal inclusion bodies composed of alpha-synuclein and ubiquitin protein) and Lewy neurites. The International Consensus Criteria for the clinical diagnosis of probable DLB are shown in Box 13.4.

Box 13.3 Case vignette 1

Mrs Y, aged 78, was referred to a memory clinic with a 7-month history of deteriorating memory. She lived alone and her family had become concerned as she appeared less able to care for herself. She was more forgetful: misplacing things, forgetting appointments and meals. She had started to leave sweets around the house, and when asked about this she said that children often visited her during the day. She also spoke about seeing children playing in her garden. On further questioning, it emerged that Mrs Y had no grandchildren and her family thought it unlikely that any children visited her. Her confusion appeared to fluctuate, and some days it was better than others. Her sleep pattern had become quite disturbed and she frequently complained of nightmares. The family were concerned that she was having falls and appeared to be slow in her movements, having been a very sprightly woman before. There was no family history of dementia and no medical history.

Physical examination revealed bilateral cogwheel rigidity and bradykinesia. Her gait was unsteady. MMSE was 21/30 (losing 6 points on orientation and 3 points on recall). Addenbrooke's Cognitive Examination score was 69/100 (she lost 6 points on orientation and concentration, 15 points on memory, 5 points on language, and 5 points on visuospatial skills). She was referred for a DaTSCAN, which revealed low dopamine transporter uptake in the brain's basal ganglia.

Box 13.4 Revised criteria for the clinical diagnosis of probable and possible dementia with Lewy bodies (DLB)

Essential for a diagnosis of DLB is dementia, defined as a progressive cognitive decline of sufficient magnitude to interfere with normal social or occupational functions, or with usual daily activities. Prominent or persistent memory impairment may not necessarily occur in the early stages but is usually evident with progression. Deficits on tests of attention, executive function, and visuoperceptual ability may be especially prominent and occur early.

Core clinical features

Fluctuating cognition, with pronounced variations in attention and alertness, recurrent visual hallucinations, which are typically well formed and detailed, rapid eye movement (REM) sleep behaviour disorder, which may precede cognitive decline, spontaneous motor features of parkinsonism

Supportive clinical features

Severe sensitivity to antipsychotic agents;
postural instability;
repeated falls;
syncope or other transient episodes of unresponsiveness;
severe autonomic dysfunction (e.g. constipation, orthostatic hypotension, urinary incontinence; hypersomnia);
hyposmia;
hallucinations in other modalities;
systematized delusions;
apathy, anxiety, and depression

Indicative biomarkers

Reduced dopamine transporter uptake in basal ganglia demonstrated by SPECT or PET
Abnormal (low uptake) [123]iodine-MIBG myocardial scintigraphy
Polysomnographic confirmation of REM sleep without atonia

Supportive biomarkers

Relative preservation of medial temporal lobe structures on CT/MRI scan.
Generalized low uptake on SPECT/PET perfusion/metabolism scan with reduced occipital activity with or without the cingulate island sign on FDG-PET imaging.
Prominent posterior slow-wave activity on EEG with periodic fluctuations in the pre-alpha/theta range.

Probable DLB can be diagnosed if

a. Two or more core clinical features of DLB are present, with or without the presence of indicative biomarkers, or
b. Only one core clinical feature is present, but with one or more indicative biomarkers.

Probable DLB should not be diagnosed on the basis of biomarkers alone.

Possible DLB can be diagnosed if

a. Only one core clinical feature of DLB is present, with no indicative biomarker evidence, or
b. One or more indicative biomarkers is present but there are no core clinical features.

Box 13.4 (cont.)

DLB is less likely

a. In the presence of any other physical illness or brain disorder including cerebrovascular disease, sufficient to account in part or in total for the clinical picture, although these do not exclude a DLB diagnosis and may serve to indicate mixed or multiple pathologies contributing to the clinical presentation, or

b. If parkinsonian features are the only core clinical feature and appear for the first time at a stage of severe dementia.

DLB should be diagnosed when dementia occurs before or concurrently with parkinsonism. The term Parkinson's disease dementia (PDD) should be used to describe dementia that occurs in the context of well-established Parkinson's disease. In a practice setting the term that is most appropriate to the clinical situation should be used and generic terms such as Lewy body disease are often helpful. In research studies in which distinction needs to be made between DLB and PDD, the existing 1-year rule between the onset of dementia and parkinsonism continues to be recommended.

McKeith IG, Boeve BF, Dickson DW, et al. Diagnosis and management of dementia with Lewy bodies: fourth consensus report of the DLB Consortium. *Neurology* 2017; 89: 88–100. DOI: 10.1212/WNL.0000000000004058

Computed Tomography

Computed tomography has been less useful in differentiating AD from DLB. Watson and colleagues completed a review of MRI studies of patients who had DLB.[25] They found the disease to be associated with less atrophy of the medial temporal lobes and principally subcortical atrophy; there was very little difference between patients with DLB and patients with PDD. This may allow a way of distinguishing DLB from AD, where medial temporal lobe atrophy is predominant.

Functional Neuroimaging

SPECT has been considered to be the gold standard scan in the diagnosis of DLB, showing reduced dopamine transporter activity in the basal ganglia. ^{123}I-FP-CIT SPECT (DaTSCAN; Figure 13.3) uses a ligand that binds to the dopamine transporter molecule; this can highlight areas of nigrostriatal degeneration associated with DLB. Studies assessing this show specificity of up to 90% and sensitivity of 75%,[26] suggesting that a DaTSCAN is more accurate than clinical diagnosis alone. DAT imaging is also useful as a way to distinguish DLB from AD with a sensitivity of 78% and a specificity of 90%.[27]

PET reveals hypo-metabolism in the occipital cortices.[26] PiB PET shows amyloid deposition in DLB similar to that in AD, but deposition is less in PDD than in DLB. This suggests that, although amyloid deposition is part of the pathology of the disease, it may have little effect on the clinical manifestation.[28]

Earlier comparisons of ^{123}I-FP-CIT SPECT with [(18)]F-FDG PET showed that the former had a greater diagnostic accuracy and effect size, but that both were useful in the assessment of suspected DLB.[29] Even this earlier study showed 100% specificity for the 'cingulate island sign', that is relative preservation of metabolism in the mid or posterior cingulate gyrus, in the diagnosis of DLB.[29] However, the superiority of PET scanning over SPECT scans in DLB has gradually been demonstrated.[30]

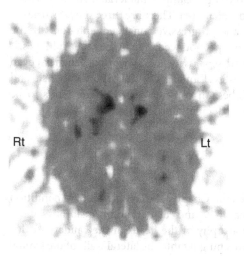

Rt   Lt

Figure 13.3 DaTSCAN for a patient with suspected dementia with Lewy bodies (DLB). The scan shows reduced tracer uptake in both putamina, with relatively normal uptake in the heads of caudate nuclei bilaterally. These findings are in keeping with DLB

Frontotemporal Dementia

The case vignette in Box 13.5 describes a typical presentation of the symptoms of FTD.

As reflected in the 2018 NICE Guideline, there are various types of FTD with their own diagnostic criteria.[3] International consensus criteria for the behavioural form of FTD have been agreed (see also Chapter 3).[31]

Box 13.5 Case vignette 2

Mr X, a 70-year-old retired accountant's clerk, was referred to the memory clinic with low mood and a 12-month history of a gradual decline in his poor short-term memory. He had been misplacing things and repeating his conversations. He had become more socially withdrawn over the preceding 6 months; his wife reported that he had lost interest in her and his friends and preferred to watch television all day. He had developed a strict routine of eating his meals at set times every day and insisting on the same food. If this routine was disrupted, he would become very irritable and would lose his temper. He had become coarser in his personality and was frequently rude to his guests. There was no family history of dementia. His medical history included hypertension and type 2 diabetes.

Physical examination was unremarkable and neurological examination was normal. MMSE score was 27/30 (losing 2 points on repetition and 1 on three-stage command). Addenbrookes Cognitive Examination score was 74/100 (losing 5 points on memory, 10 points on verbal fluency, 8 on language, and 3 on visuospatial skills). He was able to generate seven animals in 1 minute and four words beginning with 'P'. There was some evidence of perseveration on examination and he performed poorly on proverb interpretation, cognitive estimates, Luria motor sequencing, and Go–No-Go testing. MRI revealed bilateral frontal lobe atrophy.

Structural neuroimaging is generally unremarkable apart from showing cortical and subcortical atrophy in the frontal and temporal lobes, usually with enlarged ventricles.[9] FTD can be differentiated from AD by the pattern of atrophy that tends to spread from the anterior to posterior, whereas in AD the atrophy is to some extent uniform, despite a predilection for the entorhinal cortex and the hippocampus bilaterally. In some cases, the atrophy may be localized to a specific lobe or lobar area. There are three subcategories of FTD: frontal variant FTD, semantic dementia, and progressive non-fluent aphasia.[32] In the last form, atrophy of the left temporal lobe is more pronounced than in the other subtypes.[33]

Functional neuroimaging has great diagnostic sensitivity and may prove beneficial even when the structural scan shows very little. Both SPECT and PET reveal hypometabolism and hypoperfusion of the frontal and temporal lobes. In contrast, in AD there tends to be hypometabolism of the parietal lobes early on in dementia progression.

Other Dementias

Huntington's Disease

Huntington's disease (which is also discussed in Chapter 3) is a hereditary condition associated with chorea, neuropsychiatric features, and dementia of insidious onset. Computed tomography and MRI often show atrophy of the heads of the caudate nuclei. This is associated with a loss of the normal convex bulging into the lateral walls of the frontal horns.[33] Caudate atrophy is highly specific to Huntington's disease. MRI studies have also shown subcortical atrophy and atrophy of the thalamus and medial temporal lobes, which appears to correlate with the degree of cognitive impairment. SPECT and PET scans show decreased blood flow and glucose metabolism in the caudate nuclei.[33]

Creutzfeldt–Jakob Disease

Creutzfeldt–Jakob Disease (CJD) belongs to the group of transmissible spongiform encephalopathies, which also includes Gerstmann–Sträussler–Scheinker disease and fatal familial insomnia (see also Chapter 4). These prion diseases are associated with relatively rapid onset of dementia together with other neuropsychiatric symptoms such as depression, anxiety, and behavioural changes, cerebellar ataxia, and myoclonus. Variant CJD is a distinct disease from sporadic CJD and is associated with characteristic signs on MRI, which have been incorporated into the World Health Organization's diagnostic criteria.[34] MRI shows the distinctive pulvinar sign and hockey stick sign. The pulvinar sign is bilateral pulvinar hyperintensity, relative to the anterior putamen, on fluid attenuated inversion recovery (FLAIR) MRI.[35] The hockey stick sign is hyperintensity in the dorsomedial thalamic nuclei and periaqueductal grey matter.[35] Both SPECT and PET show regional brain hypometabolism and hypoperfusion, but these are fairly non-specific.

Progressive Supranuclear Palsy

Progressive supranuclear palsy is associated with FTD. MRI changes may include atrophy of the midbrain and brainstem, and third ventricle dilation, but these findings are not specific to progressive supranuclear palsy.[36] PET studies in patients with FTD show a global hypometabolism, but this is more pronounced in the frontal lobes, caudate, putamen, and thalamus.[36]

Mild Cognitive Impairment

Patients with MCI are at risk of developing dementia. It has been considered to be a prodromal stage in the development of AD: between 10% and 15% of patients with aMCI with no vascular risk factors develop AD each year.[37] Structural imaging of patients with clinical MCI has shown a reduction in the volumes of the entorhinal cortices and hippocampi, more than in the cognitively intact elderly, but less than that seen in AD.[9] Serial MRI scanning of patients with MCI showed grey matter loss in the amygdala, entorhinal cortices, and anterior hippocampus.[9] As cognition deteriorates and the clinical picture begins to resemble AD, this grey matter loss extends to incorporate the entire hippocampi and temporal and parietal lobes.[38]

In studies of MCI, SPECT and PET scans reveal changes similar to those seen in AD: hypoperfusion and hypometabolism of the temporal and parietal lobes.[38] Patients with MCI who subsequently developed AD had more significant reductions in cerebral blood flow to the medial temporal lobes than those patients who did not develop the disease.[38]

Several studies have assessed the utility of neuroimaging in the prediction of conversion from MCI to AD. These found that a smaller volume of the entorhinal cortices and hippocampi both independently predicted conversion to AD.[39] However, there was little additional benefit from this than from measuring cognitive variables and prediction based on age.

Special Groups

Intellectual Disability

The prevalence of dementia in people with intellectual disability is higher than in the general population. Down's syndrome in particular is associated with AD: about 54.5% of 60- to 69-year-olds with the syndrome have a diagnosis of dementia.[40] Intellectual disability not due to Down's syndrome is also associated with a higher prevalence of dementia: about 13% of over-50-year-olds and 22% of over-65-year-olds in this group have a form of dementia.[41] The diagnosis of dementia in people with intellectual disability can be more complex because of difficulties in detecting cognitive decline and because changes in behaviour are often attributed to the intellectual disability. Consequently, patients often present to dementia services late in the progression of the disease.[40]

The use of neuroimaging in dementia in patients with intellectual disability has not been studied to a great extent. Most of the research has focused on Down's syndrome and has involved small numbers of patients. Structural imaging (CT and MRI) has shown atrophy of the medial temporal lobes, in keeping with the changes expected in AD.[40] However, it must be borne in mind that people with Down's syndrome and other forms of intellectual disability are likely to have abnormal scans anyway, and so scans may be misinterpreted.[42] Consequently, neuroimaging may be used as a supportive tool in examining these patients for dementia, but diagnosis remains a task for experienced clinicians.

Young-Onset Dementia

A 2007 report for the Alzheimer's Society revealed that young-onset dementia (diagnosed before the age of 65) accounted for 2.2% of cases of dementia in the country.[43] AD was the most common subtype of dementia in patients of any age (see also Chapter 3 for further discussion of young-onset dementia). Late-onset dementia was slightly more common in women; among patients aged 50–65, young-onset dementia was more common in men, with FTD accounting for a substantial proportion of cases. In black and minority ethnic groups, 6.1% cases of dementia were of early onset, compared with the national average of 2.2%.

Research into neuroimaging findings in young-onset dementia is sparse, and there are very few studies that make comparisons between young-onset and late-onset findings. One study that compared MRI findings in addition to neuropsychology battery results in patients with young-onset and late-onset AD found that in young-onset disease cortical atrophy was more common in occipital and parietal lobes, whereas in late-onset disease hippocampal atrophy was more common.[44] Comparison of TC-99m HMPAO SPECT scans of patients with early- and late-onset AD showed that young-onset disease was associated with hypoperfusion predominantly in the posterior cortical association area, whereas late-onset disease was associated with medial temporal lobe hypoperfusion.[45] Although the numbers of patients in both of these studies were small, there do appear to be differences in neuroimaging findings between young-onset and late-onset dementia cases, and further research may be beneficial.

Depressive Pseudodementia

Depressive pseudodementia is a reversible cause of cognitive impairment caused by depression (see also Chapter 18). As depression is frequently comorbid with dementia, it can be difficult to distinguish between pseudodementia and a primary diagnosis of dementia. MRI findings in patients with either depression or dementia both show hippocampal atrophy, but there is a good correlation between the length of history of cognitive impairment and extent of atrophy of the entorhinal cortices.[9] For patients with cognitive dysfunction of unclear aetiology, the degree of temporal lobe atrophy on MRI could allow differentiation between dementia and depression: the former would show a greater degree of atrophy.[9]

A small study that evaluated SPECT findings in four samples – individuals with AD, those with depression without cognitive impairment, those with depressive pseudodementia, and healthy controls – found that the depressive pseudodementia group showed hypoperfusion of the temporoparietal region, similar to the findings in the AD group, but different from findings in the depression group.[46]

Discussion

The question as to whether to use neuroimaging in the investigation and diagnosis of dementia is complicated. Largely, the diagnosis of dementia is a clinical one and the diagnostic criteria for the various subcategories of dementia place neuroimaging in a supportive role.[20, 24, 47, 48]

Alzheimer's Disease

In the UK, AD is the most common form of dementia, accounting for up to 60% of cases.[49] Therefore, the utility of imaging in these cases is paramount. For AD, the findings in CT and MRI are often seen in other conditions and are not necessarily specific to AD. The characteristic signs on CT and MRI in AD are frequently absent in clinical practice and can be seen in older people without cognitive impairment. Therefore, at present, we would not suggest routinely screening patients with a clinical diagnosis of AD using CT and MRI. Although PET and SPECT in AD can be more sensitive and specific, the additional costs, invasiveness, radiation exposure, potential for allergic reactions, and relatively poor tolerability of some of these procedures in older people limit their usefulness. Some centres require a CT scan to be performed before a SPECT or PET in order to increase sensitivity and rule out other causes for memory loss such as tumour. We would recommend the use of SPECT and PET only if there is clear diagnostic uncertainty.

Vascular Dementia

For VaD there is a clearer position for structural imaging; the NINDS–AIREN diagnostic criteria include the presence of vascular insults, including infarcts, basal ganglia, and white matter lacunes or extensive periventricular white matter lesions (up to 25% of the white matter should be affected).[20] Absence of these features, according to these criteria, excludes the diagnosis. Clearly, to detect the presence or absence of these lesions, there needs to be some form of imaging performed. CT can effectively detect large vessel infarction or ischaemia, but MRI is more sensitive in detecting extensive white matter lesions. Diagnosis of VaD is often made on clinical grounds, but where there is uncertainty, CT or MRI should be used according to local resources and patient tolerability and contraindications; SPECT and PET should be used only if the diagnosis is in doubt and CT or MRI has been inconclusive.

Other Types of Dementia

For less common types of dementia, imaging may be indicated. For DLB, CT and MRI are less useful in differentiating it from other subtypes of dementia, particularly from AD. The gold standard form of imaging in these patients is a SPECT scan with a radioligand that binds to the dopamine transporter molecule (DaTSCAN) and demonstrates nigrostriatal degeneration. As SPECT has been shown to have greater diagnostic accuracy than PET in DLB, albeit the accuracy of diagnosis using PET has improved, we would recommend SPECT as an adjunct to clinical diagnosis in patients suspected of having this type of dementia.

Functional neuroimaging also plays a more important role in the diagnosis of FTD. CT and MRI findings are difficult to distinguish from changes seen in AD, whereas PET shows hypometabolism and hypoperfusion of the frontal and temporal lobes more specifically. The diagnosis is principally based on symptoms and signs, and imaging should be reserved for cases where the diagnosis is in doubt.

Huntington's disease and CJD both have characteristic imaging findings: caudate atrophy and pulvinar sign/hockey stick sign, respectively. These findings are more likely to be present on MRI and in suspected cases imaging can be used to support the diagnosis, which is in the most part dependent on genetic testing for Huntington's disease and biopsy for CJD. SPECT and PET will add little to the investigation and diagnosis of these conditions.

Recommendations

The answer to the question 'To scan or not to scan?' in suspected dementia and MCI is that routine scanning is not indicated in all patients and healthcare professionals should use their clinical judgement. The diagnosis of dementia should be made by experienced specialist clinicians, based primarily on history and mental state examination. In keeping with NICE guidance and also in our opinion, the use of diagnostic criteria can help discriminate between the subtypes of dementia. Routine imaging, in our view, such as CT and MRI should not be used. Imaging should be reserved for cases where there is uncertainty about the diagnosis. As the NICE guidance makes clear, structural imaging should be offered, but not if the diagnosis or subtype of dementia are established. Usually, PET and SPECT are relatively less well tolerated than CT among older people, so they should be reserved for complex cases, patients with suspected DLB, and in cases where further diagnostic clarity is required.

Acknowledgement

For information, the original paper on which this chapter is based was:

Sullivan V, Majumdar B, Richman A, Vinjamuri S. To scan or not to scan: neuroimaging in mild cognitive impairment and dementia. *Adv Psychiatr Treat* 2012; 18: 457–66.

Whereas Dr Victoria Sullivan was the lead author of the original paper, the chapter has been updated by Professor Sobhan Vinjamuri.

References

1. Office for National Statistics. *Living Longer: How Our Population Is Changing and Why It Matters*. ONS, 2018. Last accessed on 3 October 2019 via: www.ons.gov.uk/people populationandcommunity/birthsdeathsand marriages/ageing/articles/livinglongerho wourpopulationischangingandwhyitmat ters/2018-08-13

2. Prince M, Knapp M, Guerchet M, et al. *Dementia UK Update*. Alzheimer's Society, 2014. Last accessed on 3 October 2019 via: www.alzheimers.org.uk/about-us/policy-and-influencing/dementia-uk-report

3. National Institute for Health and Care Excellence (NICE). *Dementia: Assessment, Management and Support for People Living with Dementia and Their Carers*. NICE Guideline 97. NICE, 2018. Last accessed on 3 October 2019 via: www.nice.org.uk/gui dance/ng97/resources/dementia-assessment-management-and-support-for-people-living-with-dementia-and-their-carers-pdf-1837760199109

4. McKhann G, Drachma, D, Folstein M, et al. Clinical diagnosis of Alzheimer's disease: report of the NINCDS-ADRDA Work Group under the auspices of Department of Health and Human Services Task Force on Alzheimer's Disease. *Neurology* 1984; 34: 939–44.

5. Knopman DS, DeKosky ST, Cummings JL, et al. Practice parameter: diagnosis of dementia (an evidence-based review). *Neurology* 2001; 56: 1143–53.

6. McKhann GM, Knopmanc DS, Howard Chertkow H, et al. The diagnosis of dementia due to Alzheimer's disease: recommendations from the National Institute on Aging Alzheimer's Association workgroups on diagnostic guidelines for Alzheimer's disease. *Alzheimers Dement* 2011; 7: 263–9. DOI:10.1016/j. jalz.2011.03.005

7. Petrella JR, Coleman RE, Doraiswamy PM. Neuroimaging and early diagnosis of Alzheimer's disease: a look into the future. *Radiology* 2003; 226: 315–36.

8. O'Brien, JT, Barber, B. Neuroimaging in dementia and depression. *Advances in Psychiatric Treatment* 2000; 6: 109–19.

9. O'Brien JT (2007) Role of imaging techniques in the diagnosis of dementia. *British Journal of Radiology* 80: S71–7.

10. Davatzikos C, Bhatt P, Sha, LM, et al. Prediction of MCI to AD conversion, via MRI, CSF biomarkers and pattern classification. *Neurobiology of Aging* 2011; 32: e2322.19–27.

11. Kantarci K, Jack CR Jr. Neuroimaging in Alzheimer disease: an evidence-based review. *Neuroimaging Clinics of North America* 2003; **13**: 197–209.

12. Jagust W, Thisted R, Devous S, et al. SPECT perfusion imaging in the diagnosis of Alzheimer's disease. *Neurology* 2001; **56**: 950–6.

13. Quigley H, Colloby S, O'Brien T. PET imaging of brain amyloid in dementia: a review. *International Journal of Geriatric Psychiatry* 2010; **26**: 991–9.

14. O'Brien JT, Firbank MJ, Davison C, et al. 18F-FDG PET and perfusion SPECT in the diagnosis of Alzheimer and Lewy body dementias. *J Nucl Med* 2014; **55**: 1959–65. DOI:10.2967/jnumed.114.143347

15. Bamford C, Olsen K, Davison C, et al. Is there a preference for PET or SPECT brain imaging in diagnosing dementia? The views of people with dementia, carers, and healthy controls. *Int Psychogeriatr* 2016; **28**:1, 123–31. DOI:10.1017/ S1041610215001039

16. Herholz K, Carter SF, Jones M. Positron emission tomography imaging in dementia. *Br J Radiol* 2007; **80** (Spec No 2): S160–7.

17. Lashley T, Schott JM, Weston P, et al. Molecular biomarkers of Alzheimer's disease: progress and prospects. *Dis Model Mech* 2018; **11**(5): dmm031781.

18. Wolk DA, Sadowsky C, Safirstein B, et al. Use of flutemetamol F 18–labeled positron emission tomography and other biomarkers to assess risk of clinical progression in patients with amnestic mild cognitive impairment. *JAMA Neurol* 2018; **75**: 1114–1123. DOI:10.1001/ jamaneurol.2018.0894

19. Rabinovici GD, Gatsonis C, Apgar C, et al. Association of amyloid positron emission tomography with subsequent change in clinical management among Medicare beneficiaries with mild cognitive impairment or dementia. *JAMA* 2019; **321**: 1286–1294. DOI:10.1001/jama.2019.2000

20. Román GC, Tatemichi, TK, Erkinjuntti, T et al. Vascular dementia: diagnostic criteria for research studies. Report of the NINDS-AIREN International Workshop. *Neurology* 1993; **43**: 250–60.

21. Gold G, Giannakopoulos P, Montes-Paixao JC, et al. Sensitivity and specificity of newly proposed clinical criteria for possible vascular dementia. *Neurology* 1997; **49**: 690–4.

22. Shim YS, Yang DW, Kim BS, et al. Comparison of regional cerebral blood flow in two subsets of subcortical ischaemic vascular dementia: statistical parametric mapping analysis of SPECT. *Journal of Neurological Sciences* 2006; **250**:85–91.

23. Pascual B, Prieto E, Arbizu J, et al. Brain glucose metabolism in vascular white matter disease with dementia: differentiation from Alzheimer disease. *Stroke* 2010; **41**: 2889–93.

24. McKeith IG, Boeve BF, Dickson DW, et al. Diagnosis and management of dementia with Lewy bodies: fourth consensus report of the DLB Consortium. *Neurology* 2017; **89**: 88–100. DOI:10.1212/ WNL.0000000000004058

25. Watson R, Blamire AM, O'Brien JT. Magnetic resonance imaging in Lewy body dementias. *Dementia and Geriatric Cognitive Disorders* 2009; **28**:493–506.

26. Walker, RWH, Walker, Z. Dopamine transporter single photon emission computerized tomography in the diagnosis of dementia with Lewy bodies. *Movement Disorders* 2009; **24** (suppl 2): S754–9.

27. McKeith I, O'Brien J, Walker Z, et al. Sensitivity and specificity of dopamine transporter imaging with 123IFP-CIT SPECT in dementia with Lewy bodies: a phase III, multicentre study. Lancet Neurol 2007; **6**: 305–13.

28. Brooks DJ. Imaging amyloid in Parkinson's disease dementia and dementia with Lewy bodies with positron emission tomography. *Movement Disorders* 2009; **24** (suppl 2): S742–7.

29. Lim SM, Katsifis A, Villemang A, et al. The 18F-FDG PET Cingulate Island sign and comparison to ^{123}I-Beta-CIT SPECT for diagnosis of dementia with Lewy bodies. *J Nucl Med* 2009; **50**: 1638–45.

30. O'Brien JT, Firbank MJ, Davison C, et al. 18F-FDG PET and perfusion SPECT in the diagnosis of Alzheimer and Lewy body dementias *J Nucl Med* 2014; **55**: 1959–65. DOI:10.2967/jnumed.114.143347

31. Rascovsky K, Hodges JR, Knopman D, et al. Sensitivity of revised diagnostic criteria for the behavioural variant of frontotemporal dementia. *Brain* 2011; **134**: 2456–77. DOI:10.1093/brain/awr179

32. Hodges JR. Frontotemporal dementia (Pick's disease): clinical features and assessment. *Neurology* 2001; **56** (suppl 4): S6–S10.

33. Lovestone S. Alzheimer's disease and other dementias (including pseudodementias). In *Lishman's Organic Psychiatry: A Textbook of Neuropsychiatry* (4th ed.) (eds. A David, S Fleminger, M Kopelman, S Lovestone, J Mellers): 543–615. Wiley-Blackwell, 2009.

34. World Health Organization. *WHO Guidelines on Tissue Infectivity Distribution in Transmissible Spongiform Encephalitis (WL 300)*. WHO, 2006. Last accessed on 15 October 2019 via: www.who.int/blood products/TSEPUBLISHEDREPORT.pdf

35. Collie DA, Summers DM, Sellar RJ, et al. Diagnosing variant Creutzfeldt–Jakob disease with the pulvinar sign: MR imaging findings in 86 neuropathologically confirmed cases. *Am J Neuroradiol* 2003; **24**: 1560–9.

36. Mishina M, Ishii K, Mitani K, et al. Midbrain hypometabolism as early diagnostic sign for progressive supranuclear palsy. *Acta Neurol Scand* 2004; **110**: 128–35.

37. Ganguli M, Dodge HH, Shen C, et al. Mild cognitive impairment, amnestic type: an epidemiologic study. *Neurology* 2004; **63**: 115–21.

38. Whitwell JL, Przybelski SA, Weigand SD, et al. 3D maps from multiple MRI illustrate changing atrophy patterns as subjects progress from mild cognitive impairment to Alzheimer's disease. *Brain* 2007; **130**: 1777–86.

39. Devanand DP, Pradhaban G, Liu X, et al. Hippocampal and entorhinal atrophy in mild cognitive impairment: prediction of Alzheimer disease. *Neurology* 2007; **68**: 828–36.

40. Stanton LR, Coetzee RH. Down's syndrome and dementia. *Adv Psychiatr Treat* 2004; **10**: 50–8.

41. Moss S, Patel P. The prevalence of mental illness in people with intellectual disability over 50 years of age, and the diagnostic importance of information from carers. *Ir J Psychol Med* 1993; **14**: 110–29.

42. Strydom A, Hassiotis A, Walker Z. Clinical use of structural magnetic resonance imaging in the diagnosis of dementia in adults with Down's syndrome. *Ir J Psychol Med* 2002; **19**: 60–3.

43. King's College London, London School of Economics. *Dementia UK: The Full Report.* Alzheimer's Society, 2007. Last accessed on 15 October 2019 via: www.alzheimers.org.uk /sites/default/files/2018-10/Dementia_UK_F ull_Report_2007.pdf?fileID=2

44. Frisoni GB, Pievani M, Testa C, et al. The topography of grey matter involvement in early and late onset Alzheimer's disease. *Brain* 2007; **130**: 720–30.

45. Kemp PM, Holmes C, Hoffman SMA, et al. Alzheimer's disease: differences in technetium-99m HMPAO SPECT scan findings between early onset and late onset dementia. *J Neurol Neurosurg Psychiatry* 2003; **74**: 715–9.

46. Cho MJ, Lyoo IK, Lee DW, et al. Brain single photon emission computed tomography findings in depressive pseudodementia patients. *J Affect Disord* 2002; **69**: 159–66.

47. Neary D, Snowden JS, Gustafson L, et al. Frontotemporal lobar degeneration: a consensus on clinical diagnostic criteria. *Neurology* 1998; **51**: 1546–54.

48. Varma AR, Snowden JS, Lloyd JJ, et al. Evaluation of the NINCDS-ADRDA criteria in the differentiation of Alzheimer's disease and frontotemporal dementia. *J Neurol Neurosurg Psychiatry* 1999; **66**: 184–8.

49. Blennow K, De Leon MJ, Zetterberg H. Alzheimer's disease. *Lancet* 2006; **368**:387–403.

Supporting Self-Management in Early Dementia

A Contribution Towards 'Living Well'?

Jo Cheffey, Laura Hill and Glenn Roberts

Introduction

Social and demographic changes and advances in acute medicine are leading to an ageing population. Many, perhaps most, people will now live for significant periods with long-term health conditions and illness. There are over one million people with dementia currently living in the UK, at an estimated annual cost of £26.3 billion to society with the average cost being £32,250 per person per year. The estimated breakdown of this cost is £4.3 billion spent on healthcare, £10.3 billion on social care (publicly and privately funded), and £11.6 billion contributed by the work of unpaid carers of people with dementia.[1] It is projected that the total number of people with dementia in the UK will increase to over 2 million by 2051.

Alongside a continuing search for effective treatment and prevention, there has been a growing interest in how to live and how to 'live well' with long-term, incurable health conditions. This has been accompanied by increasing recognition of the value of enabling people to become actively involved in their own care and illness management as a route to enhanced quality of life.

Mental health services for working-age adults have embraced this with approaches emphasizing recovery, self-management, personalization, and inclusion. There is growing interest in exploring the potential benefits of applying these principles in the context of person-centred services for older people,[2] but the tools, guides, and evidence have yet to be established to support service development in dementia care. The Royal College of Psychiatrists has recently published training guidance advocating a convergence of several values-oriented approaches, including 'Recovery', as Person-Centred Care.[3]

This chapter considers the possible benefits and applicability of the recovery-oriented principle of supporting people with dementia and their carers in self-management. (See Chapter 15 for a fuller discussion of the recovery model of care.)

'Living Well' With Dementia

Dementia is a general term encompassing conditions that cause global deterioration of higher cortical functioning. Alzheimer's disease, the most common form of dementia, causes short-term memory loss with decline in speech, comprehension, judgement, and personality as the illness progresses. This leads to a decline in the ability to carry out day-to-day tasks and ultimately, through progressive deterioration, to death. There is no cure for dementia, but treatments, both medical and psychosocial, aim to reduce distress and improve quality of life.

Current policies promote personal and therapeutic approaches that focus on how to live well even in the context of an incurable and progressive disorder.[4] The importance of early diagnosis and intervention to improve care and treatment in a cost-effective way is emphasized. There has been a 56% rise in the number of people diagnosed with dementia in the UK from 2010 to 2015/16 (www.dementiastatistics.org). The introduction of drug treatments such as the acetylcholinesterase inhibitors has increased the referral rates from primary care, but there are still some people who are not aware of their diagnosis and are therefore unable to be actively involved in decisions about their care. This was recognized by Tom Kitwood, who identified the 'malignant social psychology' that dominates from the early stages of dementia and serves to disempower the person and take away their right to make choices and decisions about their condition.[5] Although taking care to avoid 'romanticising' dementia, Kitwood wanted to emphasize the 'human functioning such as relationship, emotion and sensation' that still remain important in every individual, rather than primarily focus on cognitive and other deficits when considering people with dementia.[6] He described this humanistic emphasis as a form of 'personal growth' and 'positive change' that can occur over the course of an advancing dementia.

Recovery and Dementia Care: Concepts in Conflict?

The current national mental health outcomes strategy, *No Health Without Mental Health*, is oriented around six aims, the second of which is that 'more people will recover'.[7] In clarifying what it means by 'recovery' the strategy notes that this has acquired a specific meaning in mental health, which is based on Anthony's almost universally accepted definition of personal recovery:

A deeply personal, unique process of changing one's attitudes, values, feelings, goals, skills and/or roles. It is a way of living a satisfying, hopeful and contributing life, even with limitations caused by the illness. Recovery involves the development of new meaning and purpose in one's life.[8]

The strategy also underlines the broad applicability of the values and vision of this definition across the scope of this 'all age' approach by noting that, 'Although the term is not used in relation to children and young people, the underlying principles of the recovery approach are equally applicable' (footnote to p. 16).[7] But, the question remains whether it is legitimate or helpful to talk about recovery, so defined, in dementia care.

In Chapter 15, we (L.H. and G.R.) note the close parallels between the values, principles, and practices of person-centred care in older people's mental health and those of recovery approaches commonly used in mental health services for working-age adults.[2] We also acknowledge the difficulty of reconciling the word 'recovery' with the care of people with progressive and deteriorating conditions. However, the basis for Antony's definition and the recovery approach in general centres on recognizing that you can have an illness and yet be well, and that clinical variables such as symptoms are only loosely related to personal variables such as quality of life, hope, happiness, and satisfaction. Moreover, the loose coupling between the presence of illness and experience of well-being provides a possible rationale for working to preserve or enhance well-being even for people with persistent or advancing illness. This has been a guiding principle in hospice care for many decades.

However, it may strain conceptual credulity to breaking point to call this recovery. Seeking to develop a recovery-oriented approach to dementia may risk offering false hope of cure and alienate the very people who could gain much from support for active engagement in optimizing quality of life. This does not mean that the fundamentals of the recovery approach do not apply in dementia care, as the values, principles, and many of the practices clearly do, but it does acknowledge the limits of using the word 'recovery' to describe this. Fundamentally, the important issue is in developing approaches that are useful and experienced as helpful by the people we seek to serve.

Daley et al. sought to evaluate whether a conceptual framework of recovery developed for working-age adults holds value for older people with mental health problems, including those with dementia.[9] They found that the fundamental principles of recovery had resonance with older people and that taking a recovery-oriented approach was acceptable within the limitations of the concept. They also identified similarities and differences. Working-age adults and older people similarly gave emphasis to the impact of having a mental health problem, the importance of personal responsibility, the value of coping strategies, as well as self-help information, and of feeling connected to others and their community. However, older people, including those with dementia, sought to cope with their difficulties, not so much by seeking a new sense of meaning and purpose, but through a desire for stability and a wish to 'continue being me', which was associated with the importance of holding on to an established and enduring sense of identity.

They also found that older people were much more likely to associate with and seek support from family rather than peers, and there was a routine need to consider the impact of living with coexisting mental and physical health problems and to develop coping strategies for both.[9] For people with dementia there was an additional need to include the changing experience of the condition over time and the increasing need for support from others as mediators of well-being.

Overall, there was a close correspondence between their findings[9] and the principles of recovery identified by service users in seminal papers on the subject,[10, 11] including key components of sustaining hope, maintaining control over life and symptoms, and creating opportunities to build a life beyond the illness, which are equally applicable to people living with dementia and their supporters. This ethos is also advocated by the Social Care Institute for Excellence which, when considering the needs of older adults with mental health problems, states that:

'Recovery' and well-being approaches to mental health issues developed by younger adult service users and working-age mental health services are equally applicable to older people (p. 19);[12]

and furthermore,

Recovery is [. . .] making it possible for people to have quality of life and a degree of independence and choice, even those with the most enduring and disabling conditions (p. 20).[12]

This strongly implies that specific tools and discoveries in working-age adult recovery-oriented practice may have applicability in older people's mental healthcare too.

Valuing Self-Management

Historically, much of our effort in seeking better outcomes has come through developing better treatment, where effectiveness is largely measured in terms of symptom reduction and improvement attributed to high-fidelity concordance with taking or receiving the treatment itself. More recently, there has been a growing interest in the contribution people themselves can make to their own health and well-being through becoming active

> **Box 14.1** Benefits associated with successful self-management
>
> - Increases quality of life
> - Increases social activation and promotes new friendships
> - Helps the person become more aware of resources in their social environment
> - Gives the person skills to manage their dementia
> - Helps the person with decision-making
> - Increases self-efficacy and mastery over one's life
> - Reduces the psychological distress associated with the condition through helping the person to manage the emotional consequences of the disability
> - Increases knowledge about the condition
>
> Mountain GA. Self-management for people with early dementia: an exploration of concepts and supporting evidence. *Dementia* 2006; 5: 429–46.
>
> Mountain GA, Craig CL. What should be in a self-management programme for people with early dementia? *Aging Ment Health* 2012; 16: 576–583.
>
> Reid MC, Papaleontiou M, Ong A, et al. Self-management strategies to reduce pain and improve function among older adults in community settings: a review of the evidence. *Pain Med* 2008; 9: 409–24.
>
> Laakkonen ML, Kautiainen H, Holtta E, et al. Effects of self-management groups for people with dementia and their spouses: randomized controlled trial. *J Am Geriatr Soc* 2016; 64:752–760.

participants rather than passive recipients. The Salzburg Global Seminar went as far as to describe actively participating patients as 'the greatest untapped resource in healthcare'.[13] Enabling people to take an active stance to ward their own health and well-being through supported decision-making and self-management planning has emerged as a major emphasis in recovery-focused approaches.[14, 15, 16]

Self-management has an established role in recovery-based care and was highlighted through the NHS plan as one of the key building blocks for a patient-centred health service.[17] It features as a key component in the White Paper *Our Health, Our Care, Our Say* and in *Supporting People with Long-Term Conditions to Self Care*.[18, 19] It has been adopted at local and national levels in skills training programmes (Expert Patients Programme self-management courses) and condition-specific patient education programmes, for example, DESMOND for type 2 diabetes (www.desmond-project.org.uk). Targeted investment in self-management interventions can increase people's confidence in managing their health and well-being and improve their quality of life and, collaterally, there is a possibility of additional economic benefits for the NHS.[20, 21]

Self-management can be defined as 'the individual's ability to manage the symptoms, treatment, physical and psychosocial consequences and lifestyle changes inherent in living with a chronic condition'.[22] It focuses on empowering patients to manage their own conditions by increasing their knowledge and involvement in their care,[23] and has been associated with a range of highly desirable benefits as described in Box 14.1.

Supporting Self-Management in Dementia

Self-management strategies have been developed as a response to enabling people to live more satisfactorily with recurrent or long-term conditions. Dementia is a long-term condition, yet very little is known about the efficacy of using self-management approaches with this population. Mountain, in a review of issues about selfmanagement and dementia, argues that in order to adapt self-management for people with dementia, several issues would need to be considered such as problem-solving, information-sharing, locating local resources, making an early diagnosis, supporting the impact of the diagnosis, and focusing on the person's changing needs.[24]

In a randomized controlled trial (RCT) of 136 couples in Finland, the effect of self-management group rehabilitation for people with dementia and their spouses was investigated.[27] The groups met over eight sessions and the aim was to enhance self-efficacy and problem-solving skills and to provide peer support. This group-based psycho-social intervention focusing on promotion of self-management skills for people with dementia and their spouses demonstrated beneficial effects on the Health Related Quality of Life (HRQoL) scale for spouses. It also had a positive impact on the cognition of people with dementia (using a verbal fluency test and the clock drawing test) comparing data at baseline with three and nine months post-intervention. These effects were achieved without extra costs over 24 months of follow-up. This research suggests a new model of support for people with dementia and their families post-diagnosis.[i] Future studies should explore the long-term effects of this intervention.

Mountain and Craig described the development of a six-week self-management group.[25] They started with a consultation process with five people with dementia and their main carers and identified seven themes: understanding dementia, rethinking dementia, living with dementia (strategies to manage memory), relationships, keeping mentally well, experiencing well-being, and keeping physically well. The final session also included a discussion on 'what next?' A group was then developed based on these themes and was attended by a mix of people with dementia and carers.

The group was delivered through a 'menu-based approach' where participants were offered choices from a number of themes and interventions tailored to the expressed needs of the group. This was highly valued by participants. Evaluation of the group also supported the need for skilled facilitation of the group by a professional with expertise in dementia care. The authors conclude: 'self-management for people with dementia . . . involves moving beyond a medical construct of treatment and care to one that adopts a holistic view of the person and their needs.'[25]

Claire Craig then went on to develop an occupational therapy–based self-management manual for facilitators working with people with dementia.

Journeying through Dementia is an intervention that has been developed in partnership with people with dementia. The intervention focuses on ways of enabling individuals to continue to engage in activities that they find meaningful as their condition progresses.[28]

Referring back to the original research that underpins this work,[25] Craig stated:

During this research people with dementia were clear that they wanted to continue to be active, to engage in groups that did not just talk about the diagnosis but offered practical advice and support on how to continue to live well with the condition.[28]

---

[i] We are grateful to an anonymous reviewer for alerting us, in connection with this point, to the Scottish Government's commitment since 2013 to anyone receiving a diagnosis of dementia being entitled to a minimum of a year's post-diagnostic support from a named link worker using the five pillars model of post-diagnostic support (see www.alzscot.org/our-work/campaigning-for-change/current-campaigns/5-pillar-model-of-post-diagnostic-support last accessed on 16 January 2020).

> **Box 14.2** Situations in dementia care where supported self-management might help
>
> - Negotiating understanding and disclosure of diagnosis
> - How to share this diagnosis with people
> - Giving people information about their condition
> - Increasing people's awareness of support services
> - Care planning, including carers' perspectives
> - Eliciting, preserving and remembering personal preferences
> - End-of-life planning

The National Dementia Strategy re-emphasized the importance of providing more information regarding external support services, putting service users at the centre of their care plan, delivering care according to individual need, and helping the person and carer to live alongside the dementia.[29] There are recurring dilemmas in dementia care which might be better addressed by engaging people in supported decision-making about their own care and treatment (Box 14.2).

The aim of self-management approaches in dementia is to enable the person to be at the centre of their care, drawing on and valuing their experience of their own condition, their preferences and capacity to express views on the relative merits of alternative forms of care and treatment in line with person-centred and recovery-principled approaches.

Adapting Self-Management Planning from Adult Services to Dementia Care

The concept of self-management in relation to health has grown from the field of long-term physical conditions, but is increasingly being used in mental health services. Internationally, the most popular self-management tool for maintaining mental health is the Wellness Recovery Action Plan® (WRAP®).[30] This has been incorporated into the Substance Abuse and Mental Health Services Administration (SAMHSA) National Registry of Evidence-based Programs and Practices in the United States, with a recommendation for wide dissemination.[31] It has also provided the core model for many subsequent self-management frameworks in adult mental health services and is therefore the best candidate to draw on and adapt to dementia care.[32]

WRAP was developed by Mary Ellen Copeland and other user-contributors who were seeking a means of regaining control of their lives and wanting to develop ways of effectively working on their health and well-being.[33] This resulted in the formulation of an accessible self-management plan based on what people found worked for them. It aimed to 'promote wellness, decrease the need for costly, invasive therapies, reduce the incidence of serious mental health difficulties, decrease traumatic life events caused by crises, and to raise hope'[33] (see also www.mentalhealthrecovery.com). Typically, this involves a focus on a 'wellness toolbox', which is a list of individually tailored resources that can be used to stay well. A daily maintenance plan helps to keep the person on track and reduce stress. WRAP also focuses on identifying early warning signs of relapse, potential triggers, and actions people can take to reduce distress and re-stabilize their health. It includes a plan to enable the person to survive a crisis with an advance directive if needed. The plan is written, owned, and used by the individual who chooses whether and when to share it with others at their own discretion.

Copeland's group have also developed, through extensive experience, an accompanying set of values and ethics through which WRAP is taught and shared. These include promoting self-determination, personal responsibility, empowerment, and self-advocacy, which are seen as the foundations for positive outcomes and are broadly concordant with an international review of key recovery processes.[34]

WRAP has arisen as a group learning experience where everyone is treated equally and people are led to support one another in developing their own mental health experience into expertise, although it can be used individually. Medical and diagnostic language is avoided in favour of plain English and experience-based descriptions.

WRAP has not been targeted at or developed in the context of dementia, but as an established model with an extensive body of experience gathered over 20 years it is a viable candidate from which to develop an illness-specific approach to self-management in dementia. A way forward would be to consider how to customize this self-management planning tool in the context of the similarities and differences between working-age adult mental health needs and those of older people with dementia. Some principles are held in common and others would require modification in the light of different needs profiles: especially the routine involvement of family and other supporters, progressive deterioration, loss of memory, and loss of capacity as a result of the neurodegenerative nature of dementia. In particular, this self-management tool must engage with the potential challenges faced by people with dementia around future planning for loss of capacity and end-of-life care, but yet be sensitive enough to be adaptive to change as the dementia progresses (Box 14.3).

Box 14.3 Developing a self-management plan for people with dementia based on the Wellness Recovery Action Plan® (WRAP®)

Features directly applicable

- A daily maintenance plan recording what needs to be done every day for the person to stay well
- A record of personal experience of what people have found works best for them
- A person-centred written plan prompting and reminding people of their options and preferences
- A structured plan describing different actions to be taken in response to successive levels of symptomatic difficulty or disability
- A 'crisis plan' or advanced statement describing personal preferences when needing others to act on the person's behalf

Differences to account for

- WRAP is characteristically developed in a group context supported by peers
- Peer experience and shared learning will be substituted by practitioners
- Shared ownership of plan with family and other carers
- An emphasis on supports for preservation of personal identity
- Combined planning for physical and mental health needs
- Routine inclusion in advance statement of enduring powers of attorney
- Fluctuations in health are set against progressive deterioration rather than episodic remission
- Eventual and permanent loss of capacity

Concerns and Limitations in Promoting Self-Management in Dementia

Some critics of recovery have worried that promoting self-management can be used as a way of cutting services for people with complex needs.[35] This criticism is likely to be unfounded in dementia care because individuals will need considerable help and support in completing and maintaining self-management plans, especially as their dementia progresses. The use and ownership of self-management plans is likely to shift over time and the responsibility for working with the plan will devolve to the people around the person with dementia when capacity is diminished. However, this can be seen as a way to sustain an awareness of personal preferences and positively link the person with dementia with various supports around them in terms of family, the third sector, mental health services, general practitioners, and care agencies. A well-formulated and regularly updated self-management plan can be used as a vehicle to support communication and an opportunity to learn continuously from experience about what an individual finds useful to enhance their well-being, particularly as the dementia progresses.

The contents of self-management plans constructed in adult mental health settings are constantly modified in the light of changing experiences of mental health and what people find works best for them. In adult services, self-management plans are typically constrained by an expectation that mental health problems will be episodic and when crises occur they will eventually resolve, with the opportunity to learn from that experience how best to avoid or cope with recurrence (i.e. 'post-crisis planning' in WRAP parlance). There is a hope, supported by a growing evidence base,[31, 36] that successful self-management will be accompanied by increasing stability, health, and well-being, and reduced use of services, particularly owing to unforeseen crises. Self-management planning with people with dementia means working with a different set of expectations and needs to be modified to account for success being defined as having the ability to live well with a deteriorating condition. However, within this declining condition there will be many fluctuations, and seeking to learn what modifies such changes and what choices can be made to optimize health and reduce symptoms are all potential benefits.

When considering using a self-management approach with someone who has dementia, it is important to consider the individual's complex and changing relationship with their condition and what coping strategies people may wish to use in accommodating a progressive illness. In the context of early psychosis, McGorry framed this as 'avoid adding insight to injury', which may be an equally applicable concern in early dementia.[37] At the time of assessment, an individual may not have insight into their condition and be minimizing or denying the extent of their difficulties. This makes giving a potential diagnosis very difficult, especially as the person's denial may preclude them from receiving medical or psychosocial interventions. Their capacity towards self-management and care will therefore be compromised if it depends on an understanding and acceptance of a diagnosis, but may still be possible if people are able to acknowledge difficulties and needs. It also raises the possibility of developing self-management strategies with carers to optimize their health as well as offering them a structure and rationale for actions and decisions made on behalf of others. These issues highlight the importance of gaining informed consent before assessment and the value of pre- and post-diagnostic counselling.

Adapting self-management to the needs of dementia also raises the issue of end-of-life care. The person with dementia may not be prepared to think about the end stages, but there needs to be some recognition that delaying consideration of this may mean that they lose mental capacity before it is discussed in a meaningful way. In these circumstances the person's wishes may not have been considered and family members may have to make difficult decisions about nursing care and end-of-life choices on their behalf. Introducing a self-management plan may be a way of broaching these sensitive and life-changing issues at a time that is right for the person.

Conclusions

The prevalence of dementia is set progressively to increase owing to many forces such as diagnostic rates increasing because of early identification in memory clinics and the older adult population growing at a projected rate of 55% over the next 30 years.[38] However, as with other long-term conditions, there may be considerable and currently unexplored potential to support people in optimizing their quality of life through developing structured support for self-management. There has been considerable interest in developing self-management in adult mental healthcare as part of developing recovery-oriented approaches, and there is a timely possibility of learning from approaches such as WRAP and considering how these could be translated and modified to the needs of people with dementia.

Giving people more information about dementia and focusing on strategies to manage memory difficulties and the emotional consequences of the condition may provide valuable gains in enhancing self-efficacy, hope, and control. This approach resonates with numerous government policy initiatives on recovery, person-centred care, inclusion, dementia, co-creating health and long-term care, as well as addressing clinical needs and service demands. There is currently a lack of research indicating whether the application of these principles to a neurodegenerative illness is acceptable or effective and what would need to be included in a self-management plan for people with dementia to optimize its value as a support for 'living well'. However, as dementia services realign to prioritize early diagnosis and intervention services, developing strategies to support self-management could provide a valuable contribution towards interventions aimed at fulfilling the national strategy.

Acknowledgement

For information, the original paper on which this chapter is based was:

Cheffey J, Hill L, Roberts G, Marlow R. Supporting self-management in early dementia: a contribution towards 'living well'? *Adv Psychiatr Treat* 2013; 19: 344–50.

The authors gratefully acknowledge the contribution of Ruth Marlow, who was involved in writing the original article.

References

1. Prince M, Knapp M, Guerchet M, et al. *Dementia UK: Update Second Edition.* King's College London and London School of Economics for Alzheimer's Society, 2014. Last accessed 13th October 2019 via: www.alzheimers.org.uk /sites/default/files/migrate/downloads/de mentia_uk_update.pdf

2. Hill L, Roberts G, Wildgoose J, Perkins R, Hahn S. Recovery and person-centred care in dementia: common purpose, common practice? *Adv Psychiatr Treat* 2010; 16: 288–98.\

3. Royal College of Psychiatrists (RCPsych). *Person-Centred Care: Implications for*

Training in Psychiatry [CR215]. RCPsych Person-Centred Training and Curriculum (PCTC) Scoping Group and the Special Committee on Professional Practice and Ethics, 2018. Last accessed on 9 September 2019 via: www.rcpsych.ac.uk/d ocs/default-source/improving-care/better-mh-policy/college-reports/college-report-cr215.pdf?sfvrsn=7863b905_2.

4. Dept of Health. *Prime Minister's Challenge on Dementia 2020*. London: Department of Health, 2015. Last accessed on 13 September 2019 via: www.gov.uk/gov ernment/publications/prime-ministers-challenge-on-dementia-2020

5. Kitwood T. *Dementia Reconsidered: The Person Comes First*. Open University Press, 1997.

6. Kitwood T. Positive long-term changes in dementia: some preliminary observations. *J of Mental Health* 1995; **4**: 133–44.

7. Department of Health. *No Health Without Mental Health: A Cross-government Mental Health Outcomes Strategy for People of All Ages*. HM Government, 2011.

8. Antony W. (1993) Recovery from mental illness: the guiding vision of the mental health service system in the 1990s. *Psychosoc Rehabil J* 1993; **16**: 11–23.

9. Daley S, Newton D, Slade M, Murray J, Banerjee S. Development of a framework for recovery in older people with mental disorder. *Int J Geriatric Psychiatry* 2013; **28**: 522–9.

10. Repper J, Perkins R. *Social Inclusion and Recovery*. Ballière Tindall, 2003.

11. Shepherd G, Boardman J, Slade M. *Making Recovery a Reality*. Sainsbury Centre for Mental Health, 2008.

12. Social Care Institute for Excellence (SCIE). *Assessing the Mental Health Needs of Older People (Adults' Services: SCIE Guide 03)*. SCIE, 2006.

13. Elwyn G. Salzburg statement on shared decision making. Salzburg Global Seminar. *BMJ* 2011; **342**: d1745.

14. Department of Health. *Independence, Choice and Risk: A Guide to Best Practice in Supported Decision Making*. Department of Health, 2007.

15. Alakeson V, Perkins R. *Recovery, Personalisation and Personal Budgets*. Centre for Mental Health, 2012.

16. Baker E, Fee J, Bovingdon L, et al. From taking to using medication: recovery-focused prescribing and medicines management. *Adv Psychiatr Treat* 2013; **19**: 2–10.

17. Department of Health. *Self Care – A Real Choice. Self Care Support – A Practical Option*. Department of Health, 2005.

18. Department of Health. *Our Health, Our Care, Our Say. A New Direction for Community Services (White Paper)*. The Stationery Office, 2006.

19. Department of Health. *Supporting People with Long-term Conditions to Self Care: A Guide to Developing Local Strategies and Good Practice*. The Stationery Office, 2006.

20. Expert Patients Programme, Community Interest Company. *Self Care Reduces Costs and Improves Health – The Evidence*. Expert Patients Programme, 2010.

21. Expert Patients Programme, Community Interest Company. *Healthy Lives Equalling Healthy Communities – The Social Impact of Selfmanagement*. Expert Patients Programme, 2011.

22. Barlow J, Wright C, Sheasby J, Turner A, Hainsworth J. Self-management approaches for people with chronic conditions: a review. *Patient Educ Couns* 2002; **48**: 177–87.

23. Jonker AAGC, Comijs HC, Knipscheer KC, Deeg DJ. Promotion of self-management in vulnerable older people: a narrative literature review of outcomes of the chronic disease self-management program (CDSMP). *Eur J Ageing* 2009; **6**: 303–14.

24. Mountain GA. Self-management for people with early dementia: an exploration of concepts and supporting evidence. *Dementia* 2006; **5**: 429–46.

25. Mountain GA, Craig CL. What should be in a self-management programme for people with early dementia? *Aging Ment Health* 2012; **16**: 576–583.

26. Reid MC, Papaleontiou M, Ong A, et al. Self-management strategies to reduce pain and improve function among older adults in community settings: a review of the evidence. *Pain Med* 2008; **9**: 409–24.

27. Laakkonen ML, Kautiainen H, Holtta E, et al. Effects of self-management groups for people with dementia and their spouses – randomized controlled trial. *J Am Geriatr Soc* 2016; **64**:752–760.

28. Craig C. Journeying through dementia: an occupational approach to supported self-management 2017. www.journeyingthroughdementia.com (accessed 18th March 2019).

29. Department of Health. *Living Well with Dementia: A National Dementia Strategy.* Department of Health, 2009.

30. Slade M. *100 Ways to Support Recovery: A Guide for Mental Health Professionals.* Rethink Recovery Series: Volume 1. Rethink, 2009.

31. Substance Abuse and Mental Health Services Administration (2010) *Wellness Recovery Action Plan.* SAMHSA's National Registry of Evidence-based Programs and Practices (http://nrepp.samhsa.gov/ViewIntervention.aspx?id=208). Accessed 13 March 2013.

32. Perkins R, Rinaldi M. *Taking Back Control: Planning Your Own Recovery.* South West London and St George's Mental Health NHS Trust, 2007.

33. Copeland ME, McKay M. *The Depression Workbook: A Guide for Living with Depression and Manic Depression.* New Harbinger Publications, 1992.

34. Leamy M, Bird V, Le Boutillier C, Williams J, Slade M. Conceptual framework for personal recovery in mental health: systematic review and narrative synthesis. *Br J Psychiatry* 2011; **199**: 445–52.

35. Mind. *Life and Times of a Supermodel: The Recovery Paradigm for Mental Health. MindThink Report 3.* Mind, 2008.

36. Health Foundation. *Evidence: Helping People Help Themselves.* Health Foundation, 2011.

37. McGorry PD. The concept of recovery and secondary prevention in psychotic disorders. *Aust N Z J Psychiatry* 1992; **26**: 3–17.

38. Office for National Statistics (ONS). *National Population Projections: 2016-based Statistical Bulletin.* ONS, 2016.

Chapter 15

What Can Person-Centred Care in Dementia Learn from the Recovery Movement?

Laura Hill, Glenn Roberts and Rachel Perkins

Introduction

This chapter explores the concept of 'recovery' and its applicability to older people with mental health problems and specifically those with dementia. A previous paper noted the complementarity, shared values and convergent evolution of recovery-focused and person-centred approaches in adult and older adult care and the considerable opportunity to learn from one another.[1] This chapter revisits the development, similarities and differences in these values-led approaches and the further developments that have arisen in the last 10 years. We propose that there continues to be a fertile and mutually supportive opportunity to share inspiration and practice. Some readers may be very familiar with this emphasis and the approach we outline and feel we are 'stating the obvious' concerning practice that is already established. We wish this were the case, but when we look beyond assent to theory, seeking well-established practice and positive outcomes, we note these philosophies still have a good way to go before they are enshrined as common practice and universally available to those who need them.

What Do We Mean by Recovery?

Recovery can ordinarily be described as 'to return to a normal state of health, mind or strength', but ideas about recovery in mental health are not viewed in terms of 'getting better' and 'cure'. In mental health care, 'recovery' has come to have a different meaning which is less about clinical perspectives on 'recovering from an illness' and more about personal perspectives on 'recovering a life'.[2] The roots of this movement in psychiatry have been traced back to humanistic philosophers, social activists and compassionate clinicians over the past couple of hundred years,[3] with a central emphasis on learning from the testimony of individuals describing their own experiences of adversity and recovery.[4]

The definition by Anthony has become widely accepted in mental health.[5] He described recovery as 'a way of living a satisfying, hopeful and contributing life even within the limitations caused by illness . . . a deeply personal and unique process'. He said,

recovery involves the development of new meaning and purpose in one's life as one grows beyond the catastrophic effects of illness. . . . Successful recovery from a catastrophe does not change the fact that the experience has occurred, that the effects are still present, and that one's life has changed forever. Successful recovery does mean that the person has changed, and that the meaning of these facts to the person has therefore changed.

This redefinition of recovery has opened opportunities for people previously seen as suffering from severe mental illness to enter an open-ended process of seeking to discover how best to live well, even in the context of continuing symptoms and disabilities.

Until relatively recently ideas about recovery have typically focused on younger adults. The term 'recovery' is used much less frequently in mental health services for older adults and rarely with dementia. Woods has argued that the applicability of concepts of recovery to older people with functional mental health problems is clear, but at first sight ideas about 'recovery' may seem incompatible with a progressive and ultimately fatal condition such as dementia.[6] There are reasonable concerns that using the term 'recovery' will generate unrealistic expectations in dementia. There are worries it might give credence to unlicensed remedies of dubious provenance offering cure and negate the devastating consequences of the condition. It can provoke confusion or frustration from clinicians, patients and relatives when taken at face value. Yet there are many who believe the fundamental principles in recovery of hope, choice and opportunity are equally applicable to dementia care:

Even for conditions where there is as yet no cure, as with dementia, improvements in care and treatment are achievable and can make a significant difference to older people's quality of life . . . 'Recovery' and well-being approaches to mental health issues developed by younger adult service users and working-age mental health services are equally applicable to older people. 'Recovery' does not imply 'cure', but builds on the personal strengths and resilience of an individual 'to recover optimum quality of life and have satisfaction with life in disconnected circumstances'. Recovery is about the development of coping skills, and about social inclusion, making it possible for people to have quality of life and a degree of independence and choice, even those with the most enduring and disabling conditions.[7]

The Parallels Between Person-Centred Care and 'Recovery'

Person-centred care (PCC) is an approach which focuses on the needs of the person in the context of their life experience. It is liked, accepted and understood by old age practitioners and the majority find it a useful guiding framework when supporting older adults with mental health difficulties. It has origins in client-centred therapy and was described by Rogers as '. . .the releasing of an already existing capacity in a potentially competent individual'.[8] Kitwood built on this understanding when he used the term person-centred in the context of dementia, applying the values and principles of humanistic psychotherapy to dementia.[9]

'Recovery-focused practice' (RFP) may be a less familiar concept to clinicians but there are striking similarities between it and a person-centred approach.

As Table 15.1 illustrates, both approaches are fundamentally about a set of values related to human living, applied to the pursuit of health and wellness. There is a strong emphasis on holistic care which is individualized and responsive to people's needs, values and wishes. There is an expectation that people are treated with respect, dignity and compassion, and that they are genuinely involved in their care and treatment so that their strengths can be supported and goals can be identified and achieved. Both PCC and recovery would strongly endorse the emerging emphasis across the whole of health care on 'personalization' and are being widely adopted by health and social care services as a support for hope, purpose and direction for future services.

The similarities offer common ground and a common purpose for clinicians working to support people across the age spectrum. The old age practitioner will find value in understanding the recovery approach and those working with younger adults are increasingly looking to the principles of PCC to guide service development. There has been an

Table 15.1 Comparing recovery focused and person-centred approaches

Recovery-focused practice (RFP)	Person-centred care (PCC)
Recovery is fundamentally about a set of values related to human living applied to the pursuit of health and wellness	A value base that asserts the absolute value of all human lives regardless of age or cognitive ability
The helping relationship between clinicians and patients moves away from being expert/patient to being 'coaches' or 'partners' on a journey of discovery	The need to move beyond a focus on technical competence and to engage in authentic humanistic caring practices that embrace all forms of knowing and acting, in order to promote choice and partnership in care decision-making
Recovery is closely associated with social inclusion and being able to take on meaningful and satisfying roles in society	People with dementia need an enriched environment which both compensates for their impairment and fosters opportunities for personal growth
People do not recover in isolation. Family and other supporters are often crucial to recovery and should be included as partners wherever possible	Recognizes that all human life, including that of people with dementia, is grounded in relationships
Recovery approaches give positive value to cultural, religious, sexual and other forms of diversity as resources and supports for well-being and identity	An individualized approach – valuing uniqueness. Accepting differences in culture, gender, temperament, lifestyle, outlook, beliefs, values, commitments, taste and interests

Hill L, Roberts G, Wildgoose J, Perkins R, Hahn S. Recovery and person-centred care in dementia: common purpose, common practice? *Adv Psychiatr Treat* 2010; 16: 288–298.

emergent ambition to reset the whole of psychiatric practice on a foundation of PCC and an aspiration that our training curriculum, across all specialities, is revised accordingly such that it supports forms of practice that are 'values-led, person centred and recovery focused'.[10] It would seem the language describing the underlying principles can be used relatively interchangeably, but it is inaccurate to assume PCC and recovery are identical. PCC has evolved as, and remains, a professional-led approach to care. Recovery is about the individual's personal experience, but those in professional roles can adopt a stance that attempts to support this journey of recovery for the individual – RFP. Despite different origins, the values described by Kitwood and those of a recovery approach invite clinicians to consider what is useful and necessary to support an individual on their journey through ill health. Atul Gawande, a US surgeon, captures this in his book *Being Mortal* where he battles with the ethical dilemma of medicine endlessly striving for cure at the expense of the individual's quality of life.[11] In the fourth of his 2014 Reith Lectures, 'The Future of Medicine', he said:

We think our job is to ensure health and survival. But really it is larger than that. It is to enable well-being – and well-being is ultimately about *sustaining the reasons one wishes to be alive*...[12]

Key Aspects of Recovery with Implications for Person-Centred Care

Issues of Identity

The process of sustaining or developing a sense of self separate from the diagnosis and establishing a positive sense of personal identity is central to both RFP and PCC. There is a characteristic risk in severe illness and disabilities of all kinds that diagnosis eclipses an awareness of the person who has the problem in a context, providing an alternate and defining identity.

Kitwood has described being appalled by the misleading image of dementia as 'death that leaves the body behind' and the negative discourse used to describe people with dementia such as 'victims', 'dements' or 'elderly mentally infirm'.[9] He stated the time had come to recognize men and women with dementia in their full humanity describing the frame of reference as 'PERSON-with-dementia' rather than 'person-with-DEMENTIA'. National charities have followed this lead, highlighting the importance of upholding an emphasis on the person rather than the disease to reduce the stigma experienced by so many. The Alzheimer's Society was previously known as the Alzheimer's Disease Society until 1999 when members voted to change the name.

Specific work exploring recovery in older people has also recognized the importance of identity. Daley et al performed 'grounded theory analysis' on interview data from people with dementia and other mental health problems to build a bottom-up framework for understanding the process of recovering a life with a diagnosis of dementia.[13] They found recovery was connected to the extent to which the pre-existing sense of identity could be maintained or regained, that is, the experience of 'continuing to be me', which is integral to living well with dementia.[14]

Gaining or sustaining a secure sense of the identity of the people who become patients is potently supported by narrative approaches that are common to both recovery and PCC. Stories convey meaning, worries, hopes and ambitions and emphasize the importance of the individual journey of recovery. They form the foundation of reminiscence work, which is hugely valued by those working with people with dementia particularly as the illness progresses. Too often it has been assumed that people with dementia cannot speak for themselves but increasingly vocal groups of people with dementia have begun to emerge. Many of them have come together in the Dementia Engagement and Empowerment Project, which is discussed in greater detail towards the end of this chapter. People in prominent public positions have also challenged stigma, emphasized their own identity and raised awareness of mental health difficulties and diagnoses, for example popular author Terry Pratchett, best known for his satirical Discworld novels, disclosed his diagnosis of posterior cortical atrophy (PCA) in 2007.

Social Exclusion and the Need for Inclusion

No man is an island, entire of itself; every man is a piece of the continent, a part of the main. If a clod be washed away by the sea, Europe is the less, as well as if a promontory were, as well as if a manor of thy friend's or of thine own were. Any man's death diminishes me, because I am involved in mankind; and therefore never send to know for whom the bell tolls; it tolls for thee.

John Donne 1623, Meditation XVII, From Devotions upon Emergent Occasions

Donne's iconic observation concerning our essential interconnectedness arose following his recovery from a time of severe illness which he thought he would not survive and which was accompanied by a painful sense of separation from his fellow man. This finds rich resonance in contemporary concerns over social inclusion and end-of-life care such as pioneered by the hospice movement, and the startling finding that many people with 'severe mental illness' consider their experience of social exclusion as worse than the struggles associated with their diagnosed condition.[15]

Traditional approaches to illness and treatment are almost exclusively focused on individual clinical variables such as symptom changes in response to drug or psychotherapeutic treatment, and virtually the whole of what we regard as 'evidence' is individualistic. In contrast both recovery and PCC reemphasize contextual and relational issues. Kitwood[9] shares with Anthony[5] advocacy for the central significance of a core emphasis on 'personhood', defining it as 'a standing of status that is bestowed upon one human being, by others, in the context of relationship and social being. It implies recognition, respect and trust.' He acknowledged the particular difficulties in dementia care where declining mental powers challenge interconnectedness.

Involvement in local communities rather than segregated services is central to the recovery philosophy. Traditionally, people with severe mental illness were segregated, excluded and isolated. There has been increasing popular recognition that human connection and disconnection may be core mediating influences in the experience and outcome of illness and health. Participating in valued activities provides opportunity for social contact that is central to the health and well-being of people living with dementia. Perkins described a number of initiatives developed to reduce loneliness and isolation:[14]

- Individual or one-to-one interventions such as befriending and mentoring.
- Group services and networks – day centres, lunch clubs, dementia cafés, self-help groups.
- Wider community engagement including a range of initiatives to increase participation in existing activities such as sport, libraries and museums.

The capacity to maintain connection to patterns of ordinary living, suitably customized to the extraordinary needs of people struggling with severe mental health challenges, may be a major mediator of 'living well'.

Many alternative care settings based on the principles of PCC and recovery offer hope and potential for ordinary living in mainstream housing or suitable non-stigmatizing but supportive accommodation. There are national and international examples of specific housing for people with dementia and there is a drive to support people with dementia to remain living in their own homes with the community adapting to support them. Dementia-friendly communities encompass this ideal.[16] There are five domains which need to be addressed as part of developing a dementia friendly community:

- The physical environment (how easy it is and finding your way around)
- The attitudes of the people with whom those living with a diagnosis of dementia come into contact
- The resources available for support (formal and volunteer)
- The networks (friends, relatives, neighbours, community leaders, local businesses)
- The person with dementia and the message that *it is possible* to live well with dementia

Opportunities for Co-working

Recovery approaches recontextualize professional helpers as mentors, coaches, supporters, advocates and ambassadors with an operational stance of being 'on tap not on top'.[17] This shift towards co-working is mirrored in PCC where clinicians attempt respectfully to understand the world from the perspective of the person with dementia. Both approaches ensure the person is at the centre of decisions about their support and treatment, promoting choice and partnership. The National Institute for Health and Care Excellence is preparing guidance on shared decision-making reflecting the importance of this across all of healthcare.[18] There has also been specific work looking at shared decision-making in dementia which showed that doctors nominated people with dementia as the decision-maker in memory clinic consultations regardless of cognitive impairment.[19] Nevertheless, there was evidence in the same study that medication was often prescribed in the face of up to 80% of patients passively resisting treatment, which suggests further work is needed in this area.

The issue and experience of diagnosis has been a particularly problematic concern from a recovery perspective and there has been much debate about the 'delivery' of dementia diagnoses. Person-centred and recovery approaches emphasize the importance of understanding the individual's perspective and adapting the delivery accordingly. There are some people whose preference is not to receive the diagnosis or have their personal mental health struggles languaged in medical terminology. Others seek an early diagnosis which facilitates future planning and enables people truly to participate in decisions about their care and treatment. Unfortunately, the delivery of the diagnosis and prevailing message is frequently pessimistic. A diagnosis of dementia can be devastating and it is not surprising that many people feel hopeless and inclined to give up on themselves and their opportunities. Recovery approaches, driven by people with dementia and their families, can change this narrative. Central and North West London NHS Foundation Trust have captured this with a collection of personal accounts from people living with dementia.[20] They acknowledge the challenge of a dementia diagnosis but show how it is possible to grow beyond the diagnosis and continue to live a meaningful and valued life as part of family and community. They state: *'Life changes, but life goes on. . .and that life can be a good life.'*

The co-working role is equally applicable for informal carers who almost universally struggle with their altered experiences and expectations. Family carers may become overprotective because of the history of their relationship with the person, but frequently it is only they who understand the person and retain an awareness of their life and story. Relatives and people close to the person have a central role in enabling their loved one with the diagnosis to preserve a positive sense of identity beyond that of 'dementia'. In the early stages of dementia individuals are able to take personal responsibility for managing their illness and work out coping strategies, but as the dementia progresses, carers are able to reinforce a sense of personal identity through continuity and ensure that recovery continues to take place; that is, that the person is able to 'continue to be me' as illustrated in Figure 15.1.[13]

It is vital to acknowledge the huge role relatives, carers and friends have in supporting their loved one and to appreciate how devastating it can be when the person with dementia is verbally or physically abusive or no longer recognizes them. These 'supporters' have their own journey of recovery. This is a repairing process of mind, spirit and relationship with the person with the diagnosis. The interconnectedness is essential for all involved. So although each individual, whether 'patient' or 'carer', needs to 'recover', there will also be a 'family journey of recovery'.

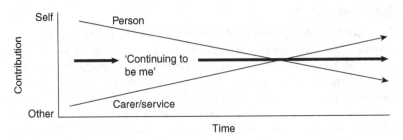

Figure 15.1 Continuing to be me (from [13] with permission)

The Value of Peer Support

Peer supportive relationships between people with lived experience of mental health problems and services are fundamental in recovery. Talking with others who have faced similar challenges and experiences can be empowering. It can enable people to feel less alone and work out ways of dealing with difficulties. Importantly, these contacts also foster images of hope and possibility. Many services now offer peer support workers (PSWs) with lived experience of dementia. This is of great benefit to those who use services:

Talking to someone who really understands makes me realize I am not alone.
   I no longer feel isolated and alone. I have made many new friends, including many who support me, and of course, others with dementia. We are a great bunch of people. [21]

Additionally, it can be a fulfilling, affirming experience for those working in these roles:

I volunteer as a peer-support worker at the memory service. I was very, very pleased, it lifted me up tremendously, knowing that I was some value and that I was going to be useful (www .mentalhealth.org.uk/stories/patricias-story-if-you-think-old-you-will-be-old-if-you-think-young-youll-stay-young).

There are many examples of peer support including sharing stories, e-based peer support and a range of groups and networks. There are now more than 40 Recovery Colleges in the UK and many include courses co-produced and run by professionals and people with dementia. Cheffey et al. explored some of these issues in a co-produced course with a person with dementia, a carer, a psychiatrist and a psychologist, and demonstrated that though there are challenges when working with someone with significant short-term memory problems, these are far outweighed by the rewards. [22]

Empowerment of Self-Management

There is increasingly recognition that self-management can reduce severity of symptoms and improve life control and satisfaction. Personal recovery is often described as pivoting upon people discovering agency and opportunity to make choices on the basis of 'what works for me' and recovery approaches place great value on all aspects of self-management. One of the most widely accepted and utilized tools in mental health for younger adults is the Wellness Recovery Action Plan or WRAP, [23] a structured framework for coping with mental illness. This can be easily adapted for people with mild cognitive impairment and dementia, with an increasingly collaborative approach with family and friends as the illness progresses to ensure people can 'continue to be me' (see Chapter 14 for fuller discussion of WRAP). There is evidence for the use of self-management techniques for people with mild cognitive impairment [24] and those with early dementia [25], and it is likely there will be increasing growth in this area over the coming years.

The Challenge of Putting Principles into Practice

There are many challenges for practitioners in applying principles of PCC and RFP particularly at the further end of morbidity and disability. There are also very positive implications for practitioners themselves. Both approaches carry reminders and recognition that practitioners are people too and that their well-being, morale, creativity, optimism and hope may be key mediators in their capacity to offer such forms of practice. Good practice therefore includes appropriate care for the practitioners too, for you cannot give what you do not have.[26]

Maintaining Hope

The reality of both severe mental illness and progressive dementia are often such as to defeat hope. Holding hope for cure in such circumstances may be naïve or mistaken. However, those trying to uphold recovery or person-centred values will hope to sustain a personal perspective on living well for all those they support.

Alzheimer's disease and other dementias are progressive disorders which will decline regardless of quality of care. The inevitability of this decline can be very difficult for those providing support; but developing an awareness of recovery principles can enable clinicians to be more in tune with the experiential reality of living with dementia. They can become more intimately connected with the person and the changing realities of their existence leading to genuinely PCC. They can also get alongside carers, understanding their feelings of sadness and despair, prompting more rewarding conversations. The paradox of RFP and PCC is to value the enhanced sense of intimacy that such personal approaches permit so as to remain in touch with the losses and face the full tragedy of the illness but find hope and sustenance in the quality of the interaction and connection. In contrast with the prevalent and pessimistic preoccupation centred on loss and deterioration these approaches uphold the aspiration that people may 'live as well as they are able' until they die.

Transforming Risk Management to Safety Planning

Responding to risk is of central significance to all forms of psychiatric practice and how we respond has long-term implications for people's experience of services and quality of life. Historically, psychiatry has mirrored dominant social trends in being characterized as 'risk averse' and it has been a sobering consideration that the limitations we impose on people's lives, apparently for their own good, may also have been accompanied by adverse consequences which are experienced as an impediment to their recovery.

Recovery-focused approaches have regarded changing how we approach risk as a major mediator of well-being and, whilst reasserting the need to assess risk carefully, have suggested that profession-centred risk management can be creatively and constructively transformed into collaborative person-centred safety planning.[27] This is at an early stage of implementation in adult and forensic services but could also have major implications for older adult care.

Paradoxically, there may be circumstances where a high degree of restriction is more supportive of recovery, for example, technological advances such as electronic tagging for people with dementia. This has provoked much debate but potentially offers the individual greater freedom, independence and dignity, and reduces the worry of carers.

It is also important to consider whether distress or disruptive behaviour is a form of communication. In advanced dementia people may be unable to express their wishes verbally and 'dementia care mapping' offers an approach to enabling others to understand what a person is trying to communicate.[28] The information gained can then be used as the basis for person-centred planning (see Chapter 24).

Cultural Shift

Few would argue against recovery and person-centred philosophies in principle, but changing years of ingrained practice poses a challenge to policy advisors, managers and clinicians and there are many organizational, environmental and societal obstacles to navigate. Superficial or tokenistic engagement is a common pitfall, as is the unexamined belief that 'we are doing it already'.

Involving people with mental health problems and dementia is essential in finding a way forward. The Dementia Engagement and Empowerment Project (DEEP) has been instrumental in getting the voice of people with dementia heard.[29] They have been actively involved in lobbying government ministers, talking to the media about dementia and advising on dementia projects. They have produced a number of DEEP guides – some designed for groups or individuals with dementia, others for organizations wanting to work well with people living with dementia. Importantly this is not just about involving people with dementia, it is about providing opportunities for them to shape the agenda and set health, social and political priorities. There is also a need to support people with dementia to continue to contribute as their needs change so that even those with advanced dementia continue to have a voice. One of the primary revisionary processes in both RFP and PCC is a fundamental focus on seeing patients as people, and what's more, *people like me and my family*, as a support for empathic connection and compassionate care.

Conclusion

There has been a long-standing need for a new story. PCC and RFP have occupied very different spheres but the parallel and overlapping developments have led us to observe a curious process of convergent evolution. Both are characterized by increased engagement in more hopeful and compassionate approaches. They are guided by a new narrative strongly focused upon the life experience of the person. They demand a creative, collaborative and self-directed approach which shifts the focus from itemizing deficits to recognizing strengths and possibilities. Equally important is that both resist the endemic depersonalizing and dehumanizing tendency for people to become over-identified with and eclipsed by their diagnoses.

The term 'recovery' remains awkward and uncomfortable in the context of old age psychiatry and the risks of misunderstanding what is intended may make it unhelpful to attempt incorporation without further qualification. Old age practitioners will need to retain an awareness of this, remembering that preferred terms are far less important than the values they support. Rather than use the unqualified term 'recovery', we suggest 'recovering a life' and an overarching emphasis on 'living well with' are more realistic and useful for people with dementia and those trying to support them. Regardless of the need for clarification and exploration of definition and meaning, commitment to the underlying principles has profound implications for what it means to be a patient or practitioner, and for establishing and maintaining the relationship between the two. This is more than 'new practice'. This points towards a paradigm shift, one that has the potential to transform the experience of care, treatment and outcomes, and simultaneously benefit our patients, their families and ourselves as humanistic practitioners.

Acknowledgements

For information, the original paper on which this chapter is based was:

Hill L, Roberts G, Wildgoose J, Perkins R, Hahn S. Recovery and person-centred care in dementia: common purpose, common practice? *Adv Psychiatr Treat* 2010; 16:288–298.

We gratefully acknowledge the contribution of Joanna Wildgoose and Susan Hahn who were involved in writing the original article.

References

1. Hill L, Roberts G, Wildgoose J, Perkins R, Hahn S. Recovery and person-centred care in dementia: common purpose, common practice? *Adv Psychiatr Treat* 2010; **16**: 288–298.

2. Roberts G, Boardman J. Understanding 'recovery'. *Adv Psychiatr Treat* 2013; **19**: 400–409.

3. Davidson L, Rakfeldt J, Strauss J. *The Roots of the Recovery Movement in Psychiatry: Lessons Learned.* Wiley-Blackwell, 2010.

4. Deegan PE. Recovery as a journey of the heart. *Psychiatr Rehabil J* 1996; **19**: 91–97.

5. Anthony WA. Recovery from mental illness: the guiding vision of the mental health service system in the 1990s. *Psychosoc Rehabil J* 1993; **16**: 11–23.

6. Woods R. Recovery: is it relevant to older people? *Signposts* 2007; **12**: 2–3.

7. Social Care Institute for Excellence (SCIE) *Practice Guide 2: Assessing the Mental Health Needs of Older People.* SCIE, 2006.

8. Rogers CR. *Client-Centred Therapy: Its Current Practices, Implications and Theory.* Houghton Mifflin, 1951.

9. Kitwood TM. *Dementia Reconsidered: The Person Comes First.* Open University Press, 1997.

10. PRAXIS. Training in psychiatry: making person-centred care a reality. *BJPsych Bull* 2019; **43**: 136–140.

11. Gawande A. *Being Mortal: Illness, Medicine and What Matters in the End.* Profile Books, 2014.

12. Gawande A. Reith Lectures *The Future of Medicine,* 2014. Last accessed on 4 May 2020 via: www.bbc.co.uk/pro grammes/b04v380z

13. Daley S, Newton D, Slade M, Murray J, Banerjee S. Development of a framework for recovery in older people with mental disorder, *Int J Geriatr Psychiatry* 2013; **28**: 522–529.

14. Perkins R, Hill L, Daley S, Chappell M, Rennison J. 'Continuing to be Me' – Recovering a Life with a Diagnosis of Dementia. *ImROC*, 2016. Last accessed on 23 September 2019 via: https://imroc.org/r esources/12-continuing-recovering-life-diagnosis-dementia/

15. Office of the Deputy Prime Minister. *Mental Health and Social Exclusion.* Social exclusion unit report. ODPM Publications, 2004.

16. Local Government Association and Innovations in Dementia. *Developing Dementia Friendly Communities. Learning and Guidance for Local Authorities,* Local Government Association, 2012.

17. Shepherd G, Boardman J, Slade M. *Making Recovery a Reality*. Sainsbury Centre for Mental Health, 2008.

18. National Institute for Health and Clinical Excellence & Social Care Institute for Clinical Excellence (NICE). *Shared Decision Making*, 2018. Last accessed on 23 September 2019 via: www.nice.org.uk/about/what-we-do/our-programmes/nice-guidance/nice-guidelines/shared-decision-making

19. Dooley J, Bass N, Livingston G, McCabe R. Involving patients with dementia in decisions to initiate treatment: effect on patient acceptance, satisfaction and medication prescription. *Br J Psychiatry* 2019; **214**: 213–217.

20. Harman G, Sims K, Perkins R. *Living Well with Dementia. Life Changes, but Life Goes On. . . and that Life Can Be a Good Life*. Central and North West London NHS Foundation Trust, 2019.

21. Mental Health Foundation. *Still Going Strong*. Mental Health Foundation, 2005.

22. Cheffey J, Hill L, McCullough C, McCullough C. Can I facilitate a project when my memory lets me down? The challenges and rewards of co-producing a 'Living Well with Dementia' course. *Psychology of Older People: FPOP Bull* 2017; **137**: 19–25.

23. Copeland ME. *Wellness Recovery Action Plan*. 1997. Last accessed on 23 September 2019 via: www.mentalhealthrecovery.com

24. The Health Foundation. *Shine 2014 Final Report: A Study of the Use of Self-Management Techniques in Patients with Mild Cognitive Impairment*, Devon Partnership NHS Trust, 2015.

25. Quinn C, Toms G, Jones C, et al. A pilot randomized controlled trial of a self-management group intervention for people with early-stage dementia (The SMART study). *Int Psychogeriatr* 2016; **28**: 787–800.

26. Care Services Improvement Partnership, Royal College of Psychiatrists & Social Care Institute for Excellence (CSIP, RCPsych & SCIE). *A Common Purpose – Recovery in Future Mental Health Services* (Joint Position Paper 08). SCIE, 2007.

27. Boardman J, Roberts G. *Risk, Safety and Recovery*. ImROC, 2014.

28. Bradford Dementia Group. *DCM 8 User's Manual: The DCM Method*, 8th edition. Bradford, University of Bradford, 2005.

29. Litherland R. *Developing a National User Movement of People with Dementia. Learning from the Dementia Engagement and Empowerment Project (DEEP)*. Joseph Roundtree Foundation, 2015.

Psychosocial Interventions in Dementia

Andrew Kiridoshi

Introduction

This article is an update on the overview in *Advances in Psychiatric Treatment* by Patel and colleagues which summarized the evidence base for psychosocial interventions in dementia.[1] Since then there has been a large number of further studies examining the effectiveness of a wide range of non-pharmacological interventions. There has been great interest in exploring novel methods of enhancing the quality of life of people with dementia in recent years, particularly given the increased awareness of the significant harm being caused by the use of antipsychotics to manage the so-called behavioural and psychological symptoms of dementia (BPSD).

The discussion sections of the studies consistently draw attention to the need for greater standardization in measuring the effects of the various interventions. The ability to produce robust evidence has been a persistent issue in this area. Results have proved to be difficult to quantify reliably and 'definitive evidence for the effectiveness of interventions has been lacking'.[2] None the less, the results continue to show that psychosocial interventions are a fruitful area which should continue to be investigated as benefits have been demonstrated for both people with dementia and their carers. With increasing emphasis on supporting carers through the challenges of helping loved ones through the experience of dementia, the aim is to allow people to stay at home in familiar surroundings for as long as possible.

The availability of psychosocial interventions in dementia is gradually improving. As interest in ensuring people are diagnosed earlier and more accurately has grown, the provision of psychosocial interventions has generally lagged behind. While memory clinics have been established throughout the UK in each health locality since 2009, making the initial process of assessment and receiving diagnosis easier, the network of psychosocial support often remains more disorganized and harder to access. However, as the value of these interventions has become increasingly recognized, the quality and variety of psycho-social interventions has improved.

In the post-diagnosis period, psychosocial interventions play an important role in helping people adjust to their new diagnosis, helping to provide strategies to reduce the impact of symptoms of dementia, as well as enhancing remaining cognitive ability and level of functioning.[3] Especially given the limited efficacy of current pharmacological treatments for dementia, there is a pressing need to employ the use of all possible treatments effectively. The key to effective psychosocial interventions is therefore to stimulate the remaining cognitive skills and level of functioning by promoting social participation and relationships, activating creative skills, while retaining meaningful occupations and interests.[4]

Part of the shift in attitude towards managing dementia involves adopting a person-centred approach, whereby the individual's personhood is acknowledged to remain throughout the experience of dementia (see Chapter 24). Following from this, agitation and distress are considered to be forms of expressing unmet need rather than being meaningless 'symptoms' of dementia.

For the purposes of this chapter, a literature search has been completed for psychosocial interventions in dementia, with 285 studies being retrieved. A summary of the findings follows and the various interventions are grouped into creative, sensory, activity-based, psychological, carer-based and environmental categories.

Creative Interventions

Art

Evidence for the effectiveness of art therapy in dementia has gradually increased since the late 1990s, with activities such as painting, making collages and cutting shapes frequently used. Lately there has been greater diversification in the forms of art therapy used and visual arts activities, where people with dementia appreciate works of art in museums, combined with producing art, have shown benefits in terms of expressing feelings, sharing stories through art, and improving people's mental states. Four RCTs have reported 'clinically relevant outcomes in treating behavioural, social, cognitive and emotional problems of dementia patients and their caregivers'.[5]

A systematic review, however, reported 'very low'-quality evidence from 60 participants and found no significant difference in outcome measures between the art therapy group and the control group which carried out 'simple calculation activities' over 12 weeks.[6]

A museum staff education programme in the Netherlands, called 'Unforgettable', was evaluated and it was found that museum staff's attitudes towards people with dementia improved significantly and helped towards participation of people with dementia in the programme.[7]

Reminiscence

Reminiscence therapy is a popular tool used for people with dementia and encourages discussion of past events and life experiences in order to evoke personal memories and stimulate conversation.

A Cochrane systematic review of reminiscence therapy analysed evidence from 1,749 participants and included four large multicentre studies and several smaller studies of reasonable quality. Effects on quality of life, depression, communication, and cognition were found to be small and inconsistent. Individual approaches were associated with improved mood and cognition while group approaches were associated with improved communication.[8] The impact on quality of life was most promising in care home settings. As in other areas, the diversity of approaches in utilizing reminiscence therapy has made direct comparison of studies difficult.

Music/Dance Therapy

Therapies using music, dancing and singing have been incorporated into the schedules of many care homes and hospital wards caring for people with dementia, the basis for this being that recall memory is not an essential part of creativity and, in addition, gaining enjoyment from such activities is beneficial. The communal nature of these activities aims to improve communication and engagement between caregivers and patients. A systematic review of 12 studies demonstrated the efficacy of music therapy in reducing depression, agitation, and anxiety although it commented on the heterogeneity of interventions, methodological designs and evaluation tools.[9]

A meta-analysis incorporating three randomized controlled trials (RCTs) demonstrated sustained improvement in anxiety at three- and six-month follow-up in people with dementia who were anxious and had participated in a programme of music therapy combined with cognitive behavioural therapy.[10] Significant improvements in agitation, aberrant motor behaviour and dysphoria were found in a RCT with 73 participants who had moderate dementia and were care home residents.[11]

Individualized music playlists, which residents in homes (for instance) can listen to via headphones, have become very popular and there is anecdotal evidence that they are effective at decreasing agitation and the use of medication (e.g. see www.playlistforlife.org.uk). In a systematic review using critical synthesis it was shown that playlists of this nature can have a beneficial effect even without a therapist, but the effects were not universally positive, suggesting the need for further research.[12]

Sensory Interventions

Light Therapy

Sleep disorders and disruptive behaviour overnight are commonly associated with dementia. The relatively new concept of the glymphatic system, which acts as a toxic metabolite clearance system in the central nervous system operating predominantly during sleep and inactive during wakefulness, has provided further clues as to the importance of sleep across all biological species. The abnormal deposition of beta-amyloid peptide throughout the brain has been identified as a key component in the pathogenesis of Alzheimer's disease (AD). The fact that beta-amyloid is cleared by the glymphatic system suggests that abnormal sleep may be a risk factor in the development of AD rather than merely a consequence of it.[13] The theory behind light therapy is that in our increasingly digitalized and artificially lit environments our natural circadian rhythms have been disturbed and require to be 'reset'. In bright light therapy a person sits in front of a light box, which emits approximately thirty times more light than an average office light, in order to promote wakefulness during the day and better-quality sleep at night.

In one study with 17 participants, sleep disturbances were improved in patients with AD but not in other forms of dementia.[14] A systematic review of 32 articles found that light therapy has shown mixed results in treating sleep and circadian disturbances in AD although generally the trend was for positive effects and no significant adverse effects.[15]

Aromatherapy

Phytotherapy adopts an empirical approach to the use of medicinal herbs, building on traditional knowledge. Aromatherapy is an important area within phytotherapy and uses essential oils extracted from various organs of aromatic plants that are applied either topically, including with massage, or administered via inhalation. The mechanism of action of aromatic plants is not currently clear. However, the olfactory nervous system, which transmits the aromatic stimulus to the hippocampus, limbic system and amygdala with consequent release of neuromediators, and the early presence of neurofibrillary tangles in the entorhinal cortex in AD suggest a putative link with olfaction.[16] Indeed, early olfactory dysfunction has been associated with a number of neurodegenerative conditions. In one Taiwanese study with 186 participants, aroma-acupressure and aromatherapy were found to be significantly beneficial for agitation in dementia, with aroma-acupressure being superior to aromatherapy alone.[17]

Multisensory Stimulation

Lack of sensory enrichment is a common feature in the lives of people with dementia as they often become passive recipients of care, with limited variation in daily routine, and have co-morbid visual and hearing impairment. The aim of multisensory stimulation is to provide greater diversity of sensory stimulation in a variety of different modalities, without the need for higher cognitive processing. Multisensory rooms have been adopted in settings such as care homes and are typically soothing spaces with relaxing music and lights, and interesting textures to touch. Increased alertness, reduced apathy, positive effects on mood and increased social engagement have been reported following the use of such spaces.[18]

SENSE-Cog is a European, multicentre RCT currently being undertaken with 354 participants who have dementia and visual or hearing impairment which is examining whether a home-based multipart sensory intervention is effective in improving quality of life and other key outcomes (www.sense-cog.eu).

Animal-Assisted Therapy

Animals bring innate pleasure to humans from a very early age and the literature has frequently reported benefits for people with dementia of contact with animals of various sorts. In a study with 19 people with moderate to severe dementia in Germany, significantly increased pleasure and social interaction were reported following a six-month period of weekly group sessions with dogs, compared to a control group.[19] However a systematic review which included six RCTs and four quasi-experimental studies found evidence (albeit of very low certainty) that dog-assisted therapy had no effect on daily life activities, mood, agitation, quality of life or cognitive impairment. One small study in this systematic review found an apparent beneficial effect on apathy.[20]

Activity-Based Interventions

Exercise Therapy

The benefits of exercise appear to be intuitive and there is well-established evidence for the reduction of vascular risk factors generally. Evidence has also been found for increase in hippocampal volume, improved spatial memory, as well as the induction of brain neurotrophic factors in multiple animal studies.

There is conflicting evidence from various recent systematic reviews, however, on the effects of exercise on progression of dementia. The National Institute for Health Research commissioned the Dementia and Physical Activity trial to inform this debate and found that moderate to high intensity aerobic and strength exercise training programmes did not slow the rate of cognitive decline in people with mild to moderate dementia. Improvements in physical fitness were noted but not in any other clinical outcomes.[21] A two-year prospective study is currently being conducted to examine whether long-term exercise programmes prevent the onset of dementia in people at risk over the age of 50.[22]

A meta-analysis including 10 trials and 682 participants found benefits in overall sense of wellbeing for walking programs compared to control groups.[23] A systematic review of 197 studies indicated that medium-to longer-term moderate-to high-intensity exercise improves global physical and cognitive functions as well as skills in activities of daily living.[24]

Individual Activity Programmes

Participating in valued activities, whether for work, leisure or family, is an important aspect of self-identity.[25] As cognitive function declines in dementia, abilities developed over a lifetime also decline contributing to a sense of loss of self. Ensuring that people with dementia continue to find meaning and purpose in their daily life and feel empowered is the key component of individual activity programmes. Depending on the interests and current abilities of the individual, the activity or occupation would vary. A number of studies are currently being undertaken to evaluate the effectiveness of such activities, but no further evidence appears to be available since the previous review, which found weak evidence but undeniable signs of a sense of connection, well-being, belonging, self-autonomy and identity.[1]

Psychological Interventions

Doll Therapy

The use of dolls for people with dementia appears to provide a sense of security and familiarity. An increase in displays of pleasure was found at week three of a RCT involving 35 residents of a care home in Australia. There appeared to be no improvement in anxiety, agitation or aggression compared to the control group.[26] Care home staff's perceived benefits for residents of the doll therapy, however, were of emotional comfort, a calming effect and the provision of a purposeful activity. A reduction in BPSD was found on relevant rating scales as well as in caregiver-related stress in a care home for residents living with severe dementia, suggesting that this is a promising approach.[27]

With improvements in technology there have been advances in the dolls used. PARO robotic seals, for instance, are advanced, interactive, therapeutic animal dolls designed to stimulate people with dementia. Reductions in agitation and medication use have been demonstrated in care home residents, although use of a plush toy had similar effects while providing marginally greater value for money.[28] Considerable variation in responses to the PARO dolls have also been found.[29]

Cognitive Interventions

Many studies on psychosocial interventions focus on cognitive interventions as the results have been generally positive. In terms of the evidence base, there has perhaps been the greatest improvement shown in trials of cognitive interventions since the previous review.[1] This is reflected in cognitive stimulation therapy groups becoming a fairly standard part of post-diagnostic support offered in the UK. Overall, the most recent studies examining the effect of cognitive stimulation therapy and cognitive training have found positive outcomes in improving anxiety, mood, language comprehension, quality of life and carer burden. Cognitive training in conjunction with the use of cholinesterase inhibitors (ChEIs) was found to be significantly better at improving cognition than use of ChEIs alone, as assessed by MMSE scores.[23] Group cognitive stimulation shows consistent positive results for cognitive function, social interaction and integration, as well as quality of life.[24]

Carer-Focused Interventions

In an acknowledgement of the difficulties in caring for a loved one with dementia, there have been a large number of studies examining the ways in which effective support can be offered to carers. A range of different interventions has shown positive effects on carers, including for face-to-face, telephone and group support sessions, with significant improvements, which were sustained at 12 months, in terms of depression, feelings of burden and irritation.[30] Individual multicomponent caregiver therapy has been shown to be effective in reducing feelings of guilt, distress and overload, with group therapy beneficial for guilt and sadness, albeit the evidence has been of a very low grade.[31]

The Meeting Centre Support Programme (MCSP) for people with dementia and their carers was adapted and implemented in Italy, Poland and the UK as part of the MEETINGDEM network launched in 2018. Data were collected both before and after the MCSP. There were no statistically significant differences in terms of competence, mental health, emotional distress or loneliness between the 93 who received the MCSP and the 74 controls who received usual care.[32] In Italy, however, Meeting Centre caregivers showed significantly better general mental health and less caregiver distress. Most of the caregivers said they felt less burdened and more supported by participating in the programme.[32] Inevitably, there was a call for further research. Peer-led discussion is effective in terms of self-efficacy and the ability to manage disturbing symptoms associated with dementia.[33] Focusing on supporting carers of people with dementia appears, potentially, to be a fruitful and highly beneficial psychosocial intervention as a way to reinforce resilience and delay institutionalization.

Environmental Interventions

One way to support people with dementia is to modify the physical environment and architectural features of buildings so as to facilitate engagement with activities, reduce the risk of accidents and optimize level of functioning. In addition to this, the psychosocial environment is important to maintain a sense of self and quality of life. The Dutch dementia village, De Hogeweyk, is a particularly pioneering example of an environmental intervention which provides 24-hour nursing care.[34] It is said that, compared to traditional care facilities, the residents appear to be more active and require less pharmacological intervention. Such a facility would appear to be an ideal environment for those with dementia unable to live at home. A number of other countries, including in the UK, have planned to develop similar villages.

A large systematic review involving 72 studies identified that environmental strategies supported orientation in space, as well as eating and drinking, whereas aspects of self-care such as dressing, toileting and brushing teeth were less supported by environmental changes. Most of the studies in this review, however, looked at overall activity of daily living skills and found that environmental strategies had clear positive effects in assisting people with dementia to perform a range of everyday tasks.[35]

Conclusions

There has been a large number of studies looking at a wide range of psychosocial interventions in dementia in the last five years. Encouraging results have been found in many of these and provide promise for further research and for informing strategies for health authorities and local councils to support people with dementia and their carers. In the interests of optimizing quality of life and to reduce burden on social care systems, this is an area which requires ongoing attention and innovation.

A systematic review of systematic reviews has provided an overview of non-pharmacological interventions in dementia.[36] This identified that the majority of studies showed great variation in how interventions were defined and applied, in the duration of follow-up and in the type of outcomes measured. The modest sample sizes in the studies, in addition to the significant heterogeneity in study design, therefore mean that the results must be viewed with caution. The overall trend in this review, however, provides further evidence for the usefulness of non-pharmacological interventions, particularly for music therapy and behavioural management techniques.

Meanwhile, a systematic review of RCTs has recommended the most appropriate interventions for care homes to implement should include the use of person-centred care, communication skills training and adapted dementia care mapping as these have shown immediate and sustained benefits in reducing agitation.[37] This supports the view that agitation is often an expression of unmet need and frustration caused by impaired communication and function. Adopting an empathic and skilled approach in communication when interacting with people with dementia should therefore not be underestimated in its power and must be a standard requirement for all those involved in providing care.

A further systematic review found that most practices are acceptable, have no harmful effects and require minimal to moderate investment.[38] Given the well-established possible adverse effects from pharmacological interventions and the increasing acceptance that finding meaning in the individual's expression of distress is worthwhile, psychosocial interventions provide the greatest promise in terms of improving the quality of life of people with dementia.

Most studies have drawn attention to the persisting problem of being able reliably to quantify evidence and carry out high-quality studies with large samples. There was a lack of definitive evidence of effectiveness for most interventions and further studies with stronger methodology would strengthen the evidence base. None the less, there is sufficient promise in the benefits from these interventions; and the lack of adverse effects means they should continue to be explored.

Acknowledgement

For information, the original paper on which this chapter is based was:

Patel B, Perera M, Pendleton J, Richman A, Majumdar B. Psychosocial interventions for dementia: from evidence to practice. *Adv Psychiatr Treat* 2014; 20: 340–349.

The author is grateful to Dr Anna Richman, Consultant in Old Age Psychiatry, Mersey Care NHS Foundation Trust, for encouraging him to undertake this piece of work and to her co-authors of the original paper, which inspired the process.

References

1. Patel B, Perera M, Pendleton J, Richman A, Majumdar B. Psychosocial interventions for dementia: from evidence to practice. *Adv Psychiatr Treat* 2014; **20**: 340–349.

2. Clarkson P, Hughes J, Xie C, et al. Overview of systematic reviews: effective home support in dementia care, components and impacts-Stage 1, psychosocial interventions for dementia. *J Adv Nurs* 2017; **73**: 2845–2863.

3. Guss R, Middleton J, Beanland T, et al. *A Guide to Psychosocial Interventions in Early Stages of Dementia*. British Psychological Society, 2014.

4. Innes A, Szymczynska P, Stark C. Dementia diagnosis and post-diagnostic support in Scottish rural communities: experiences of people with dementia and their families. *Dementia* 2012; **13**: 233–247.

5. Chancellor B, Duncan A, Chatterjee A. Art therapy for Alzheimer's disease and other dementias. *J Alzheimer's Dis* 2014; **39**: 1–11.

6. Deshmukh S, Holmes J, Cardno A. Art therapy for people with dementia. *Cochrane Database of Systematic Reviews*. 2018. DOI:10.1002/14651858.CD011073.pub2

7. Hendriks I, Meiland F, Gerritsen D, Dröes R. Implementation and impact of unforgettable: an interactive art program for people with dementia and their caregivers. *Int Psychogeriatr* 2018; **31**: 351–362.

8. Woods B, O'Philbin L, Farrell E, Spector A, Orrell M. Reminiscence therapy for dementia. *Cochrane Database of Systematic Reviews*. 2018. DOI:10.1002/14651858. CD001120.pub3

9. Aleixo M, Santos R, Dourado M. Efficacy of music therapy in the neuropsychiatric symptoms of dementia: systematic review. *J Bras Psiquiatr* 2017; **66**: 52–61.

10. Noone D, Stott J, Aguirre E, Llanfear K, Spector A. Meta-analysis of psychosocial interventions for people with dementia and anxiety or depression. *Aging Ment Health* 2018; **23**: 1282–1291.

11. Ho R, Sing J, Lee P, et al. A music intervention in managing agitation and aberrant motor behaviour among elders with dementia. *Gerontologist* 2016; **56** (Suppl_3): 206–206.

12. Garridoa S, Dunne L, Chang E, et al. The use of music playlists for people with dementia: a critical synthesis. *J Alzheimers Dis* 2017; **60**: 1129–1142.

13. Iliff J. The Glymphatic System in Alzheimer's Disease. Presentation at: Knight Cardiovascular Institute, Oregon. Last accessed on 16 October 2019 via: www.alz.washington.edu/NONMEMBER/FALL15/DIR/Iliff.pdf Also see: Iliff JJ, Chen MJ, Plog BA, et al. Impairment of glymphatic pathway function promotes tau pathology after traumatic brain injury. *J Neurosci* 2014; **34**: 16180–16193. DOI:10.1523/JNEUROSCI.3020-14.2014

14. Sekiguchi H, Iritani S, Fujita K. Bright light therapy for sleep disturbance in dementia is most effective for mild to moderate Alzheimer's type dementia: a case series. *Psychogeriatrics* 2017; **17**: 275–281.

15. Mitolo M, Tonon C, La Morgia C, et al. Effects of light treatment on sleep, cognition, mood, and behavior in Alzheimer's disease: a systematic review. *Dement Geriatr Cogn Disord* 2018; **46**: 371–384.

16. Jimbo D, Inoue M, Taniguchi M, Urakami K. Specific feature of olfactory dysfunction with Alzheimer's disease inspected by the Odor Stick Identification Test. *Psychogeriatrics* 2011; **11**: 196–204.

17. Yang M-H, Lin L-C, Wu S-C, et al. Comparison of the efficacy of aroma-acupressure and aromatherapy for the treatment of dementia-associated agitation. *BMC Complement Altern Med* 2015; **15**: 93. DOI:10.1186/s12906-015-0612-9

18. Jakob A, Collier L. Sensory enrichment for people living with dementia: increasing the benefits of multisensory environments in dementia care through design. *Design Health* 2017; **1**: 115–33.

19. Wesenberg S, Mueller C, Nestmann F, Holthoff-Detto V. Effects of an animal-assisted intervention on social behaviour,

emotions, and behavioural and psychological symptoms in nursing home residents with dementia. *Psychogeriatrics* 2018; **19**: 219–27.

20. Zafra-Tanaka JH, Pacheco-Barrios K, Tellez WA, Taype-Rondan A. Effects of dog-assisted therapy in adults with dementia: a systematic review and meta-analysis. *BMC Psychiatry* 2019; **19**: 41. DOI:10.1186/s12888-018-2009-z

21. Lamb SE, Sheehan B, Atherton N, et al. Dementia and Physical Activity (DAPA) trial of moderate to high intensity exercise training for people with dementia: randomised controlled trial. *Br Med J* 2018; **361**: k1675. DOI:https://doi.org/10.1136/bmj.k1675

22. Iuliano E, di Cagno A, Cristofano A, et al. Physical exercise for prevention of dementia (EPD) study: background, design and methods. *BMC Public Health* 2019; **19**: 659. DOI:10.1186/s12889-019-7027-3

23. Duan Y, Lu L, Chen J, et al. Psychosocial interventions for Alzheimer's disease cognitive symptoms: a Bayesian network meta-analysis. *BMC Geriatr* 2018; **18**: 175. DOI:10.1186/s12877-018-0864-6

24. McDermott O, Charlesworth G, Hogervorst E, et al. Psychosocial interventions for people with dementia: a synthesis of systematic reviews. *Aging Ment Health* 2018; **23**: 393–403.

25. Travers C, MacAndrew M, Hines S, et al. The effectiveness of meaningful occupation interventions for people living with dementia in residential aged care: a systematic review protocol. *JBI Database System Rev Implement Rep* 2015; **13**: 87–99.

26. Moyle W, Murfield J, Jones C, Beattie E, Draper B, Ownsworth T. Can lifelike baby dolls reduce symptoms of anxiety, agitation, or aggression for people with dementia in long-term care? Findings from a pilot randomised controlled trial. *Aging Ment Health* 2019; **23**: 1442–1450.

27. Cantarella A, Borella E, Faggian S, Navuzzi A, De Beni R. Using dolls for therapeutic purposes: a study on nursing home residents with severe dementia. *Int J Geriatr Psychiatry* 2018; **33**: 915–25.

28. Mervin MC, Moyle W, Jones C, et al. The cost-effectiveness of using Paro, a therapeutic robotic seal, to reduce agitation and medication use in dementia: findings from a cluster–randomized controlled trial. *J Am Med Dir Assoc* 2018; **19**: 619–622.e1

29. Moyle W, Jones C, Murfield J, et al. Using a therapeutic companion robot for dementia symptoms in long-term care: reflections from a cluster-RCT. *Aging Ment Health* 2017; **23**: 329–36.

30. Czaja SJ, Lee CC, Perdomo D, et al. Community REACH: an implementation of an evidence-based caregiver program. *Gerontologist* 2018; **58**: e130–7.

31. Brooks D, Fielding E, Beattie E, Edwards H, Hines S. Effectiveness of psychosocial interventions on the psychological health and emotional well-being of family carers of people with dementia following residential care placement. *JBI Database System Rev Implement Rep* 2018; **16**: 1240–68.

32. Evans S, Evans S, Brooker D, et al. The impact of the implementation of the Dutch combined Meeting Centres Support Programme for family caregivers of people with dementia in Italy, Poland and UK. *Aging Ment Health* 2018. https://doi.org/10.1080/13607863.2018.1544207

33. Oliveira D, Orrell M, Radburn J. Health-promoting self-care in family carers of people with dementia. *Alzheimers Dement* 2018; **14**: P1320.

34. Godwin B. Hogewey: a 'home from home' in the Netherlands. *J Dement Care* 2015; **23**: 28–31.

35. Woodbridge R, Sullivan M, Harding E, et al. Use of the physical environment to support everyday activities for people with dementia: a systematic review. *Dementia* 2016; **17**: 533–72.

36. Abraha I, Rimland J, Trotta F, Dell'Aquila G, Cruz-Jentoft A, Petrovic M, et al. Systematic review of systematic reviews of non-pharmacological interventions to treat behavioural

disturbances in older patients with dementia. *The SENATOR-OnTop series. BMJ Open.* 2017; 7(3): e012759.

37. Livingston G, Kelly L, Lewis-Holmes E, Baio G, Morris S, Patel N, et al. Non-pharmacological interventions for agitation in dementia: systematic review of randomised controlled trials. *British Journal of Psychiatry.* 2014; **205**(6): 436–442.

38. Scales K, Zimmerman S, Miller S. Evidence-based nonpharmacological practices to address behavioral and psychological symptoms of dementia. *The Gerontologist.* 2018; **58**(suppl_1): S88–S102.

Palliative Care in Dementia

Issues and Evidence

Julian C Hughes, David Jolley, Alice Jordan and Elizabeth L Sampson

Introduction

Intimations of death often cause symptoms or syndromes of mental or emotional disorder, of which anxiety and depression are the most common.[1] It is entirely appropriate, therefore, for mental health services to be involved with those who care for the dying in whatever setting.[2] Old age psychiatrists have recognized their more direct role in caring for dying patients for many years.[3,4] And some years ago a particular impetus emerged behind the notion of palliative care in dementia.[5,6] This followed the early research by Ladislav Volicer and his colleagues in the dementia special care unit (DSCU) as part of the Geriatrics Research Education and Clinical Center at the E.N. Rogers Memorial Veterans Hospital in Bedford, Massachusetts.[7] Since then there has been a burgeoning both in the field and in the literature.[8] Gradually, different sorts of ways to provide palliative care for people with dementia have also emerged.

In this chapter, an updated version of our earlier paper,[9] before considering particular issues that arise in palliative care in dementia, we shall discuss two immediate questions: (a) In the context of dementia, what is palliative care? (b) Is there a need for improved palliative care in dementia?

What Is Palliative Care?

The World Health Organization (WHO) has provided a useful definition of palliative care (see Box 17.1).[10]

However, a difficult problem emerges in the context of dementia since it is often not seen as a 'life-threatening illness'. We know, for instance, from a recent study in Tasmania that, despite an interest in dementia, when asked what palliative care meant there was relatively little reference made to the relationship between palliative care and dementia.[11] Instead, palliative care was normally thought of as terminal care with more links to cancer. This was even the case for paid and family caregivers of people with dementia.[11]

Box 17.1 WHO (2002) definition of palliative care

Palliative care is an approach that improves the quality of life of patients and their families facing the problems associated with life-threatening illness, through the prevention and relief of suffering by means of early identification and impeccable assessment and treatment of pain and other problems, physical, psychosocial and spiritual.

World Health Organization (2002). *WHO Definition of Palliative Care*. Available via: www.who.int/cancer/palliative/definition/en/ (last accessed 22 October 2019)

> **Box 17.2** The spectrum of palliative care applied to dementia
>
> Palliative care approach – person-centred dementia care
> Palliative interventions – for example, management of BPSD
> Specialist palliative care – complex end-of-life care from symptom control to dealing with ethical issues

Palliative care can be regarded as a spectrum.[12] At one end (see Box 17.2), the palliative care approach equates to good-quality, person-centred dementia care. At the terminal end of the spectrum there may well be a requirement for specialist palliative care (involving more detailed knowledge and skills to do with, for example, pain relief).

In between, palliative interventions (which in cancer care could involve palliative radiotherapy for bone pain) might conceivably comprise the raft of psychosocial and pharmacological approaches used to treat the (so-called) behavioural and psychological symptoms of dementia (BPSD). ('So-called' because (a) these phenomena – agitation, shouting, depression and the like – are perhaps better called 'signs' rather than 'symptoms', because symptoms are things people complain of, rather than things that are observed; and (b) this terminology – 'BPSD' – begs the question whether these signs are signs *of* dementia or signs of the inhospitable and confusing psychosocial environment in which the person finds him or herself. Perhaps a better term than 'BPSD' would be 'distress behaviours' or 'needs-driven behaviours', terms which emphasizes the importance of understanding unmet needs and recognizing that distress behaviours are a sign of unmet need. (See Chapter 24 for examples of this approach.))

One conceptual and practical issue concerns whether these potential components of care in dementia can (and should) be usefully packaged together under the umbrella of 'palliative care'. A pragmatic response might be that if conceptual packaging in this way leads to improvements in patient care, perhaps through advance care planning (ACP), then the enterprise would seem worthwhile.

Is There Evidence That Palliative Care in Dementia Needs Improving?

There is compelling evidence that the care of people with dementia, especially towards the end of their lives, is less than optimal. Retrospective case-note studies have demonstrated inadequate palliative care in both psychiatric and acute hospital wards.[13] Life expectancy is more emphatically curtailed for dementia than it is by other psychiatric syndromes.[14] Yet the evidence for suboptimal care persists, especially in the terminal phase, with studies in the United States and Israel, among others, confirming the somewhat dismal picture.[15,16]

In a retrospective survey of carers in England, McCarthy et al. (1997) reported a host of common symptoms and signs experienced by people with dementia in the last year of life: confusion (83%), urinary incontinence (72%), pain (64%), low mood (61%), constipation (59%) and loss of appetite (57%).[17] The study found similar frequencies of such symptoms in cancer patients, but dementia patients experienced the symptoms for longer. Out of 170 people with dementia, none had died in a hospice.[17] A sensible reaction to this would be to point out that the study is now old. But sadly, despite greater awareness and provision of care, the situation persists for many.

Table 17.1 Morbidity and mortality in nursing home residents with advanced dementia (n = 323)[18]

Condition	Probability (%)	Adjusted 6-month mortality (%)
Pneumonia	41.1	46.7
Fever	52.6	44.5
Eating problem	85.8	38.6

For instance, in a study from the United States published in 2009, involving 323 nursing home residents with advanced dementia, over the course of 18 months 54.8% had died.[18] Morbidity was high too, as shown in Table 17.1.

In addition, distressing symptoms were common: dyspnoea in 46.0% and pain in 39.1%.[18] The authors also reported that in the last three months of life, 40.7% of the residents experienced at least one 'burdensome intervention', such as hospitalization, an emergency room visit, parenteral therapy or tube feeding.[18]

Meanwhile, in a recent nine-month prospective cohort study across London in the UK, out of the 85 people recruited with advanced dementia (79 living in nursing homes and 6 in their own homes), 38% had died by the end of the study.[19] The researchers found some symptoms to be common and persistent, such as pain (in 11% at rest and 61% on movement) and agitation (deemed significant in 54%). Other symptoms, i.e. aspiration (20%), dyspnoea (47%), septicaemia and pneumonia (together 17% at the final study visit), were more frequent in those who died.[19] There was little input from specialist geriatric or mental health teams and while 76% had 'do not resuscitate' statements, fewer than 40% had advance care plans. Other common psychiatric symptoms at the start of the study – depression (36%), anxiety (35%), apathy (53%), motor disturbances (33%) and night-time wakefulness or daytime sleepiness (44%) – persisted throughout, except that depression increased to 42% in those still alive and 48% in those who died, and motor disturbances increased to 48% in those still alive and to 50% among those who died by the end of the nine months.[19]

Over many years, therefore, there has been evidence of significant morbidity and mortality in people living with advanced dementia, as well as evidence of both inadequate treatment and inappropriate interventions.

As an example of an inappropriate intervention, hospitalization of people with advanced dementia is increasingly regarded as unhelpful, if not dangerous. In a prospective study in a London hospital, in 617 people over the age of 70 years consecutively admitted acutely to a medical ward, 75 (12.2%) died.[20] Overall, 42.4% had dementia, with the proportion rising with age to 48.8% of the men and 75% of the women over 90 years old. The people with dementia had higher mortality: of those without dementia, only 7.9% died; whereas over three times as many people with dementia (18%) and five times as many people (24%) with moderate to severe dementia died (MMSE scores of 0–15).[20] These associations remained strong even after controlling for age and severity of acute illness. An interesting reflection on the part of the authors was this:

We cannot judge from our data whether these admissions were necessary, but the high short-term mortality risk in people with dementia suggests that this intervention did not prolong life for a meaningful length of time. Individuals may have received better-quality care in a familiar environment if more support w[ere] available in the community.

Given the evidence of inadequate levels of care in both long-term institutions and hospitals, and given that people with dementia do not seem to access specialist palliative care services, the implication is that there are palliative needs – particularly in the last year of life – not being met.

What Is Palliative Care in Dementia?

At the time of the original paper upon which this chapter is based,[9] there was little evidence that palliative care was efficacious.[21] Things have moved on, a little. In 2010, two papers appeared reviewing the field. First, Sampson suggested that people living with dementia still had 'poor access to good quality end-of-life care'.[22] She continued:

Interventions such as antibiotics, fever management policies and enteral tube feeding remain in use despite little evidence that they improve quality of life or other outcomes.

She recommended more research to identify the effectiveness of 'holistic' palliative care, better outcome measures and the impact of dementia at the end of life on carers and families.[22] Reviewing a decade of research, van der Steen also felt that, despite some encouraging trends, there was little evidence that specific treatments were effective.[23] Studies were starting to report on 'treatment, comfort, symptom burden, and families' satisfaction with care', but most of these studies were small and retrospective.[23] Like Sampson,[22] van der Steen was able to identify emerging guidelines, which supported 'the benefits of advance care planning, continuity of care, family and practitioner education',[23] along with the development of 'assessment tools for pain, prognosis, and family evaluations of care'.[23]

An example of a community initiative in the United States at that time was the PEACE programme, standing for 'Palliative Excellence in Alzheimer Care Efforts'.[24] In a preliminary report, the researchers described how community support from an early stage seemed to have been helpful in terms of pain control, patients' wishes and the choice of place of death.[24] The study in Chicago came to an end, but in December 2018 a new trial – the 'Indiana Palliative Excellence in Alzheimer's Care Efforts (IN-PEACE)' – was registered, involving some of the same team (e.g. Professor Greg Sachs), with the aim of improving 'the care of community dwelling patients with dementia and their family caregivers'.[25]

One of the issues that emerges is that palliative care for people living with dementia is not one thing, but a collection of approaches to deal with different issues, hence Sampson's call for 'holistic' palliative care.[22] A better concept, therefore, might be that of supportive care, which has been at the centre of the PEACE initiative.[26] Supportive care can be characterized as:

... a full mixture of biomedical dementia care, with good quality, person-centred, psychosocial, and spiritual care under the umbrella of holistic palliative care throughout the course of the person's experience of dementia, from diagnosis until death and, for families and close carers, beyond.[27]

The multifaceted nature of the care that is required suggests two things: (a) that, in terms of services, palliative care for people with dementia will require a multidisciplinary team approach where an important function will be sign-posting to the services or resources not immediately available from within the team; and (b) that efficacy will depend on the component parts of the overall service or services. The component parts are becoming increasingly clear.

The Components of Palliative Care for People With Dementia

For instance, following an international conference in the UK in 2007 with 175 attendees and a half-day workshop with 50 participants from a variety of backgrounds, key issues and themes for palliative care in dementia were identified.[28] The main themes were:

- ACP – where raising awareness of ACP and facing practical matters were highlighted;
- Psychological support – both for people with dementia and for close family and friends;
- Managing acute events – by good communication, by care in the community and by sensible responses within hospitals;
- Terminal care – where the issues of identifying death, controlling symptoms, enabling the preferred place of death to be achieved, with attention to problems around decision-making and bereavement were all raised.[28]

A more sophisticated process led to the development of the European Association for Palliative Care's White Paper in 2014.[29] For the first time this defined palliative care in dementia on the basis of research in terms of 11 domains and, grouped into domains, optimal palliative care was defined by a set of 57 recommendations for practice, policy and research. Each recommendation was accompanied by an explanatory text which was based on evidence from the literature, with 265 references to back up the explanations, and by consensus derived through a Delphi study involving experts from across the globe.[29] The 11 domains are shown in Box 17.3.

Whilst these domains represent the views of experts, subsequent research has demonstrated that they are indeed relevant to the concerns of people living with a diagnosis of dementia and to their family carers.[30] One study reported that the domain of 'avoiding overly aggressive, burdensome, or futile treatment' was regarded by experts and family carers as being particularly relevant in the terminal phase, as were recommendations to do with comfort.[31] Families showed a preference for continuity of both care and place of care; but families were chary of the prospect of 'a large team of unfamiliar (professional) caregivers' becoming involved. Meanwhile, the professionals preferred a model in which 'a representative of a well-trained team has the time, authority and necessary expertise to

---

Box 17.3 Domains of optimal palliative care for people with dementia

   i. Applicability of palliative care
  ii. Person-centred care, communication and shared decision-making
 iii. Setting care goals and advance planning
 iv. Continuity of care
  v. Prognostication and timely recognition of dying
 vi. Avoiding overly aggressive, burdensome or futile treatment
vii. Optimal treatment of symptoms and providing comfort
viii. Psychosocial and spiritual support
 ix. Family care and involvement
  x. Education of the healthcare team
 xi. Societal and ethical issues

van der Steen JT, Radbruch L, Hertogh CM, et al. White paper defining optimal palliative care in older people with dementia: a Delphi study and recommendations from the European Association for Palliative Care. *Palliat Med*. 2014; 28: 197–209

> **Box 17.4** Key factors for the delivery of good end-of-life care
>
> i. Timely planning discussions
> ii. Recognition of end-of-life and provision of supportive care
> iii. Co-ordination of care
> iv. Effective working relationships with primary care
> v. Managing hospitalization
> vi. Continuing care after death
> vii. Valuing staff and ongoing learning
>
> Bamford C, Lee RP, McLellan E, et al. What enables good end of life care for people with dementia?
> A multi-method qualitative study with key stakeholders. *BMC Geriatr.* 2018; 18: 302. Available via:
> https://doi.org/10.1186/s12877-018-0983-0 (last accessed 20 October 2019)

provide care and education of staff and family to where people are and which ensure continuity of relationships with and around the patient'.[31]

Research elsewhere has shown tensions around some of the views held by different parties in connection with the domains of the White Paper. Families and people with dementia held different views about the importance of planning for the future.[30] The importance was unclear to people with dementia and seen to have little value, while family carers thought it was of some importance for particular types of plan.[30] Experts meanwhile tended to see advance planning as very important. Families felt poorly equipped to make decisions for their relatives with dementia. A key difference between the professional view and the lay view emerged around the understanding of dementia as a palliative condition.[30]

The same research programme also involved multiple stakeholder groups and an integrative analysis in order to identify key components of good end-of-life care for people with dementia.[32] Using qualitative methodology involving 116 interviews, 12 focus groups and 256 hours of observation, the researchers gathered the views of national experts, service managers, frontline staff, people with dementia and family carers. Analysis demonstrated seven key factors required for the delivery of good end-of-life care for people with dementia, as shown in Box 17.4.

Over time, therefore, and on the basis of several different sorts of study, the components of good-quality palliative care have emerged.

Does It Work?

The difficulty is that we lack definitive evidence to support the use, on any sort of scale, of a particular palliative intervention in dementia. Nevertheless, we can point to a range of interventions that have been tried on a smaller scale. Intuitively, it would seem likely that these would work on a larger scale, but the real question then is whether a particular intervention would be cost effective in comparison with standard care and with other putative palliative interventions. Still, it is worth considering the types of intervention that have been tried, albeit the studies have often been relatively small-scale and lacking in sophisticated economic analysis.

We have already mentioned the early work of Ladislav Volicer. Indeed, 25 years ago his team showed that a DSCU could lower levels of discomfort, lower numbers of transfers to acute medical settings, whilst also lowering costs.[33] In the UK, NHS long-term care units which used to look after people with advanced dementia have tended to close, or have been turned into units offering more specialist care for people with dementia (and occasionally other conditions) and behaviour that is found challenging.[34] There seems to have been little enthusiasm for the notion of hospice in-patient units catering specifically for people with dementia, despite reports of the benefits of such units.[35] Nevertheless, many hospices have started to run outreach or community services for people with dementia (and other non-cancer conditions), providing hospice-at-home and hospice-in-your-care-home services.[36] Some hospices now employ Admiral nurses – specialist dementia care nurses – to provide community end-of-life support.[37] Most of the institutional provision of care for people with advanced dementia now occurs in care homes. The focus on end-of-life (palliative) care in such homes is variable, but there are examples of excellent and innovative practice. For example, some homes have adopted the practice of Namaste Care – an approach which uses multisensory, psychosocial and spiritual components to enable staff in institutional settings 'to provide quality services that are holistic and meet the physical and emotional needs of their residents'[38] – for which an evidence base is emerging.[39]

Ten years ago, in 2009, there were two important small studies in the UK. In the first, Scott and Pace showed that there were unmet palliative care needs, but that '[a] specialist palliative care nurse under consultant supervision can provide an effective symptom control, carer support, and staff education and support service, to enable care to be provided through already existing channels'.[40] At the same time, in another part of London, Treloar and his team were providing a domiciliary service to enable people with dementia to die at home.[41] They demonstrated that good, home-based, multidisciplinary, palliative care for people with dementia could be achieved, but there were 'blockages to accessing support as a result of poor understanding of the needs of advanced dementia care as well as organizational prejudice'.[41] They also showed that bereavement issues could be helped by such a service.

A study from 2016 employed consultations, a consensus survey and three focus groups involving health professionals, the voluntary sector, older people, carers and their representatives to generate recommendations for a short-term integrated palliative and supportive care (SIPS) model.[42] The model was intended to provide 'holistic assessment, opportunity for end of life discussion, symptom management and carer reassurance'.[42] Whilst the older people and carers felt that early use of SIPS would be a good thing, other stakeholders felt that the service should only be used for complex cases. It was agreed that a key worker would be central, but it was not clear what criteria would be used to trigger the use of the key worker. This emphasizes that it is possible to agree on what might constitute a good palliative care service for people with dementia, but difficult to envisage implementation without the necessary resources and surety that the resources would be used efficiently.

At the same time, research from the UK highlighted heuristics (or rules of thumb) that might be used to help practitioners make end-of-life decisions for people with dementia.[43] The study identified four broad areas to do with (i) eating and swallowing difficulties, (ii) agitation and restlessness, (iii) ending life-sustaining treatment and (iv) providing 'routine care' at the end of life.[43] Subsequently, in the United States, a goals of care decision aid was shown to improve communication around end-of-life decisions.[44]

A study in two London nursing homes used an interdisciplinary care leader (ICL) whose role was to scope local practice and identify key people to support end-of-life care.[45] This was partly to ensure the intervention complemented rather than duplicated existing services. The project led to improvements in ACP, pain management and person-centred care. It did not seem to cause any harm and the main cost was the employment of the ICL.[45] One notable aspect was that implementation was different in the two nursing homes, suggesting how difficult it would be to standardize a service without flexibility and that for maximum effectiveness interventions should be adaptable to the local context. We also know that bringing about change in care or nursing homes can be difficult.[46]

Nevertheless, similar programmes in long-term care facilities have been tried in other countries. In Canada, over the course of a year, a study provided usual care in two long-term care facilities and a palliative intervention in two alternative facilities.[47] The intervention had five components:

(1) a training program for physicians and nursing staff;
(2) clinical monitoring of pain using an observational pain scale;
(3) implementation of a regular mouth care routine;
(4) early and systematic communication with families about end-of-life care issues with provision of an information booklet; and
(5) involvement of a nurse facilitator to implement and monitor the intervention.[47]

Using scales that assessed (i) families' perceptions of care and (ii) comfort and symptom management, there were significant improvements brought about by the intervention in comparison to normal care. Once again, it is interesting to note the role of the nurse facilitator.

The research that has accumulated, therefore, suggests that we do know what is required, even if we do not always know the best way to deliver services. In particular, it is obvious that no one type of professional is likely to have all of the answers, so the service has to be multi-professional; but it seems likely (on the basis of evidence and intuition)[31,40,42,45,47] that a useful intervention would be to have someone to co-ordinate care and provide continuity.

Predicting Death in Dementia

In the United States, where Medicare hospice benefit requires a predicted survival of under six months, studies have focused on predictors of death in dementia.[48] Many of the putative predictors have proved inaccurate. Nevertheless, Sachs et al.[49] suggest three markers of severity that at least imply discussions about hospice enrolment might be appropriate: first, Functional Assessment Staging (FAST),[50] where the person is non-ambulatory, has lost meaningful conversation and is dependent for most activities of daily living (i.e. stage 7C), especially when this is combined with complications such as weight loss of 10% or more, recurrent infections and multiple pressure sores; secondly, hip fracture or pneumonia in advanced dementia; and thirdly, the need for artificial feeding.

In the UK context, the *precise* prediction of death is less of an issue, but the need to discuss matters with families is real. The timing of such discussions will be a matter of clinical judgement. For instance, some people with dementia might wish to make advance decisions – about palliative care and where they wish to die – soon after diagnosis.

In any case, the pendulum is swinging away from prognostication as more and more studies have shown how unreliable and difficult it is. Instead, a needs-based approach is becoming more frequently mooted in the literature and supported by public policy. It seems eminently reasonable, if a person has unmet needs, for us to regard it as a duty to meet those needs. If this is true, it will be true at whatever stage the person might be in his or her dementia. A promising approach may be the Integrated Palliative care Outcome Scale for Dementia (IPOS-Dem), which is a needs assessment tool.[51] In initial studies it seems to bring about good effects by: 'improved observation and awareness of residents, collaborative assessment, comprehensive "picture of the person", systematic record keeping, improved review and monitoring, care planning and changes to care provision, and facilitated multi-agency communication'.[52] The tool seemed to improve symptom management, overall care, as well as engagement with and empowerment of families. It was found to be both feasible and acceptable to staff, but this did depend on leadership.[52] Nevertheless, in a complex context – with multiple morbidities and multiple people involved – it was encouraging to note that the intervention seemed to improve standards by improving observations, awareness and communication.

Physical Health in Advanced Dementia

The physical health of people with advanced dementia will need increasing consideration and there are specific symptoms and signs associated with dying.[53, 54] In the final stages of dementia, weight loss, loss of muscle and muscle strength become apparent. In part this reflects reduced food intake, but the degree of weight loss often seems greater than can be explained in this way. It is important to look for treatable causes of this general debility, which may include feeding approaches, in order to avoid deterioration by negligence. Low metabolic rate and physical inactivity can mean that a state of physiological homeostasis obtains, in which the body weight is low but constant; which must then be distinguished from progressive starvation. Even so, people approaching death with dementia can show continued loss of weight and body bulk. At the same time there are potential problems from contractures and skin integrity, which is compromised by poor diet and lack of mobility. Hence, there are requirements for physiotherapy and good nursing interventions.

Similarly, both bladder and bowel function are compromised in advanced dementia. Incontinence of urine is common, which itself threatens skin integrity, causing discomfort. Advice from a continence specialist will often be helpful. Constipation, which can sometimes lead to impaction or overflow incontinence, can occur when the diet or fluid intake are poor, or when medication slows bowel transit times. Immobility and reduced awareness of the call to stool make matters worse. Constipation itself impedes bladder function. Discomfort, pain or toxicity can follow. The person may become more confused or more agitated. A common sign of constipation is the tendency to lean to the side. Vigilance and prophylaxis, with good nursing observations and medical review, will help to avoid the worst consequences of both incontinence and constipation.[53]

Pain

There has been and is considerable concern that people with severe dementia might be in pain that is neither detected nor adequately treated. For some years great efforts have been made to develop an observation tool that would detect pain in people who were otherwise unable to communicate their feelings. Gradually, the psychometric properties of these measures have been established, although they all tend to be deficient in one respect or another.[55] Nevertheless, they are useful in helping to alert people to the possibility of pain (they make staff take a step back and really LOOK at the patient and THINK about them), they help to support clinical decisions about the presence of pain, and they can measure change in discomfort once treatments have been given.[56] One worry, however, is that observational pain tools do not solely pick up pain, but rather distress, of which pain might be one cause, but which might also represent psychosocial upsets.[57]

The prevalence of pain is difficult to be certain of, depending on whether we are talking about acute or chronic pain, pain at rest or pain on movement, nociceptive, neuropathic or visceral pain, bothersome or non-bothersome pain (when is discomfort painful?). But, as noted earlier, in Sampson et al.'s study of people with advanced dementia living in nursing homes or in their own homes, 11% had pain at rest and 61% had pain during movement, which did not change much over the course of the nine-month study.[19] In a study of residents in nursing homes in the North-East of England, 13 out of 79 participants (16%) were considered to be in pain.[56] In a study involving Dutch nursing homes, the prevalence of pain ranged from 30.7% to 54.1%,[58] but this depended on the use of observational tools, which can have poor specificity (i.e. higher false positives rates).[56]

In a useful narrative review, Achterberg et al. highlighted four perspectives from which to consider pain management in dementia.[59] The first is the biological perspective and they concluded:

There is conflicting evidence from neuropathological, neuroimaging, experimental, and clinical research regarding the impact of dementia neuropathology on pain processing and perception. One might speculate that atrophy of gray matter appears to lead to an increase in pain tolerance, while white matter lesions result in a decrease in tolerance. However, ... the direction of the impact of neuropathology may differ in subtypes of dementia, and even within individuals. There thus remains a great deal of uncertainty regarding the effects of neuropathological changes in dementia.[59]

The second perspective is to do with the assessment of pain, which we have already discussed. The third is to do with effective treatment. WHO's analgesic ladder is a useful way to guide treatment.[60] It suggests stepped care from non-opioid drugs (e.g. paracetamol or non-steroidal anti-inflammatories) to weak and then strong opioids, with adjuvant analgesics (e.g. neuropathic agents or psychotropic medication) being added at any step. Given the real possibility of side effects, non-pharmacological therapies, from heat or massage to transcutaneous electrical nerve stimulation or acupuncture, might also be tried. But, recalling that some *distress* may have psychosocial origins, reflecting (say) fear or anxiety,[57] responses to distress should be broad-based.

The Serial Trial Intervention (STI) combined non-pharmacological and pharmacological interventions to treat pain *and* behaviour thought to be challenging.[61] The STI was made up of the following steps, which were performed sequentially:

- A basic care needs assessment to assess if basic care needs are fulfilled (e.g. hunger, thirst, eyeglasses, hearing aids, or toileting)
- A pain and physical needs assessment
- An affective needs assessment
- Administer a trial of non-pharmacological comfort treatment(s)
- Administer a trial of analgesic agents
- Consult with other disciplines (e.g. psychiatrist) and/or administer a trial of prescribed as-needed psychotropic drugs[61]

When the STI was evaluated by the team that had developed it in the United States, it was found to decrease discomfort and behaviours found challenging in nursing homes.[62] Subsequently, a Dutch version was tested in the Netherlands and found to decrease pain in nursing home residents with advanced dementia, increasing the use of opioids, but not of paracetamol.[58] (The decrease in pain was in terms of 'observed' pain as opposed to 'estimated' pain.) Probably the most important recent study of pain was undertaken in 18 nursing homes in western Norway.[63] The study demonstrated the important links between pain and behaviours that are found challenging. The participants in the study ($n = 352$), who all had moderate to severe dementia and 'clinically relevant behavioural disturbances', received (in the intervention group) 'individual daily treatment for pain for eight weeks according to [a] stepwise protocol'. Analgesia included paracetamol, morphine, buprenorphine transdermal patches or pregabalin.[63] The outcome was that agitation was significantly reduced (on average by 17%) in the intervention group; pain also improved.[63] The study should certainly not be taken to imply that all agitation is caused by pain, nor that all agitation should be treated with analgesia; but sometimes both of these things are true. In a later report, the group suggested that verbal agitation, for example complaining, negativism, repetitive sentences and questions, constant requests for attention, cursing, or verbal aggression, responded to pain treatment. Restlessness and pacing were also felt to be responsive to analgesics.[64] The suggestion is only that these sorts of behaviour should trigger consideration of pain as a possible cause; but it should be added that individuals will respond in a variety of ways and not always in accordance with statistical predictions. Clinical judgement, therefore, remains crucial for both diagnosis and treatment.[65]

Infections and Fevers

For a variety of reasons, including impaired immunological responses, but also because of immobility, people with advanced dementia are vulnerable to intercurrent infections. It was Ladislav Volicer's group who, in 1990, demonstrated no difference in mortality between people receiving antibiotics and those receiving only palliative care.[66] They later showed, in a controlled, but non-randomized study, that treatment with antibiotics, as opposed to the use of simple antipyretics and analgesia, was associated with a worsening of dementia.[67]

However, van der Steen et al. found that in a group of people with dementia and pneumonia in whom antibiotics were withheld there was more discomfort than in those treated with antibiotics.[68] However, the same patients had higher rates of discomfort before the pneumonia and peak rates of discomfort were observed at baseline. Discomfort also seemed to be higher shortly before death when pneumonia was the final cause of death compared to when death had another cause. This might belie the notion that pneumonia is the 'old man's friend'. Breathing problems were noted to be the most prominent signs. This would be predictable in pneumonia and raises two issues: first, the importance of a more global assessment of distress; second, the possibility that treatment other than antibiotics might have been beneficial (e.g. morphine).

The upshot is that the efficacy of antibiotics in a given situation needs to be judged in individual specific circumstances taking into account the severity of the dementia, comorbidity, immobility, nutritional status and the person's response to the infection. In other branches of palliative care, antibiotics are sometimes used in a specifically palliative manner to ease the distress caused by infected bronchial secretions.[69] Evidence, again from van der Steen and her colleagues in The Netherlands, suggests that physicians tend to treat most pneumonias: 69% with curative intent and 8% for palliative reasons.[70] In the 23% where antibiotic treatment was withheld, the patients tended to have more severe dementia, more severe pneumonia, poorer food and fluid intake, and were more often dehydrated.[70] When patients are thus very close to death a natural concern is that antibiotics might simply delay death, but leave the patient open to further suffering from decubitus ulcers or other consequences of very advanced inanition.

Later, van der Steen's group compared death in people with advanced dementia from pneumonia and death from intake problems (leading to dehydration and cachexia).[71] Both types of death were associated with distress. However, antibiotic treatment in those with pneumonia, which was mostly oral, was associated with less discomfort before death. They also found that invasive rehydration led to more discomfort.[71]

Subsequently, however, in a study involving both van der Steen and Volicer, the situation looked far from clear because they found (in male nursing home residents with advanced dementia) that mortality was high despite the use of antibiotics and that, if antibiotics prolonged life, for many it was only for a few days.[72] The worry was that antibiotics were merely prolonging the dying process. It may have been that the effectiveness of the antibiotics depended on fluid intake. In any event, it is difficult to make definitive statements about the use of antibiotics in someone with advanced dementia: in some, they may be curative; in some they may have a good palliative effect; in others they may simply prolong distress. It may be different for different types of infection, depending on the severity and depending on the person's more general physical status. As van der Steen and colleagues concluded, 'For many dementia patients, whether or not to treat [lower respiratory tract infections] with antibiotics remains a treatment dilemma'.[72]

Artificial Nutrition and Hydration

Several things happen to a person's feeding as dementia worsens. First, just as it is common for appetite and the enjoyment of food to be reduced in terminal conditions, so too in dementia there is a loss of appetite, a loss of the experience of hunger and of the need for a routine of regular meals.[73] Second, there can be dyspraxic and sequencing problems that cause difficulties with the process of feeding. Third, swallowing problems become increasingly noticeable. Aspiration pneumonia becomes a concern in the severer stages of the condition. It is particularly with this risk in mind that attention turns to the potential use of nasogastric (NG) and percutaneous endoscopic gastrostomy (PEG) tubes.

However, research over many years has found no good evidence that tube feeding is beneficial in advanced dementia.[74,75] Moreover, there are adverse effects of tube feeding which have not been fully researched.[74,75] Ethical commentary also suggests that, other than in special situations (e.g. where the dysphagia is likely to be a temporary phenomenon caused by something other than the general progression of the dementia), tube feeding should not be used routinely in advanced dementia.[76,77] Instead, the emphasis should be on conservative management of dysphagia following expert assessment (usually by a speech and language therapist) using food thickeners, with appropriate posture and careful hand-feeding techniques. There is evidence that older people themselves would support such an approach.[78]

As in the case of antibiotic use, the individual's particular medical state, the course of the dementia and judgements about quality of life are key to decision-making around feeding and drinking in advanced dementia. Such decisions should involve the family,[79] and may be helped by decision-aids.[80]

Resuscitation

In advanced dementia cardiopulmonary resuscitation (CPR) is unlikely to be successful.[81] The success rate is akin to that found in people with metastatic cancer.[82] Hence, a consensus has emerged that it is inappropriate to attempt CPR in people with advanced dementia.[81,83] As in all decisions regarding people who are unable to make decisions for themselves, close friends, family and other carers should be consulted (see Chapter 22).

Indeed, family and carers have a pivotal role to play in palliative care for people with dementia and may experience their own difficulties as a consequence. We have not considered this in further detail here, but our earlier paper considered families and carers;[9] and the issues and effects of being a family carer for someone with dementia are covered excellently elsewhere.[84]

Spiritual and Religious Needs

Again, whereas in the earlier iteration of this work we highlighted the psychosocial needs of people with dementia,[9] space does not allow us to pursue these matters further. Chapter 16 of this volume deals with psychosocial interventions, many of which will be relevant to palliative care in dementia. A palliative approach may also be relevant to behaviours that are challenging in dementia.[85] But we shall say something now about spirituality because the literature in this field has grown.

Until relatively recently, the personal dimensions of spirituality and faith have tended to be ignored by medical practitioners. Palliative care has helped to lead to a returning awareness and respect for such issues. Spiritual perspectives help to illuminate the nature of personhood in dementia.[86] Spirituality is often conceived in terms of meaning, purpose, connectedness; whereas religion is our way of making formal, by way of concepts, symbols, rituals and the like, our response to spiritual inclinations and yearnings.[87] Many people experience dementia within the context of religious belief in ways that appear helpful.[88] People with dementia and their carers seem to benefit from spiritual support.[89] Dementia can raise deep, existential issues to do with our lives and relationships,[90] so the possibility of spiritual or religious advice and support should be open to all.

Certainly the interest in spirituality and dementia has increased and provides a rich source of inspiration.[91] Namaste Care, mentioned earlier, itself draws from a spiritual background: the spirit within.[38]

One initial problem is that many of us have a limited vocabulary and understanding when it comes to spiritual and religious matters. This has been explored to some extent by two studies from Norway. In the first it was shown that carers tended to conceptualize spirituality in terms of meaning.[92] The study demonstrated the importance of developing more knowledge around how spiritual needs are expressed by people with dementia living in care homes and how staff might pick up such needs. The second study suggested it would be important to find space and time for nurses to 'reflect upon and discuss their professional understanding of spiritual care'.[93] Meanwhile, a study from the Netherlands helps to confirm that the right sort of communication is necessary in order to encourage talk about spirituality and religious needs in people with dementia admitted to long-term care facilities.[94]

In a thought-provoking review, Kevern has considered (among other things) how spirituality can be maintained and encouraged when cognitive capacities and communications skills have been impeded by dementia.[95] He concludes:

If we are to affirm that there is any sense at all in talking of the spirituality of a person with late-stage dementia, we must understand spirituality as essentially involving the dimension of time and/or social space. One option is to stress the longitudinal, habitual dimension of spirituality: that the values, meaning and practices most deeply ingrained at the heart of 'who we are' are those which have been repeated and reinforced over and over again from our infancy. The other is to stress the character of spirituality as held in common with others who, collectively, share the task of defining, maintaining and celebrating our individual identity. . . . The practical lessons to be drawn from this study are that the spirituality, and by extension the personhood, of somebody in late-stage dementia cannot be separated from their embeddedness in a particular social and historical milieu; and that the preservation of personhood thus rests on, as far as possible, the preservation of personal history and social context. ... The consideration of spirituality among people with dementia presents a challenge not just to common constructions of spirituality, but to the way in which this dimension of human life is fostered and supported in contemporary western society as a whole.[95]

Advance Care Planning

It seems important to end with ACP both because, in the UK at least, it has become public policy that it is a good thing and because there is some chance it will encourage and enable good palliative care. We know, however, that relatively few people have engaged with ACP: in a survey in the UK to which 1,832 had replied (34% of the total surveyed), with a median age of 73 years, only 308 (17%) had taken part in some type of formal ACP (mostly (13%) advance statements of preferences, with a few (4%) advance decisions to refuse treatment).[95]

Ambivalence and uncertainty around ACP exist among professionals too.[96,97] Hertogh has aptly spoken of 'the misleading simplicity of advance directives'.[98] ACP would seem to be a good idea, but not if people are ignorant of what it entails, suspicious of the process or do not trust it works.

Initiating ACP in dementia is complex and depends on characteristics of the professionals, the people with dementia and the families involved.[99] We know that ACP can reduce family uncertainties when they are faced by decisions to be made for their relatives with dementia.[100] This would suggest that education and good communication are key to improving uptake of ACP.

But does it work? This will partly depend on what is being aimed at. We have evidence involving people with dementia, however, that it is more likely you will die where you would prefer if it is specified that you only want to receive symptomatic care; it is less likely if you have specified that you wish to be resuscitated.[101] In 2018, a systematic review of the literature concluded that, although the evidence base was still limited, 'ACP is likely to be relevant and applicable to people with dementia and that ACP may, in some circumstances, be associated with a range of positive end-of-life outcomes'.[102] The review suggested improvements for further research, such as broader outcome measures to take account of the views of people with dementia and their families, research in the community as well as in institutions, and more rigorous evaluation using better methodologies.[102]

Conclusion

Palliative care is an approach that squares well with the aims of person-centred dementia care. The standards of care for many people with advanced dementia are poor. Still, there are a number of areas in relation to caring for people with severe dementia where a palliative approach seems beneficial and gradually the evidence is emerging to support such an approach. Clinical decisions have to be made on an individual basis, applying the evidence within a palliative framework. Good communication and continuity of care, probably provided by a key worker with the appropriate skills and knowledge, seem centrally important. ACP is likely to encourage this process, but this needs to be built into conversations at appropriate moments, ideally with someone who knows the person and family well. To conclude, there is certainly a moral imperative behind the idea that care at the end of life for people with dementia should be improved.

But now there is a new challenge emerging, namely the needs of prisoners with dementia. The population of people in prisons is growing and ageing. England and Wales have 86,000 prisoners (figures from 2015), which is the highest prison population in Western Europe, and 14% are over the age of 50 years.[103] People are also dying in prison, including from old age and from dementia. But there are challenges to providing palliative care to prisoners. It is difficult to find enough staff to accompany them if they leave the prison to receive care elsewhere (and in any case they then have to be handcuffed); but it can also be difficult to have enough staff in the prisons to give drugs or to provide suitable care (e.g. if the person is incontinent) especially at night. The effects are practical – staff leave because they cannot cope – and emotional for all involved: other prisoners, prison officers, clinical staff, as well as for the people who are dying.[103] Thus, the need for good-quality palliative care for people living with dementia expands. So our conclusion is the same: the moral imperative extends to those most marginalized too.

Acknowledgement

For information, the original paper on which this chapter is based was:

Hughes JC, Jolley D, Jordan A, Sampson EL. Palliative care in dementia: issues and evidence. *Adv Psychiatr Treat* 2007; 13: 251–260.

References

1. Barraclough J. ABC of palliative care. Depression, anxiety, and confusion. *Br Med J* 1997; **315**: 1365–1368.

2. Spiess JL, Northcott CJ, Offsay JD, Crossett JH. Palliative care: something else we can do for our patients. *Psychiatr Services* 2002; **53**: 1525–1526, 1529.

3. Black D, Jolley D. Slow euthanasia? The deaths of psychogeriatric patients. *Br Med J* 1990; **300**: 1321–1323.

4. Black D, Jolley D. Deaths in psychiatric care. *Int J Geriatr Psychiatry* 1991; **6**: 489–495.

5. Addington-Hall J. *Positive Partnerships: Palliative Care for Adults with Severe Mental Health Problems.* National Council for Hospice and Specialist Palliative Care Services, 2000.

6. Hughes JC, Robinson L, Volicer L. Specialist palliative care in dementia. *Br Med J* 2005; **330**: 57–58.

7. Volicer L, Rheaume Y, Brown J, et al. Hospice approach to the treatment of patients with advanced dementia of the Alzheimer type. *JAMA* 1986; **256**: 2210–2213.

8. Volicer L. The development of palliative care for dementia. *Ann Palliat Med* 2017; **6**: 302–305.

9. Hughes JC, Jolley D, Jordan A, Sampson EL. Palliative care in dementia: issues and evidence. *Adv Psychiatr Treat* 2007; **13**: 251–260.

10. World Health Organization (2002). *WHO Definition of Palliative Care.* Available via:

www.who.int/cancer/palliative/definition/en/ (last accessed 22 October 2019).

11. McInerney F, Doherty K, Bindoff A, et al. How is palliative care understood in the context of dementia? Results from a massive open online course. *Palliat Med* 2018; **32**: 594–602.

12. Addington-Hall J. *Reaching Out: Specialist Palliative Care for Adults with Non-Malignant Disease. Occasional Paper 14.* National Council for Hospice and Specialist Palliative Care Services, 1998.

13. Sampson EL, Gould V, Lee D, Blanchard MR. Differences in care received by patients with and without dementia who died during acute hospital admission: a retrospective case note study. *Age Ageing* 2006; **35**: 187–189.

14. Jolley, D, Baxter, D. Mortality in elderly patients with organic brain disorder enrolled on the Salford Psychiatric Case Register. *Int J Geriatr Psychiatry* 1997; **12**: 1174–1181.

15. Mitchell SL, Kiely DK, Hamel MB. Dying with advanced dementia in the nursing home. *Arch Intern Med* 2004; **164**: 321–326.

16. Aminoff BZ, Adunsky A. Their last 6 months: suffering and survival of end-stage dementia patients. *Age Ageing* 2006; **35**: 597–601.

17. McCarthy M, Addington-Hall J, Altmann D. The experience of dying with dementia: a retrospective study. *Int J Geriatr Psychiatry* 1997; **12**: 404–409.

18. Mitchell SL, Teno JM, Kiely DK, et al. The clinical course of advanced dementia. *N Engl J Med* 2009; **361**: 1529–1538.

19. Sampson EL, Candy B, Davis S, et al. Living and dying with advanced dementia: a prospective cohort study of symptoms, service use and care at the end of life. *Palliat Med* 2018; **32**: 668–681.

20. Sampson EL, Blanchard MR, Jones L, Tookman A, King M. Dementia in the acute hospital: prospective cohort study of prevalence and mortality. *Br J Psychiatry* 2009; **195**: 61–66.

21. Sampson EL, Ritchie CW, Lai R, Raven PW, Blanchard MR. A systematic review of the scientific evidence for the efficacy of a palliative care approach in advanced dementia. *Int Psychogeriatr* 2005; **17**: 31–40.

22. Sampson EL. Palliative care for people with dementia. *Br Med Bull* 2010; **96**: 159–174.

23. van der Steen JT. Dying with dementia: what we know after more than a decade of research. *Journal of Alzheimer's Disease* 2010; **22**: 37–55.

24. Shega JW, Levin A, Hougham GW, et al. Palliative excellence in Alzheimer care efforts (PEACE): a program description. *J Palliat Med* 2003; **6**: 315–320.

25. IN-PEACE clinical trial details available via: https://clinicaltrials.gov/ct2/show/NCT03773757 (last accessed 22 October 2019).

26. Shega JW, Sachs GA. Offering supportive care in dementia: reflections on the PEACE programme. In *Supportive Care for the Person with Dementia* (eds. JC Hughes, M Lloyd-Williams, GA Sachs): 33–44. Oxford University Press, 2010.

27. Hughes JC, Lloyd-Williams M, Sachs GA. The principles and practice of supportive care in dementia. In *Supportive Care for the Person with Dementia* (eds. JC Hughes, M Lloyd-Williams, GA Sachs): 301–307. Oxford University Press, 2010.

28. Hughes JC, Jordan A, Ransom P, et al. Palliative care and dementia: consensus in North Tyneside. *Eur J Palliat Care* 2010; **17**: 92–95.

29. van der Steen JT, Radbruch L, Hertogh CM, et al. White paper defining optimal palliative care in older people with dementia: a Delphi study and recommendations from the European Association for Palliative Care. *Palliat Med* 2014; **28**: 197–209.

30. Poole M, McLellan E, Bamford C, et al. End of life care: a qualitative study comparing the views of people with dementia and family carers. *Palliat Med* 2018; **32**: 631–642.

31. van der Steen JT, Dekker NL, Gijsberts M-JHE, Vermeulen LH, Mahler MM, The BA-M. Palliative care for people with dementia in the terminal

phase: a mixed-methods qualitative study to inform service development. *BMC Palliative Care* 2017; **16**: 28. Available via: doi 10.1186/s12904-017-0201-4 (last accessed 25 October 2019).

32. Bamford C, Lee RP, McLellan E, et al. What enables good end of life care for people with dementia? A multi-method qualitative study with key stakeholders. *BMC Geriatr* 2018; **18**: 302. Available via: https://doi.org /10.1186/s12877-018-0983-0 (last accessed 20 October 2019).

33. Volicer L, Collard A, Hurley A, Bishop C, Kern D, Kanon S. Impact of special care units for patients with advanced Alzheimer's disease on patient discomfort and costs. *J Am Geriatr Soc* 1994; **42**: 597–603.

34. Jenkinson J. *Development of a Quality Specialist Continuing Care Service for Older Adults* (Unpublished PhD Thesis). King's College London, 2018.

35. Tapley M, Regan A, Jolley D. Hospice: putting the heart back into dementia care. *J Dement Care* 2013; **21**: 14–15.

36. Wigan and Leigh Hospice. 'Hospice in Your Care Home'. Available via: www .wlh.org.uk/hospice-services/hospice-in-your-care-home/ (last accessed 26 October 2019).

37. St. Cuthbert's Hospice, Durham, England. 'Supporting People with Dementia, Their Families and Carers'. Available via: www .stcuthbertshospice.com/215/2/St-Cuthberts-Hospice-Dementia-Support (last accessed 26 October 2019).

38. Simard J, Volicer L. Namaste care and dying in institutional settings. In *Supportive Care for the Person with Dementia* (eds. JC Hughes, M Lloyd-Williams, GA Sachs): 291–299. Oxford University Press, 2010.

39. Stacpoole M, Hockley J, Thompsell A, Simard J, Volicer L. Implementing the Namaste Care Program for residents with advanced dementia: exploring the perceptions of families and staff in UK care homes. *Ann Palliat Med* 2017; **6**: 327–339.

40. Scott S, Pace V. The first 50 patients: a brief report on the initial findings from the Palliative Care in Dementia Project. *Dementia* 2009; **8**: 435–441.

41. Treloar A, Crugel M, Adamis D. Palliative and end of life care of dementia at home is feasible and rewarding: results from the 'Hope for Home' study. *Dementia* 2009; **8**: 335–347.

42. Bone AE, Morgan M, Maddocks M, et al. Developing a model of short-term integrated palliative and supportive care for frail older people in community settings: perspectives of older people, carers and other key stakeholders. *Age Ageing* 2016; **45**: 863–873.

43. Davies N, Mathew R, Wilcock J, et al. A co-design process developing heuristics for practitioners providing end of life care for people with dementia. *BMC Palliat Care* 2016; **15**: 1–11.

44. Hanson LC, Zimmerman S, Song MK, et al. Effect of the goals of care intervention for advanced dementia: a randomized clinical trial. *JAMA Intern Med* 2017; **177**: 24–31.

45. Moore KJ, Candy B, Davis S, et al. Implementing the compassion intervention, a model for integrated care for people with advanced dementia towards the end of life in nursing homes: a naturalistic feasibility study. *BMJ Open* 2017; **7**: 1–15.

46. Boogaard JA, de Vet HCW, van Soest-Poortvliet MC, et al. Effects of two feedback interventions on end-of-life outcomes in nursing home residents with dementia: a cluster-randomized controlled three-arm trial. *Palliat Med* 2018; **32**: 693–702.

47. Verreault R, Arcand M, Misson L, et al. Quasi-experimental evaluation of a multifaceted intervention to improve quality of end-of-life care and quality of dying for patients with advanced dementia in long-term care institutions. *Palliat Med* 2018; **32**: 613–621.

48. Schonwetter RS, Han B, Small BJ, et al. Predictors of six-month survival among patients with dementia: an evaluation of hospice Medicare guidelines. *Am J Hosp Palliat Care* 2003; **20**: 105–113.

49. Sachs G, Shega J, Cox-Hayley D. Barriers to excellent end-of-life care for patients with

dementia. *J Gen Intern Med* 2004; **19**: 1057–1063.

50. Reisberg B, Sclan SG, Franssen E, Kluger A, Ferris S. Dementia staging in chronic care populations. *Alzheimer Dis Assoc Disord* 1994; 8[Suppl 1]: S188–S205.

51. Ellis-Smith C, Evans CJ, Murtagh FEM, et al. Development of a caregiver-reported measure to support systematic assessment of people with dementia in long-term care: the integrated palliative care outcome scale for dementia. *Palliat Med* 2017; **31**: 651–660.

52. Ellis-Smith C, Higginson IJ, Daveson BA, Henson LA, Evans CJ, BuildCARE. How can a measure improve assessment and management of symptoms and concerns for people with dementia in care homes? A mixed-methods feasibility and process evaluation of IPOS-Dem. *PLoS One* 2018; **13**: e0200240. Available via: https://jour nals.plos.org/plosone/article?id=10.1371/j ournal.pone.0200240 (last accessed 26 October 2019).

53. Regnard C, Huntley ME. Managing the physical symptoms of dying. In *Palliative Care in Severe Dementia* (ed. JC Hughes): 22–44. Quay Books, 2006.

54. Jolley D, Hughes J, Greaves I, Jordan A, Sampson E. Seeing patients with dementia through to the end of life. *Geriatr Med* 2008; (September): 461–464.

55. Zwakhalen SM, Hamers JP, Abu-Saad HH, Berger MP. Pain in elderly people with severe dementia: a systematic review of behavioural pain assessment tools. *BMC Geriatrics* 2006; **6**: 3. Available via: https:// bmcgeriatr.biomedcentral.com/articles/10 .1186/1471-2318-6-3 (last accessed 26 October 2019).

56. Jordan A, Hughes J, Pakresi M, Hepburn S, O'Brien JT. The utility of PAINAD in assessing pain in a UK population with severe dementia. *Int J Geriatr Psychiatry* 2011; **26**: 118–126.

57. Jordan A, Regnard C, O'Brien JT, Hughes JC. Pain and distress in advanced dementia: choosing the right tools for the job. *Palliative Medicine* 2012; **26**: 873–878.

58. Pieper MJC, van der Steen JT, Francke AL, et al. Effects on pain of a stepwise multidisciplinary intervention (STA OP!) that targets pain and behavior in advanced dementia: a cluster randomized controlled trial. *Palliat Med* 2018; **32**: 682–692.

59. Achterberg WP, Pieper MJC, van Dalen-Kok AH, et al. Pain management in patients with dementia *Clin Interv Aging* 2013; **8**: 1471–1482.

60. World Health Organization. 'WHO's Pain Relief Ladder'. WHO, 2006. Available via: www.who.int/cancer/palliative/painlad der/en/ (last accessed on 26 October 2019).

61. Kovach CR, Noonan PE, Schlidt AM, et al. The Serial Trial Intervention: an innovative approach to meeting needs of individuals with dementia. *J Gerontol Nurs* 2006; **32**: 18–25.

62. Kovach CR, Logan BR, Noonan PE, et al. Effects of the Serial Trial Intervention on discomfort and behavior of nursing home residents with dementia. *Am J Alzheimers Dis Other Demen* 2006; **21**: 147–155.

63. Husebo BS, Ballard C, Sandvik R, Nilsen OB, Aarsland D. Efficacy of treating pain to reduce behavioural disturbances in residents of nursing homes with dementia: cluster randomised clinical trial. *Br Med J* 2011; **343**: d4065.

64. Husebo BS, Ballard C, Cohen-Mansfield J, Seifert R, Aarsland D. The response of agitated behavior to pain management in persons with dementia. *Am J Geriatr Psychiatry* 2014; **22**: 708–717.

65. Hughes JC, Ramplin S. Clinical and ethical judgement. In *Reconceiving Medical Ethics* (ed. C Cowley): 220–234. Continuum, 2012.

66. Fabiszewski KJ, Volicer B, Volicer L. Effect of antibiotic treatment on outcome of fevers in institutionalized Alzheimer patients. *Journal of the American Medical Association* 1990; **263**: 3168–3172.

67. Hurley AC, Volicer BJ, Volicer L. Effect of fever-management strategy on the progression of dementia of the Alzheimer type. *Alzheimer Disease & Associated Disorders* 1996; **10**: 5–10.

68. van der Steen JT, Ooms ME, Ader HJ, Ribbe MW, van der Wal WG. Withholding antibiotic treatment in pneumonia patients with dementia: a quantitative observational study. *Archives of Internal Medicine* 2002; **162**: 1753–1760.

69. Clayton J, Fardell B, Hutton-Potts J, Webb D, Chye R. Parenteral antibiotics in a palliative care unit: prospective analysis of current practice. *Palliative Medicine* 2003; **17**: 44–48.

70. van der Steen JT, Ooms ME, Mehr DR, van der Wal WG, Ribbe MW. Severe dementia and adverse outcomes of nursing home-acquired pneumonia: evidence for mediation by functional and pathophysiological decline. *Journal of the American Geriatrics Society* 2002; **50**: 439–448.

71. van der Steen JT, Pasman HRW, Ribbe MW, van der Wal G, Onwuteaka-Philipsen BD. Discomfort in dementia patients dying from pneumonia and its relief by antibiotics. *Scand J Infect Dis* 2009; **41**: 143–151.

72. van der Steen JT, Lane P, Kowall NW, Knol DL, Volicer L. Antibiotics and mortality in patients with lower respiratory infection and advanced dementia. *J Am Med Dir Assoc* 2012; **13**: 156–161.

73. Ikeda M, Brown J, Holland AJ, Fukuhara R, Hodges JR. Changes in appetite, food preference, and eating habits in frontotemporal dementia and Alzheimer's disease. *J Neurol Neurosurg Psychiatry* 2002; **73**: 371–376.

74. Finucane TE, Christmas C, Travis K. Tube feeding in patients with advanced dementia: a review of the evidence. *JAMA* 1999; **282**: 1365–1370.

75. Sampson EL, Candy B, Jones L. Enteral tube feeding for older people with advanced dementia (Review). *Cochrane Database of Systematic Reviews* 2009; Issue 2: Art. No.: CD007209. Available via: www.cochranelibrary.com/cdsr/doi/10.1002/14651858.CD007209.pub2/full (last accessed 28 October 2019).

76. Gillick, M. R. (2000) Rethinking the role of tube feeding in patients with advanced dementia. *New England Journal of Medicine*, **342**: 206–210.

77. Hughes JC, Baldwin C. *Ethical Issues in Dementia Care: Making Difficult Decisions.* Jessica Kingsley, 2006.

78. Low JA, Chan DK, Hung WT, Chye R. Treatment of recurrent aspiration pneumonia in end-stage dementia: preferences and choices of a group of elderly nursing home residents. *Intern Med J* 2003; **33**: 345–349.

79. The AM, Pasman R, Onwuteaka-Philipsen B, Ribbe M, van der Wal G. Withholding the artificial administration of fluids and food from elderly people with dementia: ethnographic study. *Br Med J* 2002; **325**: 1326–1330.

80. Hanson LC, Carey TS, Caprio AJ, et al. Improving decision-making for feeding options in advanced dementia: a randomized controlled trial. *J Am Geriatr Soc* 2011; **59**: 2009–2016.

81. Conroy SP, Luxton T, Dingwall R, Harwood RH, Gladman JR. Cardiopulmonary resuscitation in continuing care settings: time for a rethink? *Br Med J* 2006; **332**: 479–482.

82. Ebell MH, Becker LA, Barry HC, Hagen M. Survival after in-hospital cardiopulmonary resuscitation. A meta-analysis. *J Gen Intern Med* 1998; **13**: 805–816.

83. Volandes AE, Abbo ED. Flipping the default: a novel approach to cardiopulmonary resuscitation in end-stage dementia. *J Clin Ethics* 2007; **18**: 122–139.

84. Seeher K, Brodaty H. Family carers of people with dementia. In *Dementia* (5th ed.) (eds. D Ames, J O'Brien, A Burns): 142–160. CRC Press, Taylor Francis Group, 2017.

85. Hughes JC. Behaviours that challenge at the end of life. In *Understanding Behaviour in Dementia that Challenges: A guide to Assessment and Treatment* (2nd ed.) (eds. IA James, L Jackman): 280–292. Jessica Kingsley, 2017.

86. Allen FB, Coleman PG. Spiritual perspectives on the person with dementia:

identity and personhood. In *Dementia: Mind, Meaning, and the Person* (eds. JC Hughes, SJ Louw, SR Sabat): 205–221. Oxford University Press, 2006.

87. Sapp S. Spiritual care of people with dementia and their carers. In *Supportive Care for the Person with Dementia* (eds. JC Hughes, M Lloyd-Williams, GA Sachs): 199–206. Oxford University Press, 2010.

88. Davis R. *My Journey into Alzheimer's Disease*. Tyndale, 1989.

89. Dinning L. The spiritual care of people with severe dementia. In *Palliative Care in Severe Dementia* (ed. JC Hughes): 126–134. Quay Books, 2006.

90. Hughes J. Personhood and religion in people with dementia. In *Neurology and Religion* (eds. A Coles, J Collicutt): 149–160. Cambridge University Press, 2020.

91. Jewell A. (ed.) *Spirituality and Personhood in Dementia*. Jessica Kingsley, 2011.

92. Ødbehr L, Kvigne K, Hauge S, Danbolt LJ. Nurses' and care workers' experiences of spiritual needs in residents with dementia in nursing homes: a qualitative study. *BMC Nurs* 2014; **13**: 12. Available via: https://bmcnurs.biomedcentral.com/track/pdf/10.1186/1472-6955-13-12 (last accessed 28 October 2019).

93. Ødbehr LS, Kvigne K, Hauge S, Danbolt LJ. Spiritual care to persons with dementia in nursing homes; a qualitative study of nurses and care workers experiences. *BMC Nurs* 2015; **14**: 70. Available via: www.ncbi.nlm.nih.gov/pmc/articles/PMC4693438/pdf/12912_2015_Article_122.pdf (last accessed 28 October 2019).

94. van der Steen JT, Gijsberts M-JHE, Hertogh CMPM, Deliens L. Predictors of spiritual care provision for patients with dementia at the end of life as perceived by physicians: a prospective study. *BMC Palliat Care* 2014; **13**: 61. Available via: https://bmcpalliatcare.biomedcentral.com/track/pdf/10.1186/1472-684X-13-61 (last accessed 28 October 2019).

95. Musa I, Seymour J, Narayanasamy MJ, Wada T, Conroy S. A survey of older peoples' attitudes towards advance care planning. *Age Ageing* 2015; **44**: 371–376.

96. Robinson L, Dickinson C, Bamford C, et al. A qualitative study: professionals' experiences of advance care planning in dementia and palliative care, 'a good idea in theory but. . .' *Palliat Med* 2013; **27**: 400–408.

97. Sampson EL, Burns A. Planning a personalised future with dementia: 'the misleading simplicity of advance directives'. *Palliat Med* 2013; **27**: 387–388.

98. Hertogh CM. The misleading simplicity of advance directives. *Int Psychogeriatr* 2011; **23**: 511–515.

99. van der Steen JT, van Soest-Poortvlieta MC, Hallie-Heierman M, et al. Factors associated with initiation of advance care planning in dementia: a systematic review. *J Alzheimer's Dis* 2014; **40**: 743–757.

100. Brazil K, Carter G, Cardwell C, et al. Effectiveness of advance care planning with family carers in dementia nursing homes: a paired cluster randomized controlled trial. *Palliat Med* 2018; **32**: 603–612.

101. Wiggins N, Droney J, Mohammed K, Riley J, Sleeman KE. Understanding the factors associated with patients with dementia achieving their preferred place of death: a retrospective cohort study. *Age Ageing* 2019; **48**: 433–439.

102. Dixon J, Karagiannidou M, Knapp M. The effectiveness of advance care planning in improving end-of-life outcomes for people with dementia and their carers: a systematic review and critical discussion. *J Pain Symptom Manage* 2018; **55**: 132–150.

103. Turner M, Peacock M. Palliative care in UK prisons: practical and emotional challenges for staff and fellow prisoners. *J Correct Health Care* 2017; **23**: 56–65.

Chapter

18

Review of Treatment for Late-Life Depression

Katherine Hay, Will Stageman and Charlotte L Allan

Introduction

In 2018, Public Health England reported that one in five older people living in the community and two in five older people living in care homes are affected by depression.[1] These symptoms are associated with reduced quality of life and high morbidity,[2] and also with increased mortality through suicide and self-neglect.[3] A 2014 study showed that major depression was associated with a 43% increase in the risk of non-suicide-related mortality in adults over the age of 50.[4] Depression across all age groups has a detrimental impact on recovery from surgery, and, in older people increases the risk of coronary heart disease and stroke.[5, 6] There is a gathering body of evidence that depression is a risk factor for dementia and that in people with mild cognitive impairment the presence of depression may increase the risk of progression to dementia.[7]

Depressive disorders presenting in older people have many clinical similarities to depression in younger adults; however, biological changes related to ageing may necessitate a different approach to treatment. In this chapter, we present an evidence-based review of treatment for late-life depression, focussing on pharmacological approaches including monotherapy, combination and augmentation strategies. Selective serotonin reuptake inhibitors (SSRIs) including sertraline and citalopram are well tolerated with the advantage of a favourable side-effect profile and are good options for first-line treatment. Second-line treatment options include combination therapy with a second antidepressant, or treatment augmentation with anti-psychotic medication or lithium. We also consider evidence for non-pharmacological treatment strategies including psychological therapy and neuro-stimulation. Finally, we summarize evidence for treatment of depression in patients with dementia.

Diagnosis and Aetiology

Diagnosis of late-life depression is based on standard DSM-5 or ICD-11 criteria for mood disorders.[8, 9] There may be subtle differences in clinical presentation, with higher rates of somatic symptoms, apathy, psychomotor retardation or agitation, fatigue and executive dysfunction compared with younger age groups,[10] but these symptoms are not sufficiently different or reliable to classify this as a distinct disorder.

The aetiology of late-life depression is multifactorial, and includes biological, psychological and social factors (see Figure 18.1). These aetiological factors can lead to relapse into a depression in those with an existing vulnerability, or to the first onset of a depressive disorder in later life. Since many of the aetiological factors are age-related, there has been (and continues to be) a misconception that depression in older people is inevitable given the

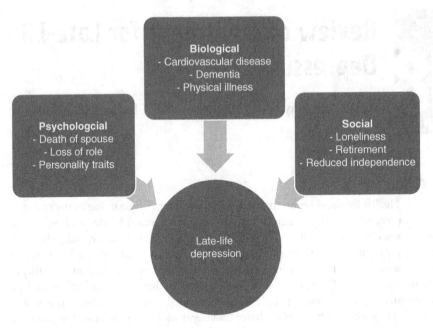

Figure 18.1 Aetiology of late-life depression

frequency of physical ill health, bereavement and loss of role in this age group. This prejudice may reduce the likelihood of help-seeking behaviour by patients and of the offer of treatment by health professionals and could be one reason why late-life depression remains an under-recognized and undertreated disorder. This may be a particularly prevalent prejudice affecting those living in nursing homes.[11] Given the significant adverse impact on patients, their families and carers, late-life depression warrants greater efforts at recognition and effective, evidence-based treatment.

Prescribing for Older Adults

Pharmacotherapy can be used effectively in late-life depression.[12] However, treatment requires a distinct approach because of age-related physiological changes, which alter pharmacokinetics and pharmacodynamics. Drug distribution within the body changes because of increased body fat and reduced volume of water. Hydrophobic compounds (e.g. antidepressants and antipsychotics) are therefore more readily distributed, whereas there is reduced distribution of hydrophilic compounds. Renal excretion is reduced, so there may be increased concentrations of active compounds that are renally excreted. These changes mean that lower doses, slow titration and careful monitoring are required.[13, 14] The increased prevalence of medical co-morbidities in this age group means that patients are more vulnerable to medication side effects. Polypharmacy is a risk, and care is needed to minimize the effects of drug interactions.[15] These considerations should not discourage the use of pharmacological treatment of late-life depression, but do necessitate a careful review of the person's past medical history before drug regimens are changed.

The Evidence Base

This chapter provides an overview of treatments for late-life depression (pharmacological, psychological and neurostimulation), based on a search of electronic databases including Medline, Embase, PsychINFO and PubMed for the terms [treatment or therapy] and [depression or depressive] and [old age or older or late-life or geriatric] between 1990 and January 2019. This is intended to summarize important and recent research findings in a format that is clinically relevant.

Pharmacological Treatment

Monotherapy

Selective Serotonin Reuptake Inhibitors

SSRIs are the most common first-line treatments for late-life depression, similar to treatment for younger patients. Sertraline has the best evidence for efficacy and tolerability and should be considered first-line for late-life depression.[18] There is also good evidence for escitalopram and citalopram in those over 65 years old; these have a low propensity for drug interactions as they have minimal impact on the cytochrome P450 system.[12, 17] All three have the advantage of a favourable side-effect profile and can be used in patients with a history of cognitive impairment and stroke.[18]

A large cross-sectional study has confirmed a modest dose-dependent QT interval increase with citalopram (10 mg to 20 mg, mean QTc increase 7.8 ms) when compared to other SSRIs.[19] The maximum recommended dose for older adults has now been reduced and citalopram should not be prescribed in conjunction with other agents which prolong the QT interval, such as antipsychotics and certain antibiotics (e.g. erthyromycin). SSRIs also carry a risk of hyponatremia which increases with age. Female gender, previous hyponatraemia or concurrent diuretic or non-steroidal anti-inflammatory drug (NSAID) prescription have all been demonstrated to confer additional risk and monitoring of urea and electrolytes should be considered in high-risk individuals.[20] SSRIs should be avoided in those with a history of gastrointestinal bleeding, especially if they are prescribed other medications which may precipitate this.

Some studies have cast doubt on the efficacy of SSRIs in late-life depression.[21] Where SSRIs are contraindicated, or poorly tolerated, other classes of antidepressants can be used as first-line treatment.

Mirtazapine and Venlafaxine

Mirtazapine is an alternative to SSRIs for first-line treatment in older adults.[12, 22] It has few cardiac side effects and a weaker association with hyponatraemia; in patients with insomnia and anorexia its side effects may be exploited for therapeutic benefit. It appears to have a faster onset of action than SSRIs, with beneficial effects found at two weeks.[23]

Venlafaxine has been proposed as a useful second-line antidepressant.[12] An open-label study demonstrated the efficacy of venlafaxine in older patients with atypical subtypes of depression including mood reactivity, hypersomnia and increased appetite.[23] Venlafaxine may, however, exacerbate hypertension and therefore close monitoring of this is needed at treatment initiation.

Agomelatine and Vortioxetine

Both vortioxetine and agomelatine have had positive placebo-controlled trials in people aged over 65 years.[24, 25] Vortioxetine, a serotonin transporter blocker, does not have a significant impact on QTc and has been found to improve cognitive tests of processing speed, verbal learning and memory in people over 65 years when compared to placebo. Nausea and vomiting can, however, be a prominent side effect in clinical practice. Agomelatine is very well tolerated but requires monitoring of liver function. A recently updated network analysis ranked agomelatine among the most efficacious antidepressants and it may be particularly useful in individuals who are prone to side effects.[26]

Tricyclics

Tricyclic antidepressants are also effective treatments in older age groups. Nortriptyline shows comparable efficacy and tolerability when compared with sertraline.[27] Adverse effects were similar in both groups, but tricyclic antidepressants should be used with caution owing to the risk of cardiac side effects, toxicity in overdose and because their anti-muscarinic effects are more likely to exacerbate cognitive impairment.

Certain antidepressants, for example dosulepin (a tricyclic) and reboxetine (a selective inhibitor of noradrenaline reuptake), are not recommended for use in older adults.[28, 29]

Next Steps

A meta-analysis of late-life depression found studies with a longer trial period (10–12 weeks) were significantly more likely to demonstrate a response, suggesting older people may take longer to respond to antidepressants – at least six weeks.[13] If there is only a modest improvement at this stage and the antidepressant is tolerated, the dose should be increased.[30] Where first-line monotherapy has been ineffective, switching to a second-line agent (in the same, or a different class) is a useful strategy, particularly for those who received minimal benefit, or could not tolerate the first-choice antidepressant.[30] If there has only been a partial response after the dose is optimized to the maximum specified or tolerated dose, augmentation should be considered.

Combination and Augmentation Therapy

Although common in clinical practice, there is little evidence that combining different anti-depressants is effective in older people.[31] Augmentation with other agents may be effective, albeit with slower and lower recovery rates; medical co-morbidity and symptoms of anxiety are associated with a poorer prognosis.[32] As in younger populations, lithium has the best evidence base as an augmenting agent with a systematic review reporting an overall response rate of 42% (95% confidence interval [CI] 21–65%).[33] For older adults, this should be accompanied by careful monitoring of renal and thyroid function, using lower doses than in younger patients.

Augmentation of antidepressant treatment with antipsychotic medication is useful for those with severe depression, particularly where there are psychotic symptoms, providing there has been careful consideration of the risks and benefits.[34] For psychotic depression in older adults, treatment with olanzapine and sertraline has been associated with significantly higher remission rates than treatment with olanzapine alone.[35] The use of olanzapine is associated with increased cholesterol and triglyceride concentrations; associated weight gain, however, may be less significant in older adults compared to younger adults.[35] In a randomized, placebo-controlled study of older patients with resistant depression, augmentation of citalopram with risperidone led to symptom resolution in a substantial number of patients, and a delay in time to relapse (56% in the risperidone group and 65% in the placebo group relapsed). [36] Though these results were non-significant, they add to evidence that suggests antipsychotics may be a clinically useful strategy, particularly for subgroups of patients with severe depression and psychotic symptoms. More recently, a high-quality randomized controlled trial (RCT) found the addition of aripiprazole to venlafaxine resulted in a 44% remission rate compared to 29% in the placebo group in 181 patients with treatment-resistant depression and a mean age of 66 years (odds ratio 2.0; 95% CI 1.1–3.7). [37] In older adults, especially in those with a history of cardiovascular disease, antipsychotics should be used cautiously and with careful monitoring to minimize side effects. If there are concerns about cognitive impairment, antipsychotics should be avoided because of the increased risk of stroke. [38]

Relapse Prevention

There is good evidence that maintenance therapy in patients over 60 years who have achieved remission is effective in preventing relapses and recurrences (number needed to treat = 3.6; 95% CI 2.8–4.8), with comparable efficacy and tolerability seen in SSRIs and tricyclics. [39] Given the high risk of relapse in older patients, pharmacotherapy should be continued for at least two years in those who have had two episodes and perhaps indefinitely in those who have suffered three or more. [30] There is limited evidence regarding the addition of psychological therapies in older adults to prevent relapse. A 2016 Cochrane review concluded that there was insufficient evidence available regarding psychological therapies preventing a relapse of depression in older people to be able to draw any conclusions or make recommendations. [40]

Non-pharmacological Therapies

There is increasing evidence that *collaborative care* is an effective non-pharmacological approach to the management of depression. In this model, structured, psychotherapeutic approaches help to increase the effectiveness of pharmacological therapy. In one study, older people with moderate to severe depression who were allocated a nurse who assessed symptoms regularly, co-ordinated care, managed medication, educated and set goals experienced a greater reduction in depressive symptoms than those receiving enhanced usual care. [41] A further study showed that the use of collaborative care delivered by a case manager, alongside usual treatment by the GP, was effective in reducing depressive symptoms at 4 months compared to usual treatment by the GP alone, albeit this difference was not maintained in the longer term. [42] This mirrors earlier studies which showed that a brief intervention combining psycho-education, support and pharmacotherapy led to improved outcomes for older adults compared to pharmacotherapy alone. [43]

The evidence for use of formal psychological approaches to treat late-life depression is increasing. Modifications to psychotherapeutic techniques include consideration of the context, maturity of patients and additional factors (e.g. physical illness and cognitive impairment) which may help to improve efficacy when used with older adults. [44] A 2015 meta-analysis of psychotherapy for older people with depression showed some evidence, but this varied a great deal depending on the type of control group used. [45] Interventions based on cognitive behavioural therapy (CBT) showed that group psychotherapy for older adults with depression had modest efficacy when compared with waiting list controls, which were maintained at follow-up. [46] In 2018, a systematic review showed evidence for the use of group therapy, specifically cognitive behavioural and reminiscence-based therapies, for the treatment of depression in older adults.[47] A meta-analysis of studies looking at problem-solving therapy (PST) as a treatment for depression in older people found that there was a significant reduction in scores on the Hamilton Rating Scale for depression with the use of PST; however, data on long-term outcomes was lacking.[48]

There is a limited evidence base for the use of more novel types of therapy in the treatment of depression in older people. An early meta-analysis of 17 studies found that a range of psychosocial treatments for depression in older adults were reliably more effective than no-treatment on self-rated and clinician-rated measures of depression. Therefore, though the evidence is weak, these may still represent important treatment modalities.[49] More recent evidence supports the use of Problem Adaptation Therapies for treatment of co-existing depression and cognitive impairment.[50] A 2018 meta-analysis showed evidence that the use of exercise as a treatment for depression in older adults is beneficial.[51] There is modest evidence for the use of creative arts therapies when delivered by qualified therapists, particularly art, drama and music therapy.[52]

Neurostimulation

Electroconvulsive Therapy

Electroconvulsive therapy (ECT) is the most effective and rapidly-acting treatment for older people with depression, with remission rates quoted from 60% to 80%; indeed increasing age may be positively correlated with ECT response.[53] It is an option both for patients who have not responded to pharmacological therapy and for patients with depressive disorder who need rapid treatment owing to the risk of self-neglect or suicide.[54] A recent study comparing ECT to medication (venlafaxine or nortriptyline) in late-life depression found remission rates of 63.8% (30/47) after 6 weeks in the ECT group and 33.3% (27/81) after 12 weeks in the medication group.[55]

The main risks of ECT are related to the use of a general anaesthetic and, therefore, careful assessment of medical and anaesthetic risks is required, with clinical examination and relevant physical investigations (e.g. ECG, venepuncture and chest X-ray) prior to first ECT, repeated at regular intervals as necessary. Another important consideration is the risk of cognitive side effects, so cognition needs to be carefully monitored prior to and during ECT.[56]

Bilateral electrode placement is faster and more effective than unilateral. However, it is associated with greater cognitive side effects.[57] Therefore, in older patients who are at risk of cognitive impairment, unilateral placement is preferred initially, unless there are urgent clinical reasons which necessitate the use of bilateral ECT. The efficacy of ECT is substantially increased by the addition of an antidepressant medication.[58]

ECT can be administered on an outpatient basis, provided that the patients are effectively supervised, particularly in the 24 hours following treatment. This is a useful treatment option for patients with severe depression who prefer to avoid hospital admission. Continuation ECT (where the interval between treatments is gradually increased) can reduce and shorten admission for older people with severe depressive disorder and this has been explored further in the PRIDE (Prolonging Remission in the Depressed Elderly) study. In this study, 128 patients who had successfully remitted following treatment three times a week with ultra-brief right-sided unilateral ECT were randomized to either medication-only or flexibly administered maintenance ECT arms.[59] At 6 months, only 13% of those in the flexible ECT group had relapsed compared to 20% in the medication arm, and the ECT-treated patients were 5 times more likely to be scored as 1 ('not ill at all') on the Clinical Global Impression (CGI) scale.

Alternatives to ECT

Alternative neurostimulation therapies which do not require repeated anaesthetic or carry cognitive risks may be beneficial in a patient group with a range of medical co-morbidities, although there is little research on older adults specifically. Transcranial magnetic stimulation has a modest antidepressant efficacy, is increasingly used in working-age adults and was recognized as a treatment by NICE in 2015 with no upper age limit.[60] Initial reports suggest increasing age may be negatively correlated with response – it is suggested – because of the increased scalp-to-cortex distance in older people. However, as the stimulation intensity is now routinely set higher (at 120%), recent meta-analysis has found no negative correlation between age and response.[61]

For both transcranial direct current stimulation and vagal nerve stimulation, there is a paucity of data in older people and the evidence base in younger age groups remains equivocal with both positive and negative systematic reviews published. They will require further evaluation, including trials in older patients, before routine use becomes more widespread.

Depression and Dementia

Estimates suggest that more than 20% of patients with dementia will have a diagnosable depression at a given time;[62] depressive illness is under-diagnosed and under-treated in nursing home residents with cognitive impairment.[63] Diagnosing depression in those with cognitive impairment can be challenging since presenting symptoms may be subtle, including behavioural change, sleep disturbance and reduced appetite.

Unfortunately, there is limited evidence for the use of antidepressants in patients with dementia.[63, 64] One of the first large studies of sertraline for the treatment of moderate depressive disorder in those with cognitive impairment showed a favourable effect,[65] yet follow-up studies have failed to replicate this. The DIADS-II[66] and the HTA-SADD[67] studies both found that sertraline was not superior to placebo in treating depression in those with dementia, regardless of the severity of depression. The HTA-SADD study also found that mirtazapine was no more effective than placebo in this patient group.

Pharmacological approaches can be used in conjunction with a range of non-pharmacological approaches (e.g. CBT, PST and reminiscence therapy) to target mood as well as cognitive symptoms. Although cognitive impairment may have an impact on the patient's ability to engage with such therapies, the treatment of any depressive symptoms in isolation from a patient's cognitive impairment risks a slower, less effective recovery.[68] A meta-analysis of RCTs using CBT, interpersonal therapy, counselling or multimodal interventions found evidence that use of these therapies in those with depression and dementia reduces depressive symptoms.[69] However, there were only six studies included in the review and a need for further high-quality RCTs was highlighted. Furthermore, this meta-analysis did not include any follow-up data, so the longer-term efficacy of psychological therapy for people with depression and dementia is unclear.

Psychosocial interventions (namely tai chi, problem adaptation therapy, exercise and multicomponent interventions) have been used to treat co-existing depression and dementia.[70] However, the quality of the trials, small sample sizes and the heterogeneity of the interventions limits the clinical recommendations that can be made based on these.

Finally, it is important to note that depressive presentations can mimic cognitive impairment, so care must be taken to avoid diagnosing dementia in someone who has a treatable depressive illness. Clinicians should also be alert to the difficulties of differentiating subcortical vascular disease from depression. A history of treatment-resistant depression should prompt the use of neuroimaging to investigate vascular pathology e.g. lacunar infarcts. MRI is the preferred option for this, but vascular changes may also be visible on CT scans. Treatment approaches for subcortical vascular disease involve use of a strict behavioural approach and a highly structured daily routine.

Conclusions

Late-life depression is a common disorder, which is under-recognized and under-treated. It is associated with high morbidity and mortality and therefore needs to be correctly diagnosed and treated appropriately. There is an increasing evidence base for the use of an integrated approach to treatment of depression in older people in a primary care setting. SSRIs are a good first-line strategy, with particularly strong evidence for sertraline in terms of efficacy and tolerability. It is important to continue first-line treatment for a sufficient duration before increasing the dose or augmenting it. Antipsychotic medication and lithium are good options for augmentation. The collaborative care model increases the effectiveness of treatments, and psychological approaches can be modified for older people, providing useful non-pharmacological therapeutic options.

Acknowledgements

For information, the original paper on which this chapter is based was:

Allan CL, Ebmeier KP. Review of treatment for late-life depression.*Adv Psychiatr Treat* 2013; 19: 302–309.

The authors wish to express many thanks to Professor Klaus P. Ebmeier for his work on the original paper.

References

1. *Better Mental Health for All: A Public Health Approach to Mental Health Improvement* (2018) London: Faculty of Public Health and Mental Health Foundation.

2. Sivertsen H, Bjorklof GH, Engedal K et al. Depression and quality of life in older persons: a review. *Dement Geriatr Cogn Disord* 2015; **40**: 311–339.

3. Djernes JK, Gulmann NC, Foldager L et al. 13 Year follow up of morbidity, mortality and use of health services among elderly depressed patients and general elderly populations. *Aust N Z J Psychiatry* 2011; **45** [8]: 654–662.

4. Saint Onge JM, Krueger PM, Rogers RG. The relationship between major depression and nonsuicide mortality for U.S. adults: the importance of health behaviours. *J. Gerontol B Psychol Soc Sci* 2014; **69**[4]: 622–632.

5. Ghoneim MM, O'Hara MW. Depression and postoperative complications: an overview. *BMC Surg* 2018; **18**: 5.

6. Pequignot R, Dufouil C, Prugger C et al. High level of depressive symptoms at repeated study visits and risk of coronary heart disease and stroke over 10 years in older adults: the three-city study. *J Am Geriatr Soc.* 2018; **64**[1]: 118–125.

7. Gallagher D, Kiss A, Lanctot K et al. Depression and risk of Alzheimer dementia: a longitudinal analysis to determine predictors of increased risk among older adults with depression. *Am J Geriatr Psychiatry* 2018; **26**[8]: 819–827.

8.   American Psychiatric Association. *The Diagnostic and Statistical Manual of Mental Disorders (5th edition).* 2013.

9.   World Health Organization. *The International Statistical Classification of Diseases and Related Health Problems (11th Revision).* 2018.

10. Hegeman JM, Kok RM, van der Mast RC et al. Phenomenology of depression in older compared with younger adults: meta-analysis. *Br J Psychiatry* 2012; **200**[4]: 275–281.

11. Brown MN, Lapane KL, Luisi AF. The management of depression in older nursing home residents. *J Am Geriatr Soc* 2002; **50**[1]: 69–76.

12. Cipriani A, Furukawa TA, Salanti G et al. Comparative efficacy and acceptability of 12 new-generation antidepressants: a multiple-treatments meta-analysis. *Lancet* 2009; **373**[9665]: 746–758.

13. Nelson JC, Delucchi K, Schneider LS. Efficacy of second generation antidepressants in late-life depression: a meta-analysis of the evidence. *Am J Geriatr Psychiatry* 2008; **18**[7]: 558–567.

14. Roose SP, Schatzberg AF. The efficacy of antidepressants in the treatment of late-life depression. *J Clin Psychopharmacol* 2005; **25**[4 Suppl 1]: S1–7.

15. Mark TL, Joish VN, Hay JW et al. Antidepressant use in geriatric populations: the burden of side effects and interactions and their impact on adherence and costs. *Am J Geriatr Psychiatry* 2011; **19**[3]: 211–221.

16. Cipriani A, La Ferla T, Furukawa TA et al. Sertraline versus other antidepressive agents for depression. *Cochrane Database Syst Rev* 2010; **14**[4]: CD006117.

17. Alexopoulos GS, Reynolds CF, Bruce ML et al. Reducing suicidal ideation and depression in older primary care patients: 24-month outcomes of the PROSPECT study. *Am J Psychiatry* 2009; **186**[8]: 882–890.

18. Apler A. Citalopram for major depressive disorder in adults: a systematic review and meta-analysis of published placebo-controlled trials. *BMJ Open* 2011; **1**[2]: e000106.

19. Castro VM, Clements CC, Murphy SN et al. QT interval and antidepressant use: a cross sectional study of electronic health records. *BMJ* 2013; **346**: 288.

20. Kirby D, Ames D. Hyponatraemia and selective serotonin re-uptake inhibitors in elderly patients. *Int J Geriatr Psychiatry* 2001; **16**[5]: 484–493.

21. Bose A, Li D, Gandhi C. Escitalopram in the acute treatment of depressed patients aged 60 years or older. *Am J Geriatr Psychiatry* 2008; **18**[1]: 14–20.

22. Watanabe N, Omori IM, Nakagawa A et al. Mirtazapine versus other antidepressive agents for depression. *Cochrane Database Syst Rev* 2011; **12**: CD006528.

23. Roose SP, Miyazaki M, Devanand D et al. An open trial of venlafaxine for the treatment of late-life atypical depression. *Int J Geriatr Psychiatry* 2004; **19**[10]: 989–994.

24. Katona C, Hansen T, Olsen CK. A randomized, double-blind, placebo-controlled, duloxetine-referenced, fixed-dose study comparing the efficacy and safety of Lu AA21004 in elderly patients with major depressive disorder. *Int Clin Psychopharmacol* 2012; **27**[4]: 215–223.

25. Heun R, Ahokas A, Boyer P et al. The efficacy of agomelatine in elderly patients with recurrent major depressive disorder: a placebo-controlled study. *J Clin Psychiatry* 2013; **74**[6]: 587–594.

26. Cipriani A, Furukawa TA, Salanti G et al. Comparative efficacy and acceptability of 21 antidepressant drugs for the acute treatment of adults with major depressive disorder: a systematic review and network meta-analysis. *Lancet* 2018; **391**[10128]: 1357–1366.

27. Bondareff W, Alpert M, Friedhoff AJ et al. Comparison of sertraline and nortriptyline in the treatment of major depressive disorder in late life. *Am J Psychiatry* 2000; **157**[5]: 729–736.

28. NICE. (2009a). *Depression: the treatment and management of depression in adults [update] [CG90].*

29. NICE. (2009b). *The treatment and management of depression in adults with chronic physical health problems (partial update of CG23).*

30. Rush AJ. STAR*D: what have we learned? *Am J Psychiatry* 2007; **184**[2]: 201–204.

31. Kok RM, Reynolds CF. Management of depression in older adults: a review. *JAMA* 2017; **317**[20]: 2114–2122.

32. Dew MA, Whyte EM, Lenze EJ et al. Recovery from major depression in older adults receiving augmentation of antidepressant pharmacotherapy. *Am J Psychiatry* 2007; **184**[6]: 892–899.

33. Cooper C et al, Katona C, Lyketsos K et al. A systematic review of treatments for refractory depression in older people. *Am J Psychiatry* 2011; **188**[7]: 681–688.

34. Alexopoulos GS. Pharmacotherapy for late-life depression. *J Clin Psychiatry* 2011; **72**[1]: e04.

35. Meyers BS, Flint AJ, Rothschild AJ et al. A double-blind randomized controlled trial of olanzapine plus sertraline vs olanzapine plus placebo for psychotic depression: the study of pharmacotherapy of psychotic depression (STOP-PD). *Arch Gen Psychiatry* 2009; **66**[8]: 838–847.

36. Alexopoulos GS, Canuso CM, Gharabawi GM et al. Placebo-controlled study of relapse prevention with risperidone augmentation in older patients with resistant depression. *Am J Geriatr Psychiatry* 2008; **18**[1]: 21–30.

37. Lenze EJ, Mulsant BH, Blumberger DM et al. Efficacy, safety, and tolerability of augmentation pharmacotherapy with aripiprazole for treatment-resistant depression in late life: a randomised, double-blind, placebo-controlled trial. *Lancet* 2015; **386**[10011]: 2404–2412.

38. Sacchetti E, Trifiro G, Caputi A et al. Risk of stroke with typical and atypical anti-psychotics: a retrospective cohort study including unexposed subjects. *J Psychopharmacol* 2008; **22**[1]: 39–46.

39. Kok R, Heeren T, Nolen W. Continuing treatment of depression in the elderly: a systematic review and meta-analysis of double-blinded randomized controlled trials with antidepressants. *Am J of Geriatr Psychiatry* 2011; **19**[3]: 249–255.

40. Wilkinson P, Izmeth Z. Continuation and maintenance treatments for depression in older people. *Cochrane Database Syst Rev* 2016 Issue 9; Art. No.: CD006727. DOI:10.1002/14651858. CD006727.pub3

41. Bruce ML, Sirey JA. Integrated care for depression in older primary care patients. *Can J Psychiatry* 2018; **63**[7]: 439–446.

42. Bosanquet K, Adamson J, Atherton K et al. CollAborative care for Screen-Positive EldeRs with major depression [CASPER plus]: a multicentred randomised controlled trial of clinical effectiveness and cost-effectiveness. *Health Technol Assess* 2017; **21**[67]: 1–252.

43. Sirey JA, Bruce ML, Alexopoulos GS. The treatment initiation program: an intervention to improve depression outcomes in older adults. *Am J Psychiatry* 2005; **182**[1]: 184–186.

44. Raue PJ, McGovern AR, Kiosses DN et al. Advances in psychotherapy for depressed older adults. *Curr Psychiatry Rep* 2017; **19**[9].

45. Huang AX, Delucchi K, Lunn LB et al. A systematic review and meta-analysis of psychotherapy for late-life depression. *Am J Geriatr Psychiatry* 2015; **23**[3]: 261–273.

46. Krishna M, Jauhari A, Lepping P et al. Is group psychotherapy effective in older adults with depression? A systematic review. *Int J Geriatr Psychiatry* 2011; **26**[4]: 331–340.

47. Tavares LR, Barbosa MR. Efficacy of group psychotherapy for geriatric depression: a systematic review. *Arch Gerontol Geriatr* 2018; **78**:71–80.

48. Kirkham JG, Choi N, Seitz DP. Meta-analysis of problem solving therapy for the treatment of major depressive disorder in older adults. *Int J Geriatr Psychiatry* 2018; **31**[5]: 526–535.

49. Scogin F, McElreath L. Efficacy of psychosocial treatments for geriatric depression: a quantitative review. *J Consult Clin Psychol* 1994; **62**[1]: 69–74.

50. Kiosses DN, Ravdin LD, Gross JJ et al. Problem adaptation therapy for older adults with major depression and cognitive impairment: a randomised clinical trial. *JAMA Psychiatry* 2015; 72[1]: 22–30.

51. Murri MB, Ekkekakis P, Menchetti M et al. Physical exercise for late life depression: effects on symptom dimensions and time course. *J Affect Disord* 2018; 230: 65–70.

52. Dunphy K, Baker FA, Dumaresq E et al. Creative arts interventions to address depression in older adults: a systematic review of outcomes, processes and mechanisms. *Front Psychol* 2018; 9: 2655.

53. Allan CL, Ebmeier KP. The use of ECT and MST in treating depression. *Int Rev Psychiatry* 2011; 23[5]: 400–412.

54. Spaans HP, Sienaert P, Bouckaert F et al. Speed of remission in elderly patients with depression: electroconvulsive therapy V. medication. *Br J Psychiatry* 2015; 206[1]: 67–71.

55. Kennedy SH, Milev R, Giacobbe P et al. Canadian Network for Mood and Anxiety Treatments (CANMAT) Clinical guidelines for the management of major depressive disorder in adults. IV. Neurostimulation therapies. *J Affect Disord* 2009; 117 Suppl 1: 44–53.

56. Carney S, Geddes J. Electroconvulsive therapy. *BMJ* 2003; 326[7403]: 1343–1344.

57. Sackeim HA, Dillingham EM, Prudic J et al. Effect of concomitant pharmacotherapy on electroconvulsive therapy outcomes: short-term efficacy and adverse effects. *Arch Gen Psychiatry* 2009; 66[7]: 729–737.

58. Kellner CH, Husain MM, Knapp RG et al. A novel strategy for continuation ECT in geriatric depression: Phase 2 of the PRIDE study. *Am J Psychiatry* 2018; 173[11]: 1110–1118.

59. NICE. [2015]. *Repetitive transcranial magnetic stimulation for depression (IPG542)*.

60. Blumberger DM, Hsu JH, Daskalakis ZJ. A review of brain stimulation treatments for late-life depression. *Curr Treat Options Psych* 2015; 2[4]: 413–421.

61. Livingston G, Sommerlad A, Orgeta V et al. Dementia prevention, intervention and care. *Lancet* 2017; 390[10113]: 2673–2734.

62. Volicer L, Frijters DH, Van der Steen JT. Relationship between symptoms of depression and agitation in nursing home residents with dementia. *Int J Geriatr Psychiatry* 2012; 27[7]: 749–754.

63. Farina N, Morrell L, Banerjee S. What is the therapeutic value of antidepressants in dementia? A narrative review. *Int J Geriatr Psychiatry* 2017; 32[1]: 32–49.

64. Nelson J, Devanand D. A systematic review and meta-analysis of placebo-controlled antidepressant studies in people with depression and dementia. *J Am Geriatr Soc* 2011; 59[4]: 577–585.

65. Weintraub D, Rosenberg PB, Drye LT et al. Sertraline for the treatment of depression in Alzheimer disease: week-24 outcomes. *Am J Geriatr Psychiatry* 2010; 18[4]: 332–340.

66. Drye LT, Martin BK, Frangakis CE et al. Do treatment effects vary among differing baseline depression criteria in Depression in Alzheimer's Disease Study 2 (DIADS-2)? *Int J Geriatr Psychiatry* 2011; 26[6]: 573–583.

67. Banerjee S, Hellier J, Romeo R et al. Study of the use of antidepressants for depression in dementia: the HTA-SADD trial – a multicentre, randomised, double-blind, placebo-controlled trial of the clinical effectiveness and cost-effectiveness of sertraline and mirtazapine. *Health Technol Assess* 2013; 17[7]: 1–186.

68. Wilkins V, Kiosses D, Ravdin L. Late-life depression with comorbid cognitive impairment and disability: nonpharmacological interventions. *Clin Interv Aging* 2010; 5: 323–331.

69. Ortega V, Qazi A, Spector AE et al. Psychological treatments for depression and anxiety in dementia and mild cognitive impairment. *Cochrane Database Syst Rev* 2014, Issue 1; Art. No.: CD009125. DOI:10.1002/14651858.CD009125.pub2

70. Noone D, Stott J, Aguirre E et al. Meta-analysis of psychosocial interventions for people with dementia and anxiety or depression. *Ageing Ment Health* 2018; 17: 1–10.

Chapter 19

Reducing the Healthcare Burden of Delirium
The Challenge of Developing More Cognitive-Friendly Services

David J Meagher, Henry O'Connell, Walter Cullen and Dimitrios Adamis

Introduction

Delirium is recognized as a key healthcare target for our increasingly aged society. Improved management of delirium and related neuropsychiatric presentations can allow significant improvements in outcomes but requires fundamental change in the structure of healthcare services. There is a pressing need for cognitive-friendly hospital programmes that can increase awareness of delirium, provide better education around its management, improve detection in real-world practice, and promote evidence-based management of cognitive problems in the general hospital. We outline key elements of delirium-friendly services that span interventions in our day-to-day clinical care of individual patients all the way to wider organizational practices.

Delirium: A Key Healthcare Challenge

In 1998, one in six people (15.9%) in the UK was aged over 65 years. By 2018 this had increased to almost one in every five (18.3%) and is projected to reach one in every four (24.2%) by 2038. This increasingly aged society brings with it increased multimorbidity, general frailty, cognitive impairment, and dementia. Alongside this increasing burden, resource-pressurized healthcare services are struggling to respond to the complex needs of older persons. The care challenge posed by delirium represents a particular example of how we need to adapt towards more cognitive-friendly care practices.

Delirium is a common serious neuropsychiatric disorder that occurs across healthcare settings. The impact of delirium is particularly apparent in the acute general hospital setting, where there is a concentration of vulnerable populations such as frail elderly with pre-existing cognitive impairment. Point prevalence studies indicate that delirium can be identified in 20–25% of the hospitalized elderly, with higher rates in specific groups, such as older patients with severe medical illness or pre-existing cognitive impairments, terminal illness, or those receiving intensive care facilities. One study across a complete general hospital in Ireland identified an 18% point prevalence of delirium,[1] while a point prevalence study of delirium status in 1,867 older patients across 108 acute and 12 rehabilitation wards in Italian hospitals found 23% with delirium.[2]

Delirium is also highly prevalent in community-based settings such as nursing homes. The all too common practice of early discharge of patients, often despite continued significant morbidity, to post-acute and community-based facilities means that improving delirium awareness among primary care practitioners is key. A recent point prevalence study of 71 nursing homes across Italy found that 37% had active delirium at assessment.[3] In a cohort study of 12 nursing homes in Canada, 40% developed at least one episode of delirium over three years.[4] Delirium is highly predictable by virtue of well-identified risk factors such that pre-hospital preparation can substantially reduce delirium risk during elective admissions.

Delirium is a significant independent predictor of adverse health outcomes, including longer duration of hospitalization, reduced subsequent functional independence, reduced cognitive functioning, and elevated mortality.[5] The economic impact of delirium is highly significant, with direct one-year US healthcare costs of $152 billion – comparable to cardiovascular disease ($257.6 billion).[6] In the UK, a health economic analysis of elderly acute medical patients found that 12-week costs for patients with delirium were more than double the costs of those without delirium.[7]

Delirium as a major source of health and economic burden thus has unrivalled penetration across healthcare services. The emergence of organizations (e.g. European Delirium Association, American Delirium Society) has promoted greater clinical and research effort with delirium but everyday management remains far from optimal as delirium continues to be underappreciated in healthcare planning.

O'Connell et al. described a model for improved delirium care through more cognitive-friendly hospitals.[8] This includes a multifaceted approach to reducing incidence, improving detection, and providing more targeted management focusing on seven levels of care: patient, task, staff, team, environment, organization, and institution, while addressing key barriers to cognitive-friendly practices such as inadequate assessment, inappropriate intervention, stigma, and deficiencies in staff levels and training. We revisit this model from a societal perspective, again focusing upon hospital practices but also exploring how efforts away from hospital can contribute to reducing the healthcare burden of delirium and related conditions too.

The Nosology of Delirium and Related Disorders

Historically, acute generalized disturbances of cognition have been referred to by more than 50 synonyms, each reflecting delirium occurring in particular populations or treatment settings (e.g. 'confusional state', 'encephalopathy', 'acute brain failure') and tending to confuse clinical practice. In 1980, DSM-III introduced *delirium* as the umbrella term to replace these concepts while providing systematic criteria for delirium diagnosis that have evolved to the current DSM-5 criteria.[9]

These categorize delirium as a major neurocognitive disorder based upon five key criteria (see Box 19.1) that reflect the occurrence of generalized disturbance of brain function (evidenced by cognitive and neuropsychiatric symptoms with inattention and reduced awareness being central) that is relatively recent in onset, tends to fluctuate, and occurs in the context of physical morbidity. Delirium symptoms can present as sub-syndromal illness where full syndromal criteria are lacking and in such cases outcomes are typically intermediate between delirium and non-delirium.[10]

In addition, the concept of Post-Operative Cognitive Disorder (POCD) has emerged to account for the many patients who are diagnosed with new cognitive impairments in the early post-operative period which persist beyond what is traditionally considered as delirium.[11] The incidence of POCD among older patients is approximately 26% at one week and 10% at three months following surgery.[12] Unlike delirium and dementia,

---

Box 19.1 DSM-5 criteria for delirium

A. A disturbance in attention (i.e. reduced ability to direct, focus, sustain, and shift attention) and awareness (reduced orientation to the environment).

B. The disturbance develops over a short period of time (usually hours to a few days), represents a change from baseline attention and awareness, and tends to fluctuate in severity during the course of a day.

C. An additional disturbance in cognition (e.g. memory deficit, disorientation, language, visuospatial ability, or perception).

D. The disturbances in Criteria A and C are not better explained by a pre-existing, established, or evolving neurocognitive disorder and do not occur in the context of a severely reduced level of arousal, such as coma.

E. There is evidence from the history, physical examination, or laboratory findings that the disturbance is a direct physiological consequence of another medical condition, substance intoxication or withdrawal, or exposure to a toxin, or is due to multiple aetiologies.

POCD lacks a clear definition in DSM-5 with a positive diagnosis based upon a difference in preoperative and post-operative test scores that equates with a z-score two standard deviations from the mean. There is also a lack of clarity around its relationship to both delirium and dementia – many cases are preceded by delirium but this is not invariable. Also, it remains uncertain whether POCD is part of a continuum that culminates in dementia or is a distinct entity that is, for example, relatively static compared to the conventional notion of a progressive dementia. To date, studies have linked POCD with reduced thalamic and hippocampal volumes and reduction of cerebral blood flow.[13]

In short, while dementia is a major risk factor for developing delirium (and underpins delirium in approximately 50% of cases), increasing evidence implicates delirium as not only a marker for emerging dementia, but as an aggravating factor in dementia that accelerates its course and is an independent risk factor for long-term cognitive impairment which can persist and in some cases is irreversible.

What Does Cognitive-Friendly Mean?

When applied to healthcare, cognitive-friendly refers to practices and the environment in which they occur that promote optimal cognitive functioning while minimizing the likelihood and impact of neurocognitive disorders. As such, it refers to the combined impact of both structural and functional elements in providing an environment that is sensitive to the vulnerabilities of those prone to delirium and related conditions. The lived environment is the arena where our cognitive skills, preferences, and attitudes come together to determine our ability to interact with the world.[14] Environmental design is an important contributor to cognitive functioning; the ability to form cognitive maps is a key element in the orientation process that declines with age. Cognitive-friendly environments are engaging and appropriately stimulating in a way that facilitates cognitive performance. Avoiding clutter and excessive perceptual complexity (e.g. the number of different colours in an environment), simplicity of design to ease wayfinding, and providing facilities that promote the capacity for social interaction all make the environment more navigable for cognitively impaired patients, which in turn promotes a sense of efficacy.[15] Environments should also promote physical activity, which is associated with better cognitive performance in older age. Early mobilization after procedures is one example of how promoting engagement with one's surroundings can positively impact upon cognitive outcomes.

From a functional perspective, efforts to provide cognitive-friendly services need to occur across the healthcare system, such that cognitive difficulties are also addressed both before and after periods of hospitalization. Programmes that are 'senior-friendly' flag persons with pre-existing cognitive issues at entry to hospital as at higher risk throughout their hospital journey and undertake proactive delirium prevention measures and rapid assertive intervention in the event of emerging delirium. A range of evidence-based interventions can reduce the risk of experiencing incident delirium in hospital,[16] and have demonstrated cost-effectiveness.[17]

A cognitive-friendly hospital considers the entire patient 'journey' in terms of the different clinical areas and services within the general hospital, from points of access to care (e.g. emergency department), through to areas of continuing care (e.g. medico-surgical wards, intensive or palliative care), and appropriate discharge planning. This facilitates cohesive multicomponent intervention that is tailored to particular patient needs at different points of the at-risk versus active episode versus post-episode recovery spectrum. These efforts should also link effectively with primary and community care settings, where possible before, and always after hospital admission.

The Delirium Experience, Education, and Action

Increasing staff awareness and expertise in managing patients with cognitive disorders is an essential first step in the development of a cognitive-friendly hospital programme. However, such efforts have limited impact unless they are aligned to changes in clinical practice. These include flagging patients who have known difficulties (e.g. the butterfly scheme) along with specific screening practices (e.g. cognitive vital sign monitoring), identifying specific dementia champions to promote better awareness and practices, and providing access to specialist supports such as a dementia specialist nurse to advise on specifics of care.

It is increasingly recognized that caregiver-centred detection tools such as the FAM-CAM and Sour Seven can improve delirium detection.[18] In addition to front-line medical and nursing staff, allied healthcare professionals, care attendants, and non-clinical staff with high levels of patient contact (e.g. cleaners and catering staff) can be included in efforts to identify and best manage delirious patients as subtle changes in eating and hygiene/self-care can assist in delirium detection.

Central to providing more delirium-friendly care environments is understanding and integrating knowledge derived from recovered patients. This patient perspective has been previously underappreciated owing to the erroneous belief that delirious patients lack the capacity to communicate their perspective and experiences usefully. Recent studies indicate that, even during an episode, many patients can usefully communicate that they are confused – with more than a third recognizing their own loss of functionality as feeling confused or mixed-up.[1]

Qualitative studies have identified care practices that connect best with patients, including simplicity, repetition, reassurance, and clarity of communication. Garrett provides a particularly coherent account of his experiences during a delirious episode and how a change in the environment fuelled further disturbing experiences:

On moving out to the surgical ward I became paranoid. Convinced that I was in a small, poorly funded cottage hospital, I was certain that the staff resented having me there, as I was a serious drain on their resources. They were constantly trying to get me removed and annoyed with me and the demands my condition was making on them.[19]

It can be useful to keep a diary to assist in making sense of events after recovery and to reduce the impact of negative recollections. Similarly, retrospective accounts of patients experiencing delirium during intensive care unit (ICU) stays highlight ward noise, disruptions from other patients and visitors, the sense of isolation, difficulties in communication, restricted movement, and loss of functional integrity as particularly distressing.[20] Many patients described their frustration at how staff underestimated their awareness and that in many cases added to the sense of paranoia by discussing the patient without acknowledging their presence.

A range of simple activities can promote delirium awareness: talks from expert clinicians, distribution of written material, posters, and staff emails. Once integrated into staff induction and training these activities need to be repeated on a regular basis in order to encourage discussion and appropriate treatment of cognitive impairment. However, such programmes must be underpinned by operational changes and supports to copper-fasten attitudinal gains. At the core of this issue is the need to recognize delirium as a key condition within healthcare activities and routinely monitor its impact upon outcomes. Educational interventions can assist in delirium prevention and detection in acute hospital and community settings with positive effects in respect of staff attitudes, reduced falls, and medication use.[21]

Building on a heightened awareness of delirium among all hospital staff, formal training in delirium should be targeted at all clinical and support staff. Different levels and types of education are required for different members of staff, depending on the professional background and clinical profile of patients. For example, the nurse working in the ICU will have a very different profile of patient from the physiotherapist working in the orthopaedic ward. However, a similar foundation in delirium education and training is essential for all healthcare professionals, with some specialization for different individuals, tailored to their particular field. Relevant professional bodies can support the development, approval, and monitoring of initiatives along with the efficiency of delivery.[22]

Health service managers need to be aware of the impact of delirium on clinical outcomes and financial costs.[6] They can add crucial weight behind programmes that emphasize delirium prevention and treatment. Service planning must ensure the needs of older patients are considered and their impact should be monitored by including delirium as a routine activity measure. It is advocated that all hospital staff should have mandatory training on delirium and cognitive problems in the general hospital, with such training being delivered at the commencement of employment and repeated regularly (e.g. every 6 months). The impact of staff education and training initiatives should also be monitored and evaluated on a regular basis (e.g. through surveys of staff knowledge, attitudes, and clinical practices).

Overall, success of delirium programmes is linked to systems factors that include involvement of clinical leaders, support from senior management, linking the implementation of programmes to periods of systems change, providing educational elements that are sustained and engaging, integrating mechanisms to support decision-making into everyday routines (e.g. electronic care pathways), and monitoring procedures to promote continued adherence. In general, improving delirium care is best achieved where it is supported by activities that promote enthusiasm, support implementation, remove barriers, and allow for progress monitoring.

Risk Factors and Delirium Prevention

A central element of cognitive-friendly services is to minimize exposure to factors that increase the risk of developing delirium. There is good evidence for a range of preventative strategies in reducing delirium occurrence but much less for interventions once delirium becomes established. Resources should thus be directed towards primary preventative measures. The occurrence of delirium reflects the interaction of a range of predisposing patient, illness, and treatment factors with acute precipitating insults to produce a generalized disturbance of brain function. Many of these factors are highly preventable (including many with significant iatrogenic elements)[23] such that better service organization can allow for preventative measures to produce better patient outcomes with reduced incidence and duration of delirium when it occurs. In general, interventions that are complex, multifaceted, and focused upon site-specific risk factors are most successful and can reduce the burden of delirium by more than a third.[24]

The concept of 'delirium readiness' has been long recognized. Lindroth and colleagues reviewed 23 different prediction models for delirium that share many recurring factors (severe morbidity, older age, pre-existing dementia, and exposure to opioids, benzodiazepines, or general polypharmacy).[25] Baseline risk is especially important as patients with high baseline vulnerability can develop delirium even in response to minor precipitants.

Many risk factors are modifiable while others assist in assessing risk–benefit balance of surgical and other interventions in deciding upon optimal care, especially in frail elderly patients with cognitive impairments (see Figure 19.1). Many of the strategies that are employed in delirium prevention reflect attention to ensuring a high standard of basic medical and nursing care (e.g. avoiding unnecessary polypharmacy, correcting sensory deficits, promoting self-efficacy). However, it has become necessary to protocolize many

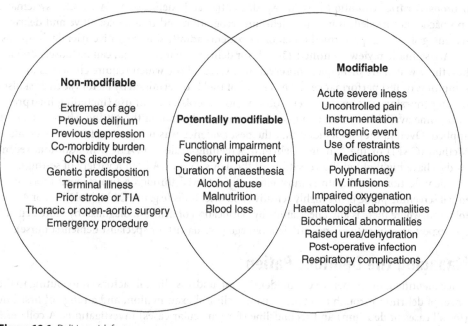

Figure 19.1 Delirium risk factors

such practices in order to ensure that they occur consistently in our increasingly chaotic and time-pressurized healthcare environments. As such, improved delirium care with more cognitive-friendly environments is a key target as we embrace the need to provide for an increasingly aged society. In addition, a range of targeted interventions can reduce delirium incidence with gathering evidence for positive impact from interventions that focus upon encouraging physical exercise[26] and music therapy.[27]

Management of Delirium

Historically, delirium care has focused on hospital-based activities. A key development has been the recognition of how common delirium is in community-based settings where primary care practitioners are the key care providers. Moreover, primary care practitioners have an important role in managing delirium risk prior to scheduled hospitalizations through so-called 'prehabilitation' as well as providing support after periods of hospital care that have involved episodes of delirium. The latter includes addressing any residual symptoms, clarifying the nature of the delirium episode, and addressing the ongoing risk of recurrence by optimizing sensory and functional integrity. They can promote manageable medication regimes that balance the likely benefits of agents with the risks of poor adherence owing to impaired executive abilities and the impact of polypharmacy as a risk factor for delirium recurrence.

Improving Detection

Delirium is poorly detected across healthcare settings with up to 72% of cases either missed or diagnosed late.[28] This reflects the heterogeneity of delirium as a condition that has a variety of different clinical presentations (e.g. hypoactive versus hyperactive subtypes) along with the inherent fluctuation and considerable phenomenological overlap and comorbidity with other neuropsychiatric conditions, such as dementia and depression. As such, systematic approaches are needed to improve delirium recognition and routine cognitive and delirium screening should be performed on all older patients admitted to cognitive-friendly hospitals.

A systematic review identified 23 tools for delirium detection that can be loosely divided into those which are principally observational versus those which require clinicians to elicit symptoms or test performance.[28] The choice of tool is determined by factors such as skillset of rater (nursing staff tend to prefer observational tools), ease of use (including interpretation), time available for screening, and accuracy of the tool in the setting where it is to be applied. Overall, they concluded that the best evidence was for the Confusion Assessment Method (CAM) or the Nursing Delirium Screening Scale (NuDESC). In addition, recent studies have highlighted the versatility of the 4-A's Test (4-AT) in a variety of settings.[7]

Identification of delirium is most efficiently achieved through a two-stepped process: an initial screening phase using highly sensitive and brief tools (e.g. the CAM, NuDESC, or 4-AT) followed, where there is any uncertainty, by clarification of delirium diagnosis by more detailed and expert assessment (e.g. geriatrician, old age psychiatrist, or specialist dementia nurse).

Managing the Delirious Patient

Once identified, the imperative is to identify and address clinical factors contributing to the onset of delirium through a detailed history, clinical examination, and a range of first-line (for all cases of delirium) and second-line (for particular cases) investigations. A collateral

> **Box 19.2** Multicomponent non-pharmacological management of symptoms of delirium
>
> Educate patient and family/carer on delirium and prognosis
> Involve family/carer in hospital care routine
> Reorientation and reassurance strategies
> Normalize sleep patterns
> Prevent complications – e.g. falls, constipation
> Ensure adequate hydration
> Ensure pain relief is adequate
> Encourage activity – mobility and ADLs
> Use visual/hearing aids to facilitate communication
> Nurse with familiar staff in relaxed environment

history clarifying baseline cognition function is central to accurate diagnosis and optimally managing delirium symptoms. A variety of programmes has emerged over recent years which facilitate gathering relevant information about baseline disposition and functioning as well as highlighting particular needs around sensory input and maintaining everyday routines.

Many patients with delirium do not require specific pharmacological treatment for their symptoms, but benefit from a multicomponent, patient-centred approach applying gerontological nursing principles to address the range of patient needs (Box 19.2). Unnecessary movement of patients between different clinical areas should be avoided, and patients should have their symptoms reviewed at regular intervals to ensure they are not deteriorating. Studies have demonstrated how nursing in a single room rather than a multi-bedded environment can reduce the delirium incidence in medical and ICU settings.[29] Targeted care practices in a delirium-friendly environment can also allow for improved care: Flaherty and Little described a specialized 'delirium room' designed to optimize cognitive and adaptive functioning while minimizing aggravating factors for delirium using comprehensive multidisciplinary care.[30] They reported reduced length of stay, functional loss, length of stay, and mortality.

Pharmacological Management of Delirium

Antipsychotic agents are commonly used in the management of delirium in everyday practice across clinical settings. This is supported by prospective studies which indicate that around two-thirds of patients treated with typical or atypical antipsychotics experience symptomatic improvement. However, more recent placebo-controlled studies are less supportive: two small studies in ICU and elderly medicine populations suggest more rapid resolution of symptoms with quetiapine, while larger studies of haloperidol and ziprasidone in ICU, and haloperidol or risperidone in palliative care indicate no benefit.[31] Worryingly, the latter study also indicated poorer survival in those treated with antipsychotics.[31] A recent meta-analysis did not support antipsychotic use in delirium treatment.[32]

As such, decisions around the use of antipsychotics for delirium treatment in everyday practice are challenging. In essence, antipsychotic use requires careful consideration of therapeutic targets supported by systematic monitoring for adverse extrapyramidal, sedative, cerebrovascular, and cardiac conduction effects. The NICE guidelines support targeted use of antipsychotics for delirium where behavioural disturbance, psychosis, and distress warrant intervention.[33] These recommendations are sensitive to the reality of everyday practice where the safety, distress, and dignity of patients frequently present a compelling argument for intervention and non-pharmacological techniques are not always effective. However, the merits of antipsychotic use in less urgent circumstances are unclear and relate to factors such as comorbid dementia status and adverse effect risk. A key target in managing delirium is to develop treatment protocols that can guide dose titration and optimize identification of adverse effects. It is important to recognize that in real-world practice antipsychotic treatment frequently continues for extended periods including beyond hospital discharge. It is thus crucial that initiation of antipsychotic treatment always includes a clear plan to limit the duration of exposure with careful assessment on a daily basis of the merits of ongoing use.

With regard to other classes of medications, a Cochrane review found insufficient evidence to support the use of benzodiazepines for the treatment of delirium and, in view of their potential to aggravate or even precipitate delirium, they should be reserved for delirium related to withdrawal states or seizures.[34] Despite theoretical potential, evidence around the use of procholinergic agents has been largely negative.

Discharge Planning and Delirium Management Post-Hospitalization

Despite the high prevalence of delirium in the general hospital and its impact on subsequent cognitive and adaptive function, delirium occurrence is frequently omitted from discharge planning and in communications with primary care and other community services. The occurrence of delirium has important implications for post-acute care where ongoing risk factors can be minimized while addressing any residual functional deficits or psychological sequelae.

Delirium is a distressing experience for patients and their caregivers. Delirium-recovered patients may be uncomfortable discussing their delirium episodes because they equate it with senility or being 'mad'. More than half of patients who recover from delirium can recall their psychotic symptoms and many are still distressed by their recollections six months later.[35] Persistent psychological disturbances are a particular target for interventions that can impact upon subsequent help-seeking behaviour. Formal follow-up visits can facilitate post-delirium adjustment by allowing discussion of the meaning of delirium and planning how to minimize future risk.

A Plan for Improved Delirium Care

A cognitive-friendly hospital environment embraces a holistic approach to the identification, prevention, and management of delirium through patient-centred clinical care. Delirium care pathways are increasingly becoming embedded into the everyday practice of all hospitals that aspire to a cognitive-friendly environment. While the general principles for optimal delirium care are well described, care pathways must consider the challenges that are specific to each setting. Seven key elements of delirium-friendly services are detailed in Table 19.1. As we embrace these challenges and provide more cognitive-friendly healthcare, we can reduce the growing burden of delirium and its adverse consequences for society.

Table 19.1 Key elements of delirium-friendly services

(1) promoting awareness of delirium by including its detection and management as a key educational component of medical and nursing programmes at undergraduate and postgraduate level

(2) ensuring that delirium risk status monitoring is embedded into daily routines across all healthcare settings, including hospitalized and community-based settings

(3) systematic application of preventative measures, particularly in high-risk patients

(4) earlier and more consistent detection of delirium through formal systematic screening in everyday practice

(5) linkage of delirium identification to evidence-based action through protocolized management based upon a more coherent understanding of how to manage specific clinical presentations of delirium optimally

(6) Close liaison between primary and secondary care to promote the active management of the post-delirium phase, including the risk for subsequent episodes and addressing secondary psychological sequelae

(7) monitoring of the frequency of delirium and its impact upon outcomes as a routine performance indicator within services.

Acknowledgement

For information, the original paper on which this chapter is based was:

O'Connell H, Kennelly S, Cullen W, Meagher D. Managing delirium in everyday practice: towards cognitive-friendly hospitals. *Adv Psychiatr Treat* 2014; 20: 380–389.

The authors wish to acknowledge with thanks the contribution of Dr Sean Kennelly to the original paper.

References

1. Ryan DJ, O'Regan NA, Caoimh RO et al. Delirium in an adult acute hospital population: predictors, prevalence and detection. *BMJ Open* 2013; 3(1).

2. Bellelli G, Morandi A, Di Santo SG et al. 'Delirium Day': a nationwide point prevalence study of delirium in older hospitalized patients using an easy standardized diagnostic tool. *BMC Med* 2016; 18: 106. DOI:10.1186/s12916-016-0649-8.

3. Morichi V, Fedecostante M, Morandi A et al. A point prevalence study of delirium in Italian nursing homes. *Dement Geriatr Cogn Disord* 2018; 46: 27–41.

4. Cheung ENM, Benjamin S, Heckman G et al. Clinical characteristics associated with the onset of delirium among long-term nursing home residents. *BMC Geriatr* 2018; 18: 39. DOI:10.1186/s12877-018-0733-3.

5. Hapca S, Guthrie B, Cvoro V et al. Mortality in people with dementia, delirium, and unspecified cognitive impairment in the general hospital: prospective cohort study of 6,724 patients with 2 years follow-up. *Clin Epidemiol* 2018; 10: 1743–1753.

6. Leslie DL, Inouye SK. The importance of delirium: economic and societal costs. *J Am Geriatr Soc* 2011; 59(Suppl 2): S241–S243.

7. MacLullich AM, Shenkin SD, Goodacre S et al. The 4 'A's test for detecting delirium in acute medical patients: a diagnostic accuracy study. *Health Technol Assess* 2019; 23: 1–194.

8. O'Connell H, Kennelly SP, Cullen W, Meagher DJ. Managing delirium in everyday practice: towards cognitive-friendly hospitals. *Adv Psychiatr Treat* 2014; 20: 380–389.

9. American Psychiatric Association. *Diagnostic and Statistical Manual of Mental Disorder* (5th edn) (DSM-5). APA, 2013.

10. Meagher D, O'Regan N, Ryan D et al. Frequency of delirium and subsyndromal delirium in an adult acute hospital population. *Br J Psychiatry* 2014; **205**: 478–485.

11. Evered L, Silbert B, Knopman D et al. Recommendations for the nomenclature of cognitive change associated with anaesthesia and surgery-2018. *J Alzheimers Dis* 2018; **66**: 1–10.

12. Moller J, Cluitmans P, Rasmussen L. Long-term postoperative cognitive dysfunction in the elderly: ISPOCD1 study. *Lancet* 1998; **351**: 857.

13. Huang C, Mårtensson J, Gögenur I, Asghar MS. Exploring postoperative cognitive dysfunction and delirium in noncardiac surgery using MRI: A systematic review. *Neural Plast* 2018; 1281657. DOI:10.1155/2018/1281657.

14. Cassarino M, Setti A. Complexity as key to designing cognitive-friendly environments for older people. *Front Psychol* 2016; **7**: 1329. DOI:10.3389/fpsyg.2016.01329.

15. Cassarino M, Setti A. Environment as 'Brain Training': a review of geographical and physical environmental influences on cognitive ageing. *Ageing Res Rev* 2015; **23** (Pt B): 167–182.

16. Siddiqi N, Harrison JK, Clegg A et al. Interventions for preventing delirium in hospitalised non-ICU patients. *Cochrane Database Syst Rev* 2016; **3**: CD005563. DOI:10.1002/14651858.CD005563.pub3.

17. Akunne A, Murthy L, Young J. Cost-effectiveness of multi-component interventions to prevent delirium in older people admitted to medical wards. *Age Ageing* 2012; **41**: 285–291.

18. Rosgen B, Krewulak K, Demiantschuk D et al. Validation of caregiver-centered delirium detection tools: a systematic review. *J Am Geriatr Soc* 2018; **66**: 1218–1225.

19. Garrett RM. Reflections on delirium – a patient's perspective. *J Intensive Care Soc* 2019; **20**: 258–262.

20. Darbyshire JL, Greig PR, Vollam S, Young JD, Hinton L. 'I can remember sort of vivid people...but to me they were plasticine.' Delusions on the intensive care unit: what do patients think is going on? *PLoS One* 2016; **11**: e0153775. DOI:10.1371/journal.pone.0153775

21. Siddiqi N, Young, J, House AO et al. Stop Delirium! A complex intervention to prevent delirium in care homes: a mixed-methods feasibility study. *Age Ageing* 2011; **40**: 90–98.

22. Morandi A, Pozzi C, Milisen K et al. An interdisciplinary statement of scientific societies for the advancement of delirium care across Europe (EDA, EANS, EUGMS, COTEC, IPTOP/WCPT). *BMC Geriatr* 2019; **19**: 253. DOI:10.1186/s12877-019-1264-2

23. Abraha I, Trotta F, Rimland JM et al. Efficacy of non-pharmacological interventions to prevent and treat delirium in older patients: A systematic overview. The SENATOR project ONTOP Series. *PLoS One* 2015; **10**: e0123090. DOI:10.1371/journal.pone.0123090

24. Khan A, Boukrina O, Oh-Park M et al. Preventing delirium takes a village: systematic review and meta-analysis of delirium preventive models of care. *J Hosp Med* 2019; **14**: E1–E7.

25. Lindroth H, Bratzke L, Purvis S et al. Systematic review of prediction models for delirium in the older adult inpatient. *BMJ Open* 2018; **8**: e019223. DOI:10.1136/bmjopen-2017-019223

26. Haley MN, Casey P, Kane RY, Dārziņš P, Lawler K. Delirium management: Let's get physical? A systematic review and meta-analysis. *Australas J Ageing* 2019; February 22. DOI:10.1111/ajag.12636

27. Guerra G, Almeida L, Zorzela L et al. and Canadian Critical Care Trials Group. Efficacy of music on sedation, analgesia and delirium in critically ill patients. A systematic review of randomized controlled trials. *J Crit Care* 2019; **53**: 75–80.

28. van Velthuijsen EL, Zwakhalen SM, Warnier RM et al. Psychometric properties and feasibility of instruments for the detection of delirium in older hospitalized

patients: a systematic review. *Int J Geriatr Psychiatry* 2016; **31**: 974–989.

29. Blandfort S, Gregersen M, Rahbek K, Juul S, Damsgaard EM. Single-bed rooms in a geriatric ward prevent delirium in older patients. *Aging Clin Exp Res* 2019; March 21. DOI:10.1007/s40520-019-01173-y

30. Flaherty JH, Little MO. Matching the environment to patients with delirium: lessons learned from the delirium room, a restraint-free environment for older hospitalized adults with delirium. *J Am Geriatr Soc* 2011; **59**(Suppl 2): S295–300.

31. Meagher D, Agar MR, Teodorczuk A. Debate article: antipsychotic medications are clinically useful for the treatment of delirium. *Int J Geriatr Psychiatry* 2018; **33**: 1420–1427.

32. Burry L, Mehta S, Perreault MM et al. Antipsychotics for treatment of delirium in hospitalised non-ICU patients. *Cochrane Database Syst Rev* 2018 June 18; **6**: CD005594. DOI:10.1002/14651858. CD005594.pub3

33. NICE (2010) Delirium: prevention, diagnosis and management. Clinical Guideline 103 2010, updated 2019. Available via: www.nice.org.uk/guidance/cg103 (last accessed 29 October 2019).

34. Lonergan E, Luxenberg J, Sastre AA. (2009) Benzodiazepines for delirium. *Cochrane Database Syst Rev* 2009; **4**: CD006379. Available via: www.cochranelibrary.com/cdsr/doi/10.1002/14651858.CD006379.pub3/full (last accessed 29 October 2019).

35. O'Malley G, Leonard M, Meagher D, O'Keefe ST. (2008) The delirium experience: a review. *J Psychosom Res* 2008; **65**: 223–228.

Chapter 20

Controlling the Confusion

Using Barrier Analysis in the Care Home Sector

Robert Colgate, Alison Turner and Danika Rafferty

Introduction

There is now very little room for doubt that care of older people will be a major consumer of health and social services resources in the UK for the foreseeable future.[1] Similar pressures, including effective coordination of care delivery with training, have also been identified in other countries.[2, 3] A perfectly valid desire to have individualized packages of care for people in their own homes contrasts strongly with the need to achieve economies of scale by providing care for more and more older adults with mental health problems in residential and nursing care settings.

There is a clear need for mental health services for older adults to be closely involved in the monitoring of mental health needs in the care home sector. Rates of depressive illness remain consistently high at around 40% in the UK,[4, 5] whilst the number of cases of dementia is rising steadily as ageing populations grow. Published reports point to widespread lack of mental health expertise in primary care and increasing societal expectations to manage increasingly complex combinations of mental and physical health needs.[6, 7, 8]

Over time, these issues have received attention from a wide variety of different sources, from conventional healthcare publications to general interest articles in magazines and mass media. The Royal College of General Practitioners has promoted good practice through a publicly available Mental Health Toolkit (www.rcgp.org.uk/clinical-and-research/resources/toolkits/mental-health-toolkit.aspx). Some idea of the range of public interest can be shown by just a few examples.

A collaboration with the BBC and the Open University by business expert Sir Gerry Robinson led to the production of a film in 2009 entitled *'Can Gerry Robinson fix Dementia Care Homes?'*, which was originally available as a DVD and promoted for use as a teaching or public education resource.[9] An anonymous personal view column in the *British Medical Journal* (Anonymous 2010) catalogued a damaging sequence of admissions and attempts at treatment involving her father before concluding that the only reliable source of practical help was 'family, friends and neighbours'.[10] The conclusion is all the more striking as the author is a hospital consultant.

Jolley et al. (1998) encouraged mental health services to 'address the situation [of mental illness in care home settings] actively' by using a genuine multidisciplinary approach to provide a 'full competent assessment'.[11] The Consumers Association magazine *Which?* has published a variety of articles, one of which described in some detail the experiences of three actors staying in four care homes in 2011.[12] The *Which?* website (www.which.co.uk) contains a downloadable checklist of points to consider when choosing a care home and sources for further information.

Bridgend Mental Health Service for Older Adults

In late 2009, the mental health service for older adults in Bridgend was reorganized to create a dedicated multi-professional team with specific responsibility for all residents in care homes in the Bridgend County Borough area. This team also maintained responsibility for providing a mental health liaison service to secondary care health services in Bridgend (based at the Princess of Wales and Maesteg General Hospitals), whilst the team consultant also provided senior psychiatric advice to a shared care ward (rehabilitation medicine and mental healthcare) on the Princess of Wales Hospital site.

The All-Party Parliamentary Group on Dementia has drawn attention to lack of expert input stating:

... specialist mental health services that could provide support and training to staff is highlighted as another barrier to workforce development (p. xii).[6]

In 2014, the Older People's Commissioner for Wales, Sarah Rochira, published 'A Place to Call Home',[13] with a follow-up report in 2017 detailing further recommendations and actions required to achieve the necessary impact in a number of areas including medication (especially antipsychotic drugs), falls prevention, befriending and dementia training.[14]

Published evaluations of care home in-reach teams have recognized the potential value of a more focused approach by nursing staff,[15] or nurses working with physiotherapists.[16] Commissioners and planners of local services in Bridgend confirmed that suitable training and education of staff was indeed a key priority area. Jolley et al. (1998) concur with this, stating that 'the need for generous and sensitive attention to the training and support of staff cannot be overestimated'.[11] Consequently, a strategic decision was taken deliberately to integrate the new liaison service with an existing educational team.

The educational team collaborated closely with the liaison team in order to identify further potential training or advisory issues within a care home. This might involve referral of a resident for advice around a specific issue or for an individual approach to care or for an intervention. It might also include supportive advice concerning design principles within the care setting, or recommended approaches to meaningful interaction – building upon material taught previously in educational sessions. Other issues that have been considered include concern about mental capacity, pain assessment, and the management, care and support of particular behaviours.

The educational team has consistently emphasized the need actively to consider the role and purpose of antipsychotic medication in dementia and it has been able to coordinate its efforts with members of the care home in-reach team. In addition, attention has been focused upon advance care planning, end-of-life plans and the role of mental health staff in providing advice and support to primary care. In selected cases, this has been undertaken with the intention of avoiding an unnecessary or disruptive hospital admission for people in the terminal stages of dementia.

The Dementia Care Training Team in Bridgend

The number of people with dementia in the UK in 2009 was around 820,000, representing about 1.3 % of the overall population.[17] A 2014 report by the Alzheimer's Society predicted the figure would increase, reaching one million by 2025 and doubling again by 2051 to just over 2 million people.[18]

Clinical Guideline 42 from NICE made specific reference to staff training, clearly stating that:

all staff working with older people in the Health, Social Care and Voluntary sectors have access to dementia-care training (skill development) that is consistent with their roles and responsibilities.[7]

This was expanded in updated guidance published in June 2018 with an emphasis upon person-centred care.[8] In 2016, the Care Council for Wales published *Good Work, the Dementia Learning and Development Framework for Wales*, which recommended training standards to facilitate competent dementia care, which in turn underpins the Welsh Government Dementia Care Plan 2018–2022.[19]

Prior to this, the need for specialist dementia care training and development had been identified locally in Bridgend through routine practice as well as operational and strategic meetings. As a result, a small dementia care training team was established in November 2002 and initially named the Residential Home Advisor team. The team consisted of a full-time registered mental health nurse and two occupational therapists jobsharing the equivalent of one whole-time post. In recognition of the importance of their work the dementia care training team has subsequently increased in size and scope.

Aims of the Team

Originally the aim of the team was to identify and then address the training needs of unqualified care staff working with people with dementia in the Bridgend County Borough area, both in the local authority facilities and throughout the independent care home sector. The team also sought to provide the care home staff with suitable specialist training and education along with an advisory role. The mandate of the team has since widened to provide training for other staff groups including local authority and independent sector domiciliary care and day centre staff, qualified social workers and community care workers, community and ward-based mental health staff and medical, surgical and orthopaedic ward staff (both registered and non-registered).

Training sessions have also been held for the carer education programme of the Alzheimer's Society, which has covered topics around 'what is dementia?', behavioural issues and management of eating and drinking in dementia. Dedicated sessions have been provided for specialist staff in the accident and emergency department, in a renal unit and for palliative care staff. Most recently relevant training has been provided for those working in the field of learning disabilities.

Training Needs

The vision of the team remains that, wherever a person with dementia is being supported and cared for within Bridgend County Borough, those working with them should be appropriately trained and suitably skilled with the expectation that this will lead to enhanced levels of care. This is consistent with recommendations that staff training is universally seen as a key feature in implementing and maintaining a good standard of care in both nursing and residential care homes.[20] Recent reports continue to highlight the vast need for training of the staff caring for people living with a diagnosis of dementia.

The All-Party Parliamentary Group on Dementia recommended that:

We need to move towards a situation where the workforce as a whole demonstrates effective knowl-edge and skills in caring for people with dementia (p. xiv).[6]

The report also recommended that in order to provide good, high-quality dementia care, the process of working between social care and healthcare must be closely integrated. 'Standardized training packages would provide quality assurance and consistency' (p. 33).[6] Effective support from specialist mental health teams should also be coordinated with the local education strategy to support training needs within the care home sector.

Training Package

The original dementia care training package was modular in nature and has been refined and developed over many years and in response to local needs and demands. It now consists of five days run over five consecutive weeks. The dementia care team is closely involved in the now mandatory dementia awareness training for all NHS Wales staff.

The first day provides an overview of dementia and the importance of person-centred care. The following days then cover a range of issues including communication, legal and ethical matters, behavioural concerns, hydration and nutrition, as well as hands-on care skills (see Box 20.1).

Professional advice and expert opinion have been sought when developing and rede-signing the days to ensure they are evidence-based, relevant and contemporary. The training was originally delivered in both care home settings and central venues, but owing to funding constraints it is now only delivered in central settings. Each day incorporates a wide variety of teaching and learning strategies that enable and facilitate care staff interaction. The package content and form are also influenced by evaluation responses.

The training package has in the past been accredited at certificate level with Swansea University. Specific 'bespoke' sessions have been written for certain staff groups – for example, an emphasis upon strategies to manage pain in dementia was required for medical, surgical and orthopaedic nursing staff.

The Dementia Care Training team completed a service evaluation project in 2011 using an action research model to investigate the question '*How does the dementia care training package impact on person-centred practice?*' The curriculum underwent a further review by Worcester University in 2016, and at present is undergoing a follow up review by Swansea University.

Box 20.1 Dementia care training package

Day 1: An Overview of Dementia

Day 2: Communication and Understanding Behaviour

Day 3: Physical and Mental Health Well-being

Day 4: Legal and Ethical Issues and End-of-Life Care

Day 5: Positive Environments and Meaningful Interactions

Barrier Analysis

The title of this chapter ('Controlling the confusion') reflects the complexity involved in providing an effective mental health service to the care home sector and at the same time

Box 20.2 Airport security	
Administrative	Printed list of prohibited items
	Warning signs and notices
Personnel	Routine enquiries from check-in staff
Physical	Checkpoints including passport control
	X-ray and screening of all luggage
Natural	Secure airfield perimeter
	Separation of open access and 'airside'

ensuring an integrated approach to training and education. As part of the design process for the service, several different interventions and innovations were deployed. The measures taken were deliberately selected from within the categories of physical and natural barriers, as described in barrier analysis.

Barrier analysis as a technique was developed in the nuclear and chemical industry during the 1990s primarily to reduce error.[21] This approach was subsequently transferred to healthcare settings, again with an emphasis on reducing mistakes. Formal teaching and training in barrier analysis was disseminated widely within the NHS in the UK by the National Patient Safety Agency (NPSA) as a component of root cause analysis.

Using the analysis, barriers can be usefully categorized into four main groups:

- Barriers dependent upon people
- Administrative or 'paper' barriers
- Physical or geographical barriers
- Natural barriers related to space or time

Standard teaching suggests that barriers reliant upon paper or upon people are weaker and less effective, while physical or natural barriers are in practice more effective as barriers.

To illustrate this further, it may be helpful to consider the process of maintaining and improving security at international airports. From first principles, it is a relatively simple task to list several measures and interventions that have progressively developed over recent years to prevent the unauthorized carriage of weapons or hazardous material onto commercial flights (see Box 20.2).

This list is not meant to be exhaustive, but it does usefully illustrate the essence of barrier analysis. If the items in this list are categorized into one of the four groups – people or paper (administrative), physical and natural – it quickly becomes clear that in this case more attention and investment has been focused upon physical or natural barriers that are traditionally felt to be more effective.

Barrier Analysis in Healthcare

While maybe not as obvious or as dramatic, it may also be helpful to compare the process of maintaining security on commercial flights with common and familiar healthcare processes such as correct site surgery and blood transfusion. In 2008, the WHO introduced a surgical safety checklist.[22] The first edition incorporated examples of both physical and natural barriers drawn directly from the basic principles of barrier analysis. Strict protocols regarding marking of the site of surgery represent a physical barrier to reduce the incidence of incorrect site surgery. The introduction of a 'time out' period before surgery commences is an excellent example of a natural barrier. Once again, emphasis upon physical and natural barriers is entirely consistent with the principles of ensuring a safe and effective process.

Similarly, the adoption of increasingly strict requirements, stipulated by NHS Wales, before a blood transfusion can go ahead represents another attempt to introduce a physical safety barrier. Recent developments include 'zero tolerance' concerning documentation at all stages of blood sampling, matching and administration of blood products, or transfusion. Incorrect spelling or missing information will result in rejection of samples for cross-matching.

While barrier analysis has traditionally been used to explore and analyse adverse incidents after they have happened, the NPSA has identified a prospective role for this technique, in which possible weaknesses or areas of vulnerability are searched for ahead of an incident. Thus, it is constructive to use the barrier analysis classifications to explore the issue of mental health supervision of residents in the care home sector.

Development of the Liaison Service to the Care Home Sector

We previously described the establishment and development of a process of referral coordination based upon a single point of access and a dedicated referral coordinator.[23] One of the core principles of this process is that patients are prioritized according to need (rather than the availability of staff). Another core principle is that specialist services retain the responsibility for specialist decisions, in this case mental health decisions about mental health need.

New referrals to the mental health service and requests for psychiatric reviews within the care home sector are still closely linked to this established referral coordination process. There is little doubt that the level of mental health need of this group will increase incrementally over time, associated with a rising older adult population.

Effective communication is maintained using standard templates and distribution of referrals via email.

In the Bridgend County Borough area, there are currently 24 residential and nursing care homes ranging from small residential care facilities to a large specialist mental health nursing home. Overall, the county has provision for more than 800 care beds. Local data has established that around one third of the residents in this care sector are prescribed antipsychotic medication and a further one third have additional mental health needs, again ranging widely from moderately severe depressive symptoms to highly complex physical and mental health needs.

Added to this level of need are the medico-legal requirements of the *Mental Health Act 1983* (see Chapter 21) and *Mental Capacity Act 2005*, especially deprivation of liberty safeguards (concerning which see Chapter 22). This substantial workload requires a systematic and robust review process that is still sufficiently flexible to adapt to rapid changes in care needs. The key to achieving this in a reliable and effective manner has been the creation of a spreadsheet for each care home listing the residents with mental health needs in each facility with sufficient basic information to determine how often the resident should be reviewed. (This logistic exercise may be viewed as a physical intervention in terms of barrier analysis.)

The Review Process

During the initial weeks following establishment of the team, arrangements were made with each home in turn for several team members to visit together to identify (and review) all the residents in the home who were already known to the mental health service. These data formed the core of the spreadsheet. In most but not all cases, the residents were either on existing community mental health nursing caseloads or regularly attending local mental health outpatient clinics.

In addition, a list of 'drugs of interest' was compiled using the British National Formulary – essentially sections on 'Psychoses and related disorders' (antipsychotic drugs and antipsychotic depot injections), 'Mania and hypomania' (specifically preparations of lithium) and 'Dementia' (drugs for dementia).[8] In a modern mental health service, prescription of antipsychotic medication, lithium carbonate (or citrate) as maintenance treatment, or any of the drugs for dementia will be associated with at least some degree of mental health need.

The list of 'drugs of interest' was given to care home managers and senior care staff with the advice that any resident receiving a regular prescription of any of these drugs of interest should either be under regular mental health follow-up or be offered a new mental health assessment. This aspect was also supported by a clinical audit cycle focusing upon antipsychotic prescribing.

In our experience, a small number of residents had reliable existing arrangements with local learning disability or general adult psychiatry services. The new liaison team did not interfere with these arrangements. However, a further small but significant number of residents with clear psychiatric needs were found not to be under any form of regular mental health follow-up. Agreement was reached without difficulty in most cases with the relevant general practitioners (GPs) and the care home staff to arrange an up-to-date mental health review by the new liaison team. Similarly, close joint working with staff in primary care has led to the adoption of detailed advance care planning in several cases after discussion with relevant family members and care home staff.

All the identified residents were then allocated a 'review frequency' which was compatible with a system of regular monthly visits. A convention was adopted for allocation of a visit in either the following month, in three or four months' time, or in six months. In order to familiarize staff new to the process, these review categories were colour coded as red, orange and green respectively (now more familiar as Red, Amber and Green or RAG rating). Some residents were discharged from regular or routine follow-up and allocated to 'see on request'. Exceptionally, residents with active or acute mental health needs or changes in treatment required more frequent review and specific or individual arrangements were made accordingly.

All these decisions and changes were entered on the spreadsheets, which were updated on a monthly basis. As the experience and familiarity of the team with this process developed, it became possible to identify in advance the level of need of each care home as a whole. Clearly a small residential care home will have a lower level of overall need than a large general nursing home, particularly if there is an adjoining nursing Older People's Mental Health (OPMH) facility, which is often the case in Bridgend.

Results of the Review Process

Comprehensive collation of all the residents with mental health needs and allocation using the red, orange and green RAG rating (or 'traffic light') categories allowed the level of need to be quantified reasonably accurately and more importantly a sufficient allocation of liaison staff to be identified for the next routine visit.

In terms of barrier analysis, a regime of predictably regular care home visits and the use of a reliable spreadsheet to anticipate the level of need are strong natural barriers, directly equivalent to the earlier examples given above. This is an inclusive process: individual residents or quiet and undemanding care homes are rather less likely to be overlooked. Spreadsheets and the like, along with structured routines, ensure there is a consistent and structured process of review. The list of 'drugs of interest', for instance, which if seen simply as guidance would be classified as a (weak) administrative or paper barrier, has over time been used much more as a physical tactic (along with the spreadsheets) to establish a clear and consistent mental health approach, to reduce uncertainty, and ensure comprehensive coverage within each care home.

To help consolidate this physical aspect, the use of a clearly written statement for each individual patient describing the role and purpose of the antipsychotic medication (including diagnosis, target signs and symptoms and a firm commitment to a further mental health review) has become established practice. When given prominence in documentation, training and service improvement initiatives, this 'antipsychotic statement' takes on the form of a natural or a physical intervention. Table 20.1 takes a wider perspective and shows in a summary grid the greater service value of these (stronger) physical and natural barriers.

The newly established liaison team identified unmet need within the care home sector for individual residents and in terms of care home staff training. This was associated with a small initial increase in appropriate admissions to hospital. However, ongoing analysis of relevant statistics has confirmed clearly more control of the total expenditure on continuing NHS care funding in this area. In turn, this is consistent with improved treatment interventions for mental illness and earlier or more effective prevention provided to this patient group by the combined liaison service and training team approach.

As experience developed, it became possible to schedule combined visits to several different care homes which are geographically close together and the team also chose to focus on a certain area during each week of the month – for example, in the third week of the month, the team visits several homes in the Porthcawl area. This can be especially efficient as it allows for frequent review or repeat assessments by other members of the team without disruption to the underlying programme of regular reviews. Following introduction of the

Table 20.1 Comparison table

Orthodox or Conventional Sectorized Old Age Psychiatry Service	
Consultation model ('they ask, we see . . .')	Personnel
No dedicated staff role for training	Personnel
Reliance upon individual ad hoc training	Personnel
Document-based advice and guidance	Administrative
Combined Education and Liaison Old Age Psychiatry Service	
Single point of access for referrals and reviews	Physical
Allocation of dedicated staff for training	Natural
Liaison model ('looking for problems . . .')	Natural
Routine of regular scheduled care home visits	Natural

team, the average rate of mental health admission from the care home sector was largely unchanged during the first two years but subsequently reduced in a sustained manner by more than a third for the next five years (less than two admissions per month for a population over 65 years of around 25,000).

Eventually, it became possible to 'fix' a four-weekly care home visit that was later relaxed to a more sustainable six-weekly cycle for six larger homes and a 12-week cycle for the remainder. The liaison team has affectionately christened this sequence as the 'hamster wheel'. This accounted for 48 weeks – the remaining four weeks each year have accordingly been identified as time off the wheel. Activities such as team building, audit and strategic review have usefully been held during these weeks, again avoiding unnecessary disruption to the cycle of monthly care home visits.

Using an electronic calendar to schedule the routine care home visits provided an unexpected opportunity to find a solution to another perennial team management problem. The permanent liaison team is composed of mental health professionals drawn from a range of specialist backgrounds: medical (psychiatry), mental health nursing, psychology, social work and occupational therapy. (The vital contribution of administrative and clerical staff must also be acknowledged here.) However, in a modern mental health service, the actual availability of individual members of staff is affected by a range of other demands. For example, mental health nursing staff are regularly called to contribute to continuing NHS healthcare assessments and decision support tool meetings to help to resolve difficult placement issues. Senior psychiatric staff are obliged to represent the Health Board at Mental Health Review tribunals often within certain specified timescales. More junior medical members of the team often have training commitments which cannot be altered and make a contribution to other rotas, such as hospital-at-night services.

With a little practice it was possible to establish a clear and coherent process using an electronic calendar to match the anticipated level of need in any given home with available staff from the liaison team. More importantly, in the event of a serious mismatch between need and the number of available staff, arrangements could be made with the care home to reschedule or to complete any remaining reviews on another occasion.

Establishing this predictable routine then allowed the training team to coordinate their own complex educational demands with the clinical staff and achieve joint educational and clinical reviews. At a workshop in Bridgend attended by care home managers, it was also identified that senior care staff and the managers themselves have been able to adjust their own duty rosters to coordinate with the liaison and training team visits – this collaborative approach received extremely positive evaluation and feedback from staff attending the workshop.

Senior colleagues have reflected positively on the processes described. Visiting older adults with mental illness (and physical illness) within the care home avoids unnecessary and often impractical outpatient attendance. In terms of safeguarding, the findings of care home in-reach team assessments provide invaluable assurance and collateral information during periods of concern.

In addition, and as expected, the same transparent approach to scheduling will facilitate joint working with specialists outside the mental health field, again ultimately to the benefit of the care home residents: examples are specialist speech and language therapy colleagues and clinicians from the local movement disorder team. Strategies which have proven useful are summarized in Box 20.3.

> **Box 20.3** Effective strategies for care home liaison
>
> DO allocate dedicated multi-professional staff with an adequate range of experience to both training and service teams
>
> DO ensure a comprehensive approach including all local care homes in service and training developments
>
> DO ensure coordination between service and training teams
>
> DO focus upon repetition and reinforcement of teaching at an individual level within the care home sector
>
> DO grasp opportunities to teach and train health and social care staff at all levels of experience in facilities that are fit for purpose
>
> DON'T rely upon an *ad hoc* teaching approach
>
> DON'T assume that general classroom teaching will meet local or individual needs in the care home setting
>
> (Note: We support strategies that map most closely to the stronger physical and natural categories in barrier analysis rather than the weaker personnel and administrative categories.)

Conclusion

As part of a reorganization of mental health services for older adults in Bridgend at the end of 2009, a new old age psychiatry liaison team has now become established with a specific remit to deliver mental health services to residents in the care home sector as well as a traditional hospital liaison role.

The level of need for mental health support locally is substantial. There is ample evidence to predict that the current level of need will increase over time in Bridgend and more widely throughout the rest of England and Wales. Running parallel with this increasing need is a steadily rising demand for effective dementia care training.

In Bridgend, the improved level of service has been carefully coordinated and integrated within an existing well-established dementia care training team. In this chapter, barrier analysis has been useful to understand and to help explain the innovations and interventions deployed during the reorganization.[24] An infographic illustration has been prepared to extend awareness of the work of both the care home in-reach service and the dementia training team more widely, especially to family and friends of care home residents.

The role of barrier analysis in reviews of adverse incidents is already well known – the authors recommend that the same approach could be of great value to any mental health service, especially during a period of restructuring or planned reorganization.

Acknowledgements

For information, the citation for the original paper on which this chapter is based is:

Colgate R, Davies K, Lambert H, Turner A. Controlling the confusion: using barrier analysis in the care home sector. *Adv Psychiatr Treat* 2012; 19: 426–433.

Dr Colgate would like to thank current and former members of the Old Age Psychiatry Liaison team and the two anonymous reviewers for their valuable contribution to the processes described in the original article. He would also like to thank Blood Bank manager

Sylvia Lees at the Princess of Wales Hospital in Bridgend for her explanation of current blood transfusion procedures and would particularly like to thank Mr Russell Warwick for his personal and professional reflections about the care home in-reach service in Bridgend. Finally, the authors wish to record their thanks to the co-authors of the original paper upon which this chapter was based, Karyn Davies and Helen Lambert,[24] and to express their respect for the ongoing work that they do in this field.

References

1. Banks V, Searle G, Jenkins R. Psychiatry in the UK: an overview. *Int Psychiatry* 2011; 8: 35–38.

2. Bernstein CA, Hershfield B, Cohen DC. Psychiatry in the USA: an overview. *Int Psychiatry* 2010; 7: 90–92.

3. Shaji KS, Dias A. Dementia care in India: a progress report. *Int Psychiatry* 2006; 4: 9–10.

4. Godfrey M, Townsend J, Surr C et al. *Prevention and Service Provision: Mental Health Problems in Later Life*. Institute of Health Sciences and Public Health Research, Leeds University and Division of Dementia Studies, Bradford University, 2005.

5. British Geriatrics Society and Royal College of Psychiatrists. *Depression among Older People Living in Care Homes OP105*. Last accessed on 11th September 2019 via: www .bgs.org.uk/sites/default/files/content/attach ment/2018-09-12/Depression%20among%2 0older%20people%20living%20in%20care% 20homes%20report%202018.pdf

6. All-Party Parliamentary Group on Dementia. *Prepared to Care: Challenging the Dementia Skills Gap*. Alzheimer's Society, 2009. Last accessed on 11th September 2019 via: www.alzheimers.org.uk/sites/default/fil es/migrate/downloads/appg_report_prepar ed_to_care.pdf

7. National Institute for Health and Clinical Excellence and Social Care Institute for Excellence. *Dementia. Supporting People with Dementia and their Carers in Health and Social Care*. NICE Clinical Guideline 42. National Collaborating Centre for Mental Health, 2006 (amended 2011).

8. National Institute for Health and Care Excellence (NICE). *Dementia: Assessment, Management and Support for People Living with Dementia and their Carers*. NICE guideline. NICE Clinical Guideline 97. NICE, 2018. Last accessed on 11th September 2019 via: www.nice.org.uk/gui dance/ng97

9. See Open University Website: www .open.edu/openlearn/body-mind/ou-on-the-bbc-can-gerry-robinson-fix-dementia-care Last accessed 13th October 2019.

10. Anonymous. Does anyone care? *Brit Med J* 2010; 341: 348.

11. Jolley D, Dixey S, Read K. Residential and nursing homes. In: *Seminars in Old Age Psychiatry* (eds. RN Butler, B Pitt): 225–246. Gaskell, 1988.

12. Which Limited. (2011) Care homes investigated. *Which?* 2011; **May**: 58–61.

13. Older People's Commissioner for Wales. *A Place to Call Home: A Review into the Quality of Life and Care of Older People living in Care Homes in Wales*. The Older People's Commissioner for Wales, 2014. Last accessed on 11th September 2019 via: www.olderpeoplewales.com/en/Reviews/R esidential_Care_Review/ReviewReport .aspx

14. Older People's Commissioner for Wales *A Place to Call Home: Impact and Analysis. Assessing Progress to Improve the Quality of Life and Care of Older People Living in Care Homes in Wales*. The Older People's Commissioner for Wales, 2017. Last accessed on 11th September 2019 via: www .olderpeoplewales.com/Libraries/Uploads/ A_Place_to_Call_Home_-_Impact_Analys is_-_Final.sflb.ashx

15. Lawrence V and Bannerjee S. Improving care in care homes: a qualitative evaluation of the Croydon care home support team. *Aging Ment Health* 2010; **14**: 416–424.

16. Szczepura A, Nelson S, Wild D. (2008) In-reach specialist nursing teams for

residential care homes: uptake of services, impact on care provision and cost-effectiveness. *BMC Health Services Research* 2008; **8**: 269. https://bmchealth servres.biomedcentral.com/track/pdf/10 .1186/1472-6963-8-269 [last accessed 11th September 2019].

17. Alzheimer's Research Trust. *Dementia 2010: The Economic Burden of Dementia and Associated Research Funding in the United Kingdom*. University of Oxford, 2010. www.alzheimersresearchuk.org/wp-content/uploads/2015/01/Dementia2010F ull.pdf [last accessed 11th September 2019].

18. Prince M, Knapp M, Guerchet M et al. *Dementia UK* (Second edition). Alzheimer's Society, 2014. Last accessed on 11th September 2019 via: http://eprints .lse.ac.uk/59437/1/Dementia_UK_Secon d_edition_-_Overview.pdf

19. Care Council for Wales. *Good Work. A Dementia Learning and Development Framework for Wales*. Care Council for Wales, 2016. Last accessed on 11th September 2019 via: https://socialcare .wales/cms_assets/file-uploads/Good-Work-Dementia-Learning-And-Development-Framework.pdf

20. Ballard C, O'Brien J, James I, Swann A. *Dementia: Management of Behavioural and Psychological Symptoms*. Open University Press, 2001.

21. Lyons M, Woloshynowych M, Adams S, Vincent C. *Error Reduction in Medicine*. The Nuffield Trust, National Patient Safety Agency, Imperial College, 2004. Last accessed on 11th September 2019 via: www .nuffieldtrust.org.uk/files/2017-01/error-reduction-in-medicine-web-final.pdf

22. World Health Organization. *Surgical Safety Checklist (first edition)*. WHO, 2008 (revised 2009). Last accessed on 11th September 2019 via: www.who.int/patient safety/safesurgery/checklist/en/

23. Colgate R, Jones S. Controlling the confusion: management of referrals into mental health services for older adults. *Adv Psychiatr Treat* 2007; **13**: 317–324.

24. Colgate R, Davies K, Lambert H, Turner A. Controlling the confusion: using barrier analysis in the care home sector. *Adv Psychiatr Treat* 2012; **18**: 426–433.

Chapter

21

Mental Health Laws from All UK Jurisdictions

Carole Burrell and Charlotte Emmett

Introduction

Mental health law in the UK operates within three legal jurisdictions: England and Wales, Scotland and Northern Ireland. This chapter provides an overview of the legal framework that governs the treatment and care of older adults with mental disorder and mental disability in the UK. It then describes the formal civil powers that exist in law to compulsorily detain and treat older people in hospital for mental disorder, and how these laws compare across the different jurisdictions of the UK.

An Overview of Mental Health Legislation in the UK

Each of the three legal jurisdictions in the UK has its own distinct laws governing the care and treatment of adults with mental disorder (see Table 21.1). Although these laws have broadly similar functions, they can be markedly different in substance and practice.

Traditionally, in each jurisdiction, the treatment and care of older people for mental disorder and mental disability have potentially fallen under two parallel yet overlapping legislative frameworks. On the one hand, mental health legislation comprising the *Mental Health Act 1983* (MHA) in England and Wales, the *Mental Health (Care and Treatment) (Scotland) Act 2003* (MHCTA) in Scotland, and in Northern Ireland the *Mental (Northern Ireland) Order 1986* (NI Order) has provided both informal and formal powers to treat 'patients' for mental disorder in hospital or in the community. The function of this legislation is broadly similar across the UK: to treat mental disorder, using compulsion if necessary, whilst minimising the risk to the patient and/or others. On the other hand, separate incapacity laws have provided a more generalised framework that regulates decision making (including medical treatment decisions) on behalf of adults who lack capacity due to mental disorder or disability (e.g. dementia, brain injury, learning disability). In England and Wales, the *Mental Capacity Act 2005* (MCA) and in Scotland, the *Adults with Incapacity (Scotland) Act 2000* are the primary statutes which govern this area, whereas Northern Ireland has operated for many years under common law or 'judge-made' principles. The underlying ethos of mental incapacity law is the empowerment of the incapacitated individual, by maximising decision-making capacity and intervening in a person's best interests, in the least restrictive way.

Whilst these frameworks are separate, with distinct functions and court systems, their use is not mutually exclusive. An older person diagnosed with advanced dementia, for example, might be treated under more than one legal regime at any one time, receiving compulsory treatment in hospital for a mental disorder using formal powers, whilst also receiving treatment for an unrelated physical condition under incapacity laws if she lacks capacity, or under common laws when capable of making that choice. The appropriate legal framework to use in each case will depend on a range of factors, including the type of treatment proposed (i.e. whether it is for mental or physical disorder), whether a person has decision-making capacity, a person's detained status and whether they agree to the administration of treatment and care.

Although, at the time of writing, this mental health/mental incapacity distinction still exists across the UK, Northern Ireland has recently enacted sweeping law reform which aims to 'fuse' mental health and mental capacity laws under one broad statute. The new *Mental Capacity (Northern Ireland) Act 2016* was passed by the Northern Ireland Assembly on 15 March 2016 and received Royal Assent on 9 May 2016. When the Act comes into full force, the authority for all mental health treatment will be based on either impairment of decision-making capacity and best interests, or will stem from the consent of the capacitated individual. Put another way, once the 2016 Act is in full force, it will no longer be possible to use separate mental health laws to compulsorily treat patients in Northern Ireland against their will when they retain capacity and refuse treatment.

Full implementation of the 2016 Act is not envisaged until late 2020, although provisions that relate to Deprivation of Liberty are due to come into force by 1 October 2019. *The Mental Health (Northern Ireland) Order 1986* will remain in place for all until full implementation, when it will be replaced, for those aged 16 and over, by the new Act.

Whether full implementation can be realised by 2020, at a time when the Northern Ireland Assembly is (at the time of writing) suspended and alongside the deepening constitutional challenges of Brexit, remains to be seen. For this reason, we retain reference to the 1986 Order in the remainder of this chapter, whilst being alive to the possibility that a new capacity-based legal framework might be implemented in Northern Ireland under the 2016 Act in the not so distant future.

Older patients who are compulsorily detained in hospital for mental health treatment in the UK fall broadly into two groups: those who develop mental illness (predominantly dementia or depression) for the first time in later life, usually, but not always, as a consequence of the ageing process; and those with so-called 'enduring mental health problems' such as schizophrenia, psychosis and personality disorder.[1] Often mental disorder sits alongside other complex and interrelated physical health needs and can be compounded by factors such as alcohol misuse or extreme frailty. Older people might typically be detained in hospital if they are refusing treatment and display challenging behaviour or serious self-neglect that poses a risk to themselves or others which warrants a period of inpatient assessment and/or treatment. However, formal powers should be used only where inpatient hospital treatment is considered necessary, and only then when no other less restrictive way of providing care and treatment is available.[2]

In spite of the alarming rise in the use of formal powers to compulsorily detain older patients across the UK,[3] most older patients will enter hospital voluntarily as 'informal' patients under civil as opposed to criminal provisions. Nevertheless, a small minority of older people are detained as a result of a court order following criminal proceedings, or might already be under sentence in prison and require transfer to hospital for psychiatric

Table 21.1 UK mental health legislation

UK jurisdiction	Mental Health Law: provides for the compulsory detention and treatment of 'patients' for mental disorder.	Mental Incapacity Law: governs decision-making on behalf of people who lack capacity, including provisions for advance care and financial planning.	Human Rights Law
England & Wales	**Mental Health Act 1983** (as amended by 2007 Mental Health Act)	**Mental Capacity Act 2005**	**European Convention on Human Rights and Fundamental Freedoms**: has direct application in UK law via **Human Rights Act 1998**.
Scotland	**Mental Health (Care and Treatment) (Scotland) Act 2003** (as amended by 2015 Mental Health (Scotland) Act)	**Adults with Incapacity (Scotland) Act 2000**	**UN Convention on the Rights of Persons with Disabilities**: ratified by UK government in 2009. Persuasive authority only in UK.
Northern Ireland	**Mental (Northern Ireland) Order 1986**	**Common Law (judge-made principles derived from case law)**	
	Mental Capacity (Northern Ireland) Act 2016 (expected to come into force in 2020)		

treatment. Whilst these numbers are very small, prisoners over 65 years represent one of the fastest-growing age groups in prison, often exhibiting high rates of psychiatric and physical co-morbidity that require mental health intervention and treatment.[4]

Outside hospital settings, there are a number of ways in which older people living in the community can be legally compelled to engage with mental health services or receive mental health treatment. In England, Wales and Northern Ireland for example, older people who satisfy certain statutory criteria can be made subject to mental health guardianship and be required, at the behest of an appointed guardian, to reside in a particular place and/or engage with mental health services in the community. Moreover, community treatment orders, introduced by the Mental Health Act 2007 amendments, now mean that certain patients in England and Wales can receive treatment in the community rather than under detention in hospital (whilst remaining subject to potential hospital recall); community-based compulsory treatment powers also exist in Scotland.

These mental health statutes and common laws are in turn supplemented by subordinate or delegated legislation and statutory and non-statutory guidance in the form of statutory codes of practice and clinical guidance issued by professional bodies and organisations. Those who operate under mental health and mental incapacity laws are required 'to have regard to' statutory guidance in the codes of practice and any departures without good reason are likely to be unlawful.[5]

Underpinning these domestic legal frameworks, various international human rights treaties or conventions exist that promote and guarantee a range of human rights and freedoms of individuals against unlawful interference by the state. It is widely recognised that older people living with dementia and other mental health problems can often be denied their human rights, despite the existence of domestic legislation which affords such protections.[6] We are concerned with two human rights conventions in this chapter: the *European Convention on Human Rights and Fundamental Freedoms* (ECHR), which is particularly important because it has direct application in UK law via the Human Rights Act 1998; and the United Nations Convention on the Rights of Persons with Disabilities (CRPD), which requires states to adopt national policies upholding the rights of people with disabilities. The UK government ratified the CRPD in 2009, and whilst not directly enforceable in UK law, it is increasingly being used by policy makers (and the courts) to shape the future development and reform of mental health and mental capacity law in the UK.[7]

Civil Detention in the UK

Compulsory civil detention under UK mental health law is only lawful when the relevant statutory criteria are satisfied and the legally defined procedures are followed and documented correctly (summarized in Table 21.2).

The Statutory Criteria and the Role of the Clinician

There are essential grounds, contained within the legislation, which must be satisfied in order to detain a patient. These statutory detention criteria differ between the categories of detention and the jurisdictions of the UK. Commonly they involve assessments being undertaken of the type and severity of the patient's mental disorder, the level of risk that the patient presents, and the need for hospital detention. For longer-term detention the availability of appropriate medical treatment also becomes an important consideration.

Central to the forms of detention outlined further is the exercise of clinical opinion, which is essential to demonstrate that the statutory criteria are made out[8] and which may be presented as 'medical recommendations' (England, Wales and Northern Ireland) or within 'mental health reports' (Scotland).

Mental Disorder

The existence or likelihood of mental disorder is key to all decisions to detain. The MHA defines this term widely as 'any disorder or disability of the mind'[9] affording medical professionals considerable discretion in determining whether the particular presentation of an older person amounts to a mental disorder.

In Northern Ireland mental disorder is 'mental illness, mental handicap, and any other disorder or disability of mind'[10] with individual statutory definitions for mental handicap and mental illness. In Scotland the definition is 'mental illness; personality disorder or learning disability'.[11] Dementia and depression fall squarely within all these definitions.

Emergency Detention

Inevitably, situations arise which call for an immediate professional response and intervention to mental distress. In contrast to other forms of detention, emergency detention is measured in hours, involves little formality and can be implemented on the opinion of a single clinician.

For example, in England and Wales the MHA authorises the registered medical practitioner or approved clinician (AC) in charge of treatment to exercise 'holding powers' in respect of an informal inpatient where that clinician is of the opinion that an application for formal admission under the MHA[12] 'ought to be made'. Use of this power prevents the patient from leaving hospital, giving the professionals who wish to undertake a MHA assessment time to do so. A similar holding power can be exercised by a medical practitioner in Northern Ireland for up to 48 hours, and in Scotland an emergency detention certificate can be granted by a medical practitioner upon certifying that the grounds are made out to do so. Where practicable, this should be with the agreement of a mental health officer (MHO) following consultation. The certificate allows removal to hospital and, as in England and Wales, lasts no more than 72 hours.

In all UK jurisdictions, certain classes of nurses can exercise time-limited powers of restraint to prevent an informal inpatient, who is receiving hospital-based treatment for mental disorder, from leaving. In England, Wales and Northern Ireland the nurses' detention power has a maximum duration of 6 hours and is applied pending the availability of a more senior clinician who then determines whether it is appropriate to apply the holding powers outlined above. In Scotland, the nurses' detention power is limited to a maximum of three hours and is exercised in order that a medical practitioner can carry out an examination for the purpose of determining whether an emergency or short-term detention certificate is warranted.

Short-Term and Longer-Term Detention

Short-term detention (for assessment) and longer-term detention (for treatment) are the most commonly used forms of detention in the UK.

In England, Wales and Northern Ireland decisions on detention of either type are made by an approved mental health professional (approved social worker in Northern Ireland)[13] and must be founded on two medical recommendations (one in Northern Ireland)[14] confirming that the statutory grounds are met. In Scotland, an approved medical practitioner[15] (AMP) can grant a short-term detention certificate following consultation with a MHO whose consent to the grant is required whilst the decision to grant a longer-term detention called a compulsory treatment order is reserved to the Mental Health Tribunal.

- Short-term detention for assessment

Broadly speaking, assessment involves clarification of the nature and degree of the patient's condition, the development of a treatment plan and deciding whether longer-term detention is indicated. Short-term detention is for a maximum non-renewable duration of 28 days (14 days in Northern Ireland).

- Longer-term detention for treatment

Longer-term detention supports the sustained treatment of a patient's mental disorder lasting up to 6 months initially, renewable[16] for a further 6 months and then annually.[17]

Table 21.2 Statutory grounds for civil detention

UK JURISDICTION	Emergency detention	Short-term detention	Longer-term detention
England & Wales MHA Part I	**S5(2)** Appears that an application for detention ought to be made in respect of informal inpatient <72 hours **S5(4)** Appears (to nurse) that degree of mental disorder in informal inpatient necessitates immediate restraint for health/safety of patient or protection of others; immediate attendance of a RMP/AC not practicable <6 hours	**S2** Has mental disorder of nature/degree warranting detention for assessment (possibly followed by medical treatment); ought to be detained in interests of patient's health/safety or protection of others <28 days	**S3** Has mental disorder of nature/degree making medical treatment appropriate; treatment necessary for health/safety of patient or protection of others and cannot be provided unless detained; appropriate treatment available 6 months and renewable
Scotland MHCTA Parts 5–7	**S36** Likelihood of mental disorder; significant impairment of ability to decide treatment; satisfied of necessity urgently to detain to determine medical treatment required; significant risk to patient's health/ safety/welfare or to safety of another if not detained; and obtaining short-term detention cert. involves undesirable delay <72 hours **S299** Appears (to nurse) that mental disorder present; immediate restraint necessary for health/safety/ welfare of patient or for safety of another; and medical examination necessary to determine grant of emergency or short-term detention cert. <3 hours	**S44** Likelihood of mental disorder; significant impairment of ability to decide treatment; detention necessary to determine/administer medical treatment; significant risk to patient's health/ safety/welfare or to safety of another if not detained; and short-term detention cert. necessary <28 days	**S57** Satisfied of mental disorder; medical treatment likely to prevent worsening of or alleviate symptoms of disorder is available; significant risk to patient's health/safety/welfare or to safety of another if treatment not provided; significant impairment of ability to decide treatment and compulsory treatment order necessary 6 months and renewable

| Northern Ireland NIO Part II | Art 7(2) Appears that application for detention ought to be made in respect of an informal inpatient <48 hours | Art 7(3) Appears (to nurse) that application for detention ought to be made in respect of an informal inpatient; immediate attendance of RMP not practicable <6 hours | Art 4 Mental disorder of nature/degree warranting detention for assessment (or assessment followed by medical treatment) and substantial likelihood of serious physical harm to patient/other if not detained <14 days | Art 12 Mental illness or severe mental impairment of a nature/degree warranting detention for medical treatment and substantial likelihood of serious physical harm to patient/other if not detained 6 months and renewable |

Unsurprisingly, the statutory grounds are more stringent than for short-term detention. In England and Wales 'appropriate medical treatment' must be available for the patient, whilst in Northern Ireland detention is dependent on the patient suffering from 'mental illness or severe mental impairment' rather than the more general 'mental disorder'.

In Scotland, the decision on a compulsory treatment order is taken by the Tribunal upon receipt of an application submitted by a MHO with two mental health reports[18] stating that the applicable criteria are met including the availability of medical treatment likely to prevent a worsening of the patient's mental disorder or alleviation of its symptoms.

Every patient subject to short-term or longer-term detention will have a designated clinician with overall responsibility for their care and treatment. This is a responsible clinician (RC) in England and Wales and a responsible medical officer (RMO) in Scotland and Northern Ireland. For patients in Scotland, the RMO will be chosen from the pool of available AMPs. In England and Wales the RC should be the available AC with the most appropriate expertise to meet the patient's main assessment and treatment needs.[19] The RC and RMO are usually medical practitioners; however, in England and Wales the RC may be a non-medical AC.

Compulsory Mental Health Treatment in Hospital

Perhaps the single most controversial aspect of mental health law relates to its compulsory treatment provisions. Until such time as the *Mental Capacity (Northern Ireland) Act 2016* comes into force, each jurisdiction in the UK reserves the power to force patients with mental disorder to accept treatment if there is a health risk to themselves or others, despite their retaining full decision-making capacity[20] (see: Part IV of the MHA, Part 16 of MHCTA and Part IV of the NI Order) (summarized in Table 21.3). In this regard, conventional mental health law sits at odds with the social model of disability advocated by the CRPD, in particular, Article 4 ('no discrimination of any kind on the basis of disability'), Article 12 (persons shall 'enjoy legal capacity on an equal basis with others in all aspects of life') and Article 14 ('the existence of a disability shall in no case justify a deprivation of liberty').[21]

Treatment Without Consent

As a general principle, treatment for mental disorder can be administered without consent under mental health legislation if it is given by or under the direction of the AC in charge of a patient's treatment (in England and Wales) or RMO (in Northern Ireland and Scotland) and is not a treatment which has been singled out as requiring separate statutory safeguards and procedures.

Before we move to look at those safeguards in more detail, it is important to note that not all detained patients will necessarily be subject to compulsory treatment powers. Under MHA, for example, only patients detained outside of the emergency provisions of the Act are subject to Part IV and can be treated without consent, with a similar approach taken in Scotland and Northern Ireland.

Furthermore, compulsory treatment powers apply only in relation to 'medical treatment for mental disorder'. Treatment of a detained patient's physical disorder, unrelated to their mental health, falls outside the compulsory provisions and cannot be administered without a patient's consent unless she lacks capacity, in which case separate incapacity laws would apply. That said, the courts have interpreted the term 'treatment for mental disorder' widely, to include treatment that not only addresses the causes of the core mental disorder itself, but also measures taken to 'alleviate the consequences of the disorder'.[22] As such, many physical treatments are administered under compulsory treatment provisions because they are considered to be 'part and parcel of', or ancillary to, the core mental health treatment itself.

Second Opinion Safeguards

Certain categories of medical treatment for mental disorder require second opinion medical approval from outside the hospital before they can be administered lawfully. In England, Wales and Northern Ireland this second opinion role is carried out by a second opinion appointed doctor (SOAD) appointed by the Care Quality Commission or in Northern Ireland by the Regulation and Quality Improvement Authority; in Scotland it is a designated medical practitioner (DMP) appointed by the Mental Welfare Commission who fulfils this role.

The treatments that attract specific safeguards are:

- Psychosurgery, including the implantation of hormones to reduce male sex drive and surgery to destroy brain tissue, which, though rarely performed, will always require the patient's consent and certification by an independent second opinion doctor (SOAD or DMP). These safeguards apply to all patients, both voluntary and detained.
- Prolonged administration of medicine beyond a certain period of time under detention (3 months in England, Wales and Northern Ireland, and 2 months in Scotland), which, in the absence of an emergency, can only be administered if the patient consents, or if authorised by an independent second opinion doctor.
- ECT which, in the absence of an emergency, can only be administered in England, Wales and Scotland with the consent of a capable patient, or where a patient lacks capacity, with second opinion medical approval. Furthermore, under the MHA, the decision to treat with ECT must not conflict with an advance decision to refuse treatment (ADRT), or decision of a donee under a Lasting Power of Attorney (LPA) or deputy of the Court of Protection. In Northern Ireland, the safeguards surrounding ECT are not so robust and ECT can be administered to a non-consenting capacitated adult if it is authorised by a SOAD.

Urgent Treatment

The above safeguards do not apply in the case of urgent treatment. Urgent treatment is defined in the MHA as treatment which is:

1. immediately necessary to save the patient's life; or
2. not being irreversible, is immediately necessary to prevent a serious deterioration in the patient's condition; or
3. not being irreversible or hazardous, is immediately necessary to alleviate serious suffering by the patient; or
4. not being irreversible or hazardous, is immediately necessary to prevent the patient from behaving violently or being a danger to himself or others.

Similar emergency treatment provisions exist in the MHCTA and Northern Ireland Order. The way urgent treatment is defined in the MHA means that some treatments which are considered 'irreversible' (e.g. psychosurgery) or 'hazardous' (such as ECT) cannot go ahead in certain situations without safeguards, even though treatment is considered urgent. As such ECT can only be given under the MHA in an emergency where the risks are very high: it is immediately necessary to save a patient's life, or is immediately necessary to prevent serious deterioration of a patient's condition. In each case, treatment can only continue for as long as is immediately necessary and when this ceases to be the case, the normal safeguards will apply.

Discharge from Civil Detention

All forms of civil detention are subject to maximum periods of duration save that renewal or extension may be possible, most notably in respect of patients subject to longer-term detention. In many cases a patient's discharge from detention occurs before the maximum detention period expires, having been brought to an end in one of a number of ways.

The RC/RMO

Those who are ultimately accountable for the patient's care and treatment are also responsible for keeping the patient's short-term and longer-term detention under review to ensure that when the grounds for detention are no longer supported the patient's detention ends. The RC has the power and duty to discharge the patient in these circumstances with the same responsibility falling on the RMO in Northern Ireland and the RMO in Scotland who is required to revoke the patient's short-term detention certificate or compulsory treatment order.

The Tribunal

To ensure compatibility with ECHR obligations, UK mental health legislation must provide a means to enable the cases of those who are detained to be reviewed by an independent and impartial court which possesses the power to discharge the patient from detention.[23] Reviews are most often triggered by patients exercising their right to challenge their detained status; however, automatic referrals also occur periodically, for example after a certain time has elapsed within which the patient's case has not come before Tribunal (England, Wales and Northern Ireland) and following the RMO's determination to extend a compulsory treatment order in Scotland.

Irrespective of how the review is initiated, once a case is before the relevant court it has the power to order the patient's discharge, which must be exercised in certain circumstances.

In England, the *First-tier Tribunal (Mental Health)* reviews MHA detention. A *Mental Health Review Tribunal* operates in both Wales and Northern Ireland. In Scotland it is the *Mental Health Tribunal for Scotland*.

The powers exercisable by the Tribunals are contained in the applicable mental health legislation,[24] supplemented by rules governing procedure.[25]

There is much common ground in terms of practice between the four Tribunals:

- a hearing is usually convened before a panel;
- the panel comprises a legal, medical and lay[26] member;
- evidence (written and/or oral) is provided by those involved in the care and treatment of the patient, including the RC/RMO, setting out their recommendations on detention;

UK JURISDICTION	Treatment without Consent?	Prolonged medication?	ECT?	Psychosurgery?
England & Wales MHA Part IV	s63 Yes, if treatment by or under direction of AC in charge of treatment unless treatment falls under s58, s58A, s57	s58 Yes, after 3 months if AC or SOAD certifies patient capable and consents, or SOAD & 2 non-medical practitioners certify that incapable or capable but refusing and medication remains appropriate (subject to urgent treatment under s62)	s58A Yes, if AC/SOAD certifies patient capable and consents or SOAD & 2 non-medical practitioners certify that patient incapable and ECT is appropriate and no conflict with ADRT, LPA or deputy or Court of Protection decision (subject to urgent treatment under s62)	s57 Yes, if patient consents and SOAD and 2 non-medical practitioners certify that patient capable of consenting and treatment appropriate (subject to urgent treatment under s62)
Scotland MHCTA Part 16	s242 Yes, where the RMO records in writing reasons for treatment in best interest of patient and the treatment does not fall under s237 or 236	S237 Yes, after 2 months if RMO/DMP certifies patient capable and consents, or DMP certifies that incapable and in patient's best interests or that patient incapable and resists treatment but necessary in patient's best interests (subject to urgent treatment under s243)	S237 Yes, if patient capable and consents or DMP certifies patient incapable and in patient's best interests, or DMP certifies that patient incapable and resists treatment but necessary to save life, prevent serious deterioration or alleviate suffering (subject to urgent treatment under s243)	S236 Yes, if patient consents and DMP and lay opinions from MWC that patient is capable and consents and treatment is in patient's best interests, or patient incapable but no objection and treatment in best interests. Treatment must be authorised by Court of Session
Northern Ireland NIO Part IV	Article 69 Yes, if treatment by or under direction of RMO unless treatment falls under Art 63 or 64	Art 64 Yes, after 3 months if RMO or SOAD certifies patient consent, or Part II doctor or SOAD certifies that incapable, or capable but refusing and treatment should be administered as likely to alleviate/prevent deterioration of condition (Subject to urgent treatment under Art 68)	Art 64 Yes, if RMO or SOAD certifies patient consents, or SOAD certifies that incapable, or capable but refusing and treatment should be administered as likely to alleviate/prevent deterioration of condition (subject to urgent treatment under Art 68)	Art 63 Yes, if patient consents and SOAD and 2 non-medical practitioners certify patient capable and consents, and that proposed treatment is appropriate (subject to urgent treatment under Art 68)

- patients can attend the Tribunal hearing and give evidence;
- patients are usually legally represented;
- following the hearing, the Tribunal makes a determination;
- if not satisfied that the grounds for detention have been made out to the relevant legal standard, the Tribunal *must* discharge (England, Wales, Northern Ireland) or revoke (Scotland) the detention order.

Aside from the power to restore the patient's liberty, Tribunals operating in England, Wales and Northern Ireland have limited powers to make recommendations. The Scottish Tribunal has greater authority including powers to vary a compulsory treatment order by amending, removing or adding to the measures specified therein.

Other Routes to Discharge

Associate hospital managers[27] periodically review a patient's detention in England and Wales, for example upon its renewal. The managers' review follows a procedure very similar to the First-tier Tribunal albeit that it does not have the status of a court. After reviewing the evidence, if all three managers are not persuaded that detention remains warranted, discharge should follow.[28] Under the MHA the nearest relative can order a patient's discharge from detention giving not less than 72 hours' notice and subject to the RC's 'barring' power, which must be on the grounds of dangerousness.

In Scotland, the Mental Welfare Commission has the power to review and revoke compulsory treatment orders[29] although in practice it is much more likely to refer the case to the Tribunal for consideration.

Conclusion

We conclude our chapter by considering the future direction of mental health law in the UK. At the time of writing (July 2019) the laws that govern the detention and treatment of mental health patients in the UK, including older people suffering from mental ill health, are the subject of widespread review and reform. Northern Ireland's new capacity-based approach to mental health treatment and care under the *Mental Capacity (Northern Ireland) Act 2016*, in particular, heralds a new and progressive approach to mental health treatment, which is more in line with the provisions of the UNCRPD and the wider international disability rights agenda. In England and Wales an independent review of the MHA 1983, chaired by Professor Sir Simon Wessely was carried out between 2017 and 2018.[30] The Review sought to tackle the rising rates of people being detained under the MHA in England and Wales and the disproportionately high numbers of detained people from black and minority ethnic groups, and aimed to bring the MHA 1983 more in line with a modern mental health system. The Review's final report was published in December 2018[31] with recommendations for government on how the MHA and associated practice should be changed.[32] Whilst not going so far as to adopt a 'fusion law', the Review recommends a series of proposals which signal a *'shift towards a more rights-based approach [to mental health treatment and care] improving respect and dignity, and ensuring greater attention is paid to a person's freely expressed wishes and preferences'.*[33] The government is expected to publish its full response by the end of 2019.

In a similar move north of the border, the Minister for Mental Health for Scotland, Clare Haughey, recently announced plans for an independent review of Scottish mental health legislation, aiming to '*improve the rights and protections of those living with mental illness in Scotland and removing barriers to those caring for their health and welfare*'.[34]

Whilst such activities do not in themselves change mental health law and practice – and considerable work still needs to be done to convince governments to implement and resource any proposals made – they are nevertheless the first step towards shaping the future direction of mental health law to ensure the rights and freedoms of individuals with mental disorder are better served and protected.

References and Notes

1. Joint Commissioning Panel for Mental Health. *Guidance for Commissioners of Older People's Mental Health Services.* London: JCPMH, 2017; SCIE: Assessing the Mental Health Needs of Older People: mental health legislation, 2003. //www.scie.org.uk/publica tions/guides/guide03/law/leg.asp (Accessed 19 March 2019).

2. Such as informal admission or via the Mental Capacity Act and Deprivation of Liberty Safeguards soon to be Liberty Protection Safeguards under the Mental Capacity (Amendment) Bill: //services.parliament.uk/ bills/2017-19/mentalcapacityamendment .html (Accessed 19 March 2019).

3. CQC. Mental Health Act: The rise in the use of the MHA to detain people in England. January 2018, p. 19. www.cqc.org.uk/sites/d efault/files/20180123_mhadetentions_re port.pdf (Accessed 19 March 2019).

4. Centre for Policy on Ageing. Rapid review: diversity in older age: older offenders. 2016. www.cpa.org.uk/information/reviews/CPA-Rapid-Review-Diversity-in-Older-Age-Older-Offenders.pdf (Accessed March 19, 2019).

5. *R (Munjaz)* v. *Ashworth Hospital Authority* [2005] UKHL 58.

6. Williamson T. *Dementia, Rights, and the Social Model of Disability: A New Direction for Policy and Practice?* London: Mental Health Foundation, 2015; BIHR. *Mental Health Advocacy and Human Rights: Your Guide.* London: British Institute of Human Rights, 2015; Mandelstam M. *How We Treat the Sick: Neglect and Abuse in Our Health System.* London and Philadelphia: Jessica Kingsley Publishers, 2011, pp. 229–300.

7. Modernising the Mental Health Act: Final report from the independent review. 6 December 2018. https://assets

.publishing.service.gov.uk/government/up loads/system/uploads/attachment_data/fil e/778897/Modernising_the_Mental_Healt h_Act_-_increasing_choice__reducing_ compulsion.pdf (Accessed 19 March 2019); Scottish Government. Review of the Mental Health Act: Future direction of mental health and mental incapacity legislation. March 2019. www.gov.scot/ne ws/review-of-the-mental-health-act/ (accessed March 2019).

8. With the exception of the MHA, holding power who can be exercised by a non-medical AC.

9. MHA s1(2).

10. NI Order s3(1).

11. MHCTA s328.

12. For short-term or longer-term detention.

13. In these jurisdictions, the patient's nearest relative also has the power to make an application but this is rarely exercised.

14. On admission the patient must be examined immediately by another doctor whose report must support detention.

15. A medical practitioner certified as having 'special experience' in the diagnosis and treatment of mental disorder (MHCTA s22).

16. 'Extendable' in Scotland.

17. Separate legal criteria must be satisfied and procedural requirements followed to lawfully renew/extend detention.

18. Each prepared by an AMP or by one AMP and the patient's general practitioner.

19. Department of Health. MHA 1983: Code of Practice. 2015. TSO. para 36.3.

20. Zigmond T. Mental health law across the UK. *BJPsych Bulletin* 2017; **41**(6): 305–307.

21. Szmukler G, Daw R, Callard F. Mental health law and the UN Convention on the Rights of Persons with Disabilities. *International Journal of Law and Psychiatry* 2014; 37(3): 245–252.

22. *Reid* v. *Secretary of State for Scotland* [1999] AC 512.

23. ECHR, Articles 5(4) & 6.

24. MHA s72; s75 lists Tribunal powers exercisable in England and Wales.

25. In England: Tribunal Procedure (First-tier tribunal) (Health, Education and Social care Chamber) Rules 2008; in Scotland: First-tier Tribunal for Scotland Mental Health Chamber Rules of Procedure 2018 (in draft); Wales: Mental Health Review Tribunal for Wales Rules 2008; in Ireland: The Mental Health Review Tribunal (Northern Ireland) Rules 1986.

26. 'General' member in Scotland.

27. These are lay people.

28. Modernising the Mental Health Act: Final report from the independent review. 6 December 2018. https://assets .publishing.service.gov.uk/government/up loads/system/uploads/attachment_data/fil e/778897/Modernising_the_Mental_Healt h_Act_-_increasing_choice__reducing_ compulsion.pdf (Accessed 19 March 2019) recommends abolishing Managers' powers of discharge at p151.

29. Mental Health (Care and Treatment) (Scotland) Act 2003, section 81.

30. Department of Health, 'Terms of Reference – Independent Review of the Mental Health Act 191983' (policy paper, 4 October 2017). www.gov.uk/govern ment/publications/mental-health-act-independent-review/terms-of-reference-independent-review-of-the-mental-health-act-1983 (Accessed 21 July 2019)

31. Modernising the Mental Health Act 1983: Final report from the Independent Review. 6 December 2018. https://assets .publishing.service.gov.uk/government/up loads/system/uploads/attachment_data/fil e/778897/Modernising_the_Mental_Healt h_Act_-_increasing_choice__reducing_ compulsion.pdf (Accessed 19 March 2019)

32. See the Royal College of Psychiatrists' summary of the recommendations in the Final Report at www.rcpsych.ac.uk/impro ving-care/campaigning-for-better-mental-health-policy/the-mental-health-act (Accessed 21 July 2019)

33. Modernising the Mental Health Act 1983: Final Report at page 17

34. Scottish Government. Review of the Mental Health Act: future direction of mental health and mental capacity legislation (news, 19 March 2019). https:// news.gov.scot/news/review-of-the-mental-health-act (Accessed 21 July 2019)

Chapter 22

Deprivation of Liberty
Where Are We Now?

Nick Brindle and Christian Walsh

Introduction

Historically 'deprivation of liberty' has been an elusive and ill-defined concept in health and social care settings. The words themselves are derived from Article 5 of the European Convention on Human Rights (ECHR): the right to liberty and security. In England and Wales, the MCA authorizes the restriction, but not the deprivation of liberty, of a person who lacks the relevant decision-making capacity. It is therefore necessary to distinguish the tipping point between permissible restrictions authorized under section 5 of the Mental Capacity Act (MCA) (limited by section 6) and when a deprivation of liberty may arise. A deprivation of liberty (a DoL) without lawful justification and due legal process for scrutiny would be a breach of the person's rights under Article 5 with associated consequences including the right to compensation.

The judgment handed down by the Supreme Court in P and Q and P (in Cheshire West)[1] in March 2014 has established a threshold to apply and a measure of clarity as to when a deprivation of liberty may arise. This threshold is perhaps lower than many anticipated and consequently has had wide-ranging effects. In relation to older people, and particularly those with dementia, this is the situation that now applies in a whole range of clinical and social care locations. There are, however, two legal considerations for practitioners; first, what constitutes a deprivation of someone's liberty? We shall discuss this in relation to some of the relevant case law along with practical considerations as to how it may be recognized in different settings. Second, how is it authorized? At the time of writing, one scheme to authorize a deprivation under the MCA, the Deprivation of Liberty Safeguards (DoLS), is to be replaced by a second scheme, the Liberty Protection Safeguards (LPS), which is not yet operational. We shall, therefore, discuss the interface between the DoLS/LPS and the Mental Health Act 1983 (MHA) and briefly discuss the anticipated amendments the LPS will introduce.

Background to the Concept of Deprivation of Liberty

The first point to note is that Article 5 of the ECHR is a 'limited right' and does not protect us from detention. There are defined circumstances when it does not apply. It expressly permits confinement of criminals, illegal immigrants, and the 'lawful detention of persons for the prevention of the spreading of infectious diseases, of persons of unsound mind, alcoholics or drug addicts or vagrants'. It does, however, protect us against 'arbitrary detention' so that deprivations are made in accordance with a procedure prescribed in law.

A pivotal case is that of Mr L in the Bournewood Hospital.[2] The facts of his case are well known and will not be repeated here, but ultimately the two important issues were as above:

first, was Mr L deprived of his liberty? The European Court of Human Rights (ECtHR) determined that HL was deprived of his liberty because clinicians took 'complete and effective control over his care and movements' and he was not 'free to leave'. The second issue was whether or not the common law (judge-made law rather than that enshrined in statute) was sufficient authority for the deprivation. The judgment was that common law was not compliant with Article 5 because it is not a 'procedure prescribed by law'.

The MHA provides the required legal mechanisms to authorize the deprivation of liberty of 'detained' mental health patients. However, it was not generally used for patients with long-term incapacity such as dementia or learning disability, particularly if they were apparently compliant with the admission to hospital, such as Mr HL. Thereafter the 'Bournewood gap' was recognized, which referred to the legal predicament of the tens of thousands of people who lacked capacity to consent to admission to psychiatric hospitals and who were deprived of their liberty but without the protection of the law. This, of course, also applied in social care settings such as care homes. The government (in England and Wales) had to plug the legal gap left in the wake of the ECtHR ruling and introduced the DoLS to the MCA 2005 (via the 2007 amendments to the MHA).

There was, and still is, no statutory definition of the concept, although there was guidance in the DoLS Code of Practice based on the available cases relating to DoL from domestic and European courts.[3] The detailed-specific nature of the cases and differences in judicial interpretation meant that concepts were not readily generalizable and without sufficient clarity the 'Bournewood gap' remained open. This uncertainty about the meaning of deprivation of liberty was demonstrated by the failure of professional groups, including experts in the field, to agree on when it may be happening.[4] Also, considerable variation in practice arose amongst practitioners and clinicians.[5] The judgment in P and Q and P (in Cheshire West), discussed subsequently, was the Supreme Court's attempt to clarify this contentious area of law.

The practical advice on the first question of how to recognize a deprivation in the DoLS Code of Practice is therefore that one should always consider 'all the circumstances of each and every case' and includes a list of factors that have been taken into account by the European and domestic courts. The Code also points out that these are merely factors to consider and not conclusive on their own. Notwithstanding the low threshold for when Article 5 is engaged by the 'acid test' (see subsequently), for any individual it will be helpful to summarize what elements of the care plan are likely to be judged as restrictions; and then consider the effects of the care arrangements on the person's individual freedoms along with their expressed intentions and thereafter seek, where possible, to reduce their impact.

The Supreme Court Judgment in P and Q and P in Cheshire West

The 'Cheshire West' judgment handed down by the Supreme Court in March 2014 established a threshold to apply (the 'acid test') and, although not without controversy, added some clarity as to when a deprivation of liberty might arise. The case concerned three individuals: two sisters who had been taken into care (P and Q) and a man (P) with severe disabilities. The features of the cases are contained in Boxes 22.1 and 22.2.

Lady Hale, in her opening statement of the judgment, made it clear what the Court had to decide: '. . . whether the living arrangements made for a mentally incapacitated person amount to a deprivation of liberty. If they do, then the deprivation has to be authorized, either by a court or by the procedures known as the deprivation of liberty safeguards.'[1]

Box 22.1 Facts of the cases of P and Q

Concerning P:
- P's learning disability is described as being either at the 'lower end of the moderate range or at the upper end of the severe range'.
- She has problems with her sight and with her hearing.
- P's communication is limited, spending much of her time listening to music on her iPod.
- In 2007, P moved into a foster home.
- P never attempted to leave the home by herself and showed no wish to do so.
- She received no medication.
- P attended a further education unit daily during term time.
- She was taken on trips and holidays by her foster mother.
- She had very limited social life.

Concerning Q:
- Q's level of disability is described as being at the 'high end of the moderate range and borders on the mild range'.
- Her communication skills are better than those of P and her emotional understanding is quite sophisticated.
- Q also has problems with her sight.
- Q exhibits challenging behaviour with 'autistic traits'.
- Q initially moved into the home of her former respite carer but owing to her aggressive outbursts, she was moved into a small specialist residential home with three others.
- Q had occasional outbursts of challenging behaviour towards the other three residents and sometimes required physical restraint.
- She also showed no wish to go out and did not need to be prevented from doing so but was accompanied by staff whenever she did.
- She attended the same education unit as P.

Box 22.2 Features of the case of P (in Cheshire West)

P in Cheshire West:
- P lived with his mother until the age of 37.
- P's mother developed health problems and he was moved under the authority of an order of the Court of Protection to 'Z' house (November 2009).
- 'Z' house described as a spacious bungalow, cosy, and pleasant atmosphere, and shared with two other residents.
- Two staff were employed during the day and one waking member overnight.
- P also received 98 hours additional one-to-one support per week to help him leave the house whenever he chose.
- He attended a day-centre 4 days a week and hydrotherapy on the fifth.
- P went to a club, pub and shops, he also saw his mother regularly who lived close to his bungalow.
- He could walk for short distances and needed a wheelchair to go further.

The majority decision in the Supreme Court was that all three individuals were deprived of their liberty. Taking the lead in the judgment, Lady Hale emphasized that the rights in the ECHR apply to everyone and underpin the UN Convention of the Rights of Persons with Disabilities (UNCRPD). She made it clear that 'if it would be a deprivation of my liberty to be obliged to live in a particular place, subject to constant monitoring and control, only allowed out with close supervision, and unable to move away without permission even if such an opportunity became available, then it must also be a deprivation of the liberty of a disabled person'.[1] Also, these conditions apply whatever the circumstances or characteristics of the living arrangements even if they 'are comfortable, and indeed make my life as enjoyable as it could possibly be'.[1]

The key phrase used in the judgment was (again) whether the person concerned was subject to 'continuous supervision and control' and 'was not free to leave'. This, along with the deprivation being the responsibility of the state, forms the basis of the 'acid test'. Other factors, which were not relevant considerations, are the person's compliance or lack of objection; the relative normality of the placement (whatever the comparison made); and the reason or purpose behind a particular placement. Exactly the same considerations should apply whether or not a person has impaired health or capacity. While there may be some debate as to the definitions of these terms, both elements of the acid test must be satisfied, the threshold applied is low, and the confinement to a particular place must be for a 'not negligible' period of time. What constitutes a non-negligible length of time is again a moot point but will depend on the individual circumstances and, where the measures of control are more intense, the shorter the period of time that can be considered 'non-negligible'.

Implications: The 'Acid Test'

The effect of the judgment and application of the 'acid test' is to widen enormously the scope for those who are now deprived of their liberty and whose care thereby requires additional legal authorization by whichever scheme. This will apply to the broad range of settings, and not just in hospitals and care homes, to which the MHA or DoLS (currently) may apply. At the time of writing there are older people outside the scope of DoLS whose deprivation of liberty requires court authorization, for example those in supported living or occasionally in their own homes.

The 'acid test' is not as clear as it might first sound. It is not possible to say for certain what the terms 'continuous supervision and control' and 'not free to leave' mean and in frontline settings they have provoked considerable debate. Indeed, some judges have unsuccessfully tried to push back on the judgment of the Supreme Court.[6] However, the limits imply that 'continuous' does not have to mean uninterrupted; and being in a situation where one is 'not free to leave' the individual may not necessarily express a desire to do so but would be stopped if they tried. A more precise definition does not exist and there seems to be little standardization. Importantly, deliberations will need to reflect the overall effects and consequences on the person's life but, in reality, there is marked variation in interpretation and practice, which is perhaps reflected in the wide variation of referrals across England and Wales.

In considering how a deprivation is authorized, it follows that there are now different legislative routes that may apply to patients who lack capacity and may also require detention in order to provide care or treatment. The routes follow the provisions of the amended MHA or the MCA. While the principles, provisions, purposes, and policy concerns of the two acts are quite distinct, there will be instances where the most appropriate choice of legal authority is unclear and the interrelationship between the Acts will be complex.

The 'Acid Test' in Psychiatric Settings

The Care Quality Commission (CQC) have observed that between 2005 and 2006 and 2015/16 the reported number of uses of the MHA increased by 40%.[7] They proposed a number of factors that might influence the rates of detention including the increase in population and some sections of the population being 'at risk' of detention, especially older people with dementia. Furthermore, there has been a striking change in policy and practice as a result of the Cheshire West judgment, as well as how criteria for detention are now applied to people with dementia. The effect of this has been that most patients with dementia who lack the capacity to consent to admission to psychiatric inpatient care are now detained under the MHA. The implications of the judgment and thereby the guidance from the MHA Codes of Practice[8,9] suggest that there is limited scope for informal admission of incapacitated individuals to psychiatric facilities. Although the revised Code of Practice reminds us (at paragraph 4.22 of the English Code) that 'if the MCA can be used safely and effectively to assess or treat a patient, it is likely to be difficult to demonstrate that the criteria for detaining the patient under the Mental Health Act are met'.[8]

For psychiatrists, the judgment draws attention to the interface between the MHA and DoLS. Determining the appropriate basis to authorize admission and treatment for mental disorder can raise difficult questions. In an earlier upper tribunal case Mr Justice Charles highlighted some of the difficulties: 'All decision makers who have to address the application of the provisions of the DoLS contained in Schedules A1 and 1A of the MCA are faced with complicated legislative provisions and their difficulties are compounded when they have to consider the relationship between the MHA and the MCA'.[10]

It is fair to say that Schedule 1A's complexity (persons ineligible to be deprived of their liberty by the MCA) is now infamous. Notwithstanding, the revised *MHA Code of Practice* does offer some guiding principles in relation to which Act to use for both physical and mental disorders and reflects this judgment and further developments in case law. The reader is referred to the English and Welsh Codes of Practice for further details, but the influence of the Supreme Court judgment can be seen, for example, in the following statement (at paragraph 13.39 in the Welsh Code) that '. . .a person who lacks capacity to consent to being accommodated in hospital for care and/or treatment for mental disorder, and who is likely to be deprived of their liberty should never be informally admitted to hospital, whether they are content to be admitted or not'.[9]

There are instances where there seems to be a genuine choice of which legal scheme to apply. For example, DoLS may be appropriate for non-objecting patients who meet the 'acid test', but who are waiting for discharge arrangements to be put in place and may not be receiving what might in other circumstances be specialist treatment for their mental disorder. The advice of the authors is to apply the guidance in the relevant *Code of Practice* in considering both decision-making capacity and the presence of an objection, while adopting a low threshold for what constitutes an objection. In addition, it may be relevant to consider how the individual's Article 5 rights to challenge the deprivation are being protected.

The 'Acid Test' in Social Care Settings

Within social care the impact of the 'acid test' on the number of individuals, for example, on those who have dementia in care homes or other residential settings, who are now deemed to be deprived of their liberty has been overwhelming.[11] This is not to suggest that the care of these residents has become more restrictive or indeed changed at all. In the six months following the judgment there was a nine-fold increase in the number of applications for DoLS.[12] Although historically there have been wide geographic variations in the numbers of applications, and this continues, average monthly applications have risen between 2013 and 2014 from 1,000 to 9,000. The enormous pressure on Local Authority DoLS Teams and on the capacity of Best Interests Assessors (BIAs) is reflected in the failure to meet statutory timescales in around half of cases.[13] The knock-on effects are the increased burden on care providers who require the security of knowing that the care they are delivering is scrutinized, lawful, and appropriately authorized,[5] and on the capacity of the CQC to monitor and enforce the safeguards.

Meanwhile, the overwhelming burden on supervisory bodies in meeting the requirements for assessments and authorizations will remain undiminished. In so doing they will need to balance budgets and, in meeting their statutory requirements in relation to deprivation of liberty, other services and responsibilities will necessarily suffer at a time when there is the additional responsibility on local authorities to implement the Care Act 2014. The pressures in health and social care are likely to escalate with increasing scrutiny from the CQC together with the peril of court proceedings and compensation for unauthorized deprivations. There is a huge responsibility placed upon local authorities to make sure that those deprived of their liberty are afforded effective access to the Court of Protection so as to secure their rights under the ECHR. Other case law continues to highlight the difficulties and complexities that local authorities face in carrying out their duties.[14]

The 'Acid Test' in General Hospitals

The judgment potentially makes for very significant problems in general hospitals. In acute hospital settings there are inevitably large numbers of patients who lack the capacity to consent to their care or treatment and rigid application of the 'acid test' means many may be deprived of their liberty. This needs legal authorization. For patients whose lack of capacity is due to such mental disorders as delirium or dementia, the MHA or DoLS could be used.

Currently, the processes of DoLS authorization do not lend themselves to many circumstances in general hospitals and the practicalities of seeking court orders in the vast array of other situations are unworkable. Despite attempts, in many instances, to embed the principles of the MCA and DoLS into the clinical practice of general hospitals, there are clearly shortfalls which derive in part from the cumbersome nature of the processes. However, there again seem to be wide variations as to how this issue is dealt with. A difficult question arises: does ignoring the legal issue relieve physically ill people of an unnecessary burden or deprive them of their basic legal rights? At the time of writing further helpful and comprehensive guidance from the Law Society regarding the deprivation of liberty in general hospitals, hospices, and a range of other situations has been published.[15]

An important departure from the Law Society guidance has been the evolution of the concept of the 'acid test' in how it was applied differently in a case in 2017.[16] The case involved an inpatient in an ICU, who was unconscious and unable to consent to medical care. The Court of Appeal decided that there was no deprivation of liberty because the care was no different to that which anyone without a mental impairment would require: 'The root cause of any loss of liberty was her physical condition, not any restrictions imposed by the hospital.' This means that deprivation of liberty may be interpreted differently depending on the situation.

One impact of this judgment was that the *Coroners and Justice Act 2009* was amended such that at a time when a person is deprived of his or her liberty under the MCA, he or she is not considered to be in state detention. There is now no requirement for natural deaths to be reported to the Coroner, as was the case, where a person is deprived under DoLS, Court of Protection authorizations, or while applications to the court are being made. Non-authorized deprivations of liberty will still have to be reported.

This judgment has further implications, for example, in dementia care settings where individuals may be under section of the MHA and receiving end-of-life care. Under such circumstances, it may be necessary to consider:

- whether the restrictions are being imposed owing to the patient's *physical* condition;
- whether the treatment would be materially different for a patient with capacity in similar circumstances; and
- whether the purpose is for the administration of life-saving treatment.

It may be that the patient's legal predicament may have changed and requirement for the use of the MHA could be reviewed. Such decisions should form part of any discussion regarding ongoing care plans and if in doubt practitioners should seek advice from the organization's legal department.

Background to the Liberty Protection Safeguards

For clarity, the DoLS has now been repealed and replaced by a new law which is to be known as the 'Liberty Protection Safeguards'. The new legislation sets out the grounds under which the liberty of individuals who cannot consent to their current residence, care, and treatment may be deprived. The law only applies to England and Wales, with Scotland and Northern Ireland adopting their own separate legislation. The *Mental Capacity (Amendment) Act 2019* is scheduled for implementation in 2020, although this will likely be dependent upon how quickly the new *Code of Practice* and the associated regulations can be written, released for feedback, and then finally published. This information (not available at the time of writing), as well as the transitional arrangements between the schemes, will be crucial for all health and social care agencies, professionals, and also service users and carers, as to how the new legislation will work in practice.

DoLS has attracted controversy among health and social care agencies, as well as those working in the judiciary, for example, judges, solicitors, and barristers. Initially, the safeguards were criticized for the low referral rates and the apparent geographical differences in authorization numbers, while also the legislation's complex processes were highlighted. The Supreme Court judgment in Cheshire West arrived just days after the House of Lords Committee on the MCA published their post-legislative report on the MCA.[17] Some of the key findings of the report concerned the DoLS. The Committee found that the evidence suggests that tens of thousands of people were being deprived of their liberty without the protection of the law and that 'the Government needs to go back to the drawing board to draft replacement provisions that are easy to understand and implement, and in keeping with the style and ethos of the MCA'.[17]

The Law Commission subsequently undertook an extensive review of the existing DoLS legislation in order to devise a scheme that was more accessible, workable, and cost-effective.

Their final report was published in March 2017 and proposed that the current DoLS legislation be replaced as soon as possible with LPS. Many of the Law Commission recommendations were not incorporated by the government into the *Mental (Amendment) Capacity Act*. This Act received royal assent on 16 May 2019, with the final stages of the process now underway.

The DoLS are complex and introduced new roles and procedures.[18] Very briefly, the safeguards cover those people aged 18 and over who are suffering from mental disorder or learning disability and lack decision-making capacity in relation to their residency in a hospital or care home and who are assessed as needing to be deprived of liberty. The deprivation of liberty must be in the individual's own best interests, as defined by the MCA 2005, in order to protect them from harm, and to ensure they receive the care and/or treatment they need. The safeguards are not to be used solely to protect other people from harm and do not apply to people who receive the necessary Article 5 safeguards by virtue of being detained in hospital under the MHA (but with certain exceptions may be used in conjunction with guardianship, community treatment orders, and section 17 leave). Provision for people deprived of liberty to challenge their deprivation in a court of law are also included. In relation to older people it is clear that the prevalence of dementia is high in all care settings for older people. In this context, between 2017 and 2018, almost 75% of all applications for DoLS were made for people aged 75 and above,[19] with the majority placed under the safeguards having a dementia diagnosis.[20]

Liberty Protection Safeguard: The Amendments

Statutory Definition

The LPS does not contain any new definition of liberty. It is still being interpreted as set out in Article 5 of the ECHR.

Responsible Bodies (RBs) (see Table 22.1)

These will replace the Supervisory Bodies that currently exist in DoLS and will now include NHS Trusts, Clinical Commissioning Groups (CCGs), and Local Authorities.

Age

LPS now covers those individuals who are aged between 16 and 17 making the legislation consistent with the MCA.

Table 22.1 Responsible Bodies (RBs) in the Liberty Protection Safeguards (LPS)

Health/care provision	LPS stipulation concerning RBs
NHS Hospital Care	The hospital managers of the NHS Trust will be responsible for authorizing any deprivation of liberty that arises in their hospitals
Continuing Health Care Funded Care	The RB will be the funding CCG
Care Homes/Hospices	The Local Authority who is meeting the person's needs or in whose area the person is ordinarily resident
Independent Hospitals	The responsible body is the 'responsible local authority' in England (normally the authority meeting the person's needs or in whose area the hospital is situated)

Arrangements

LPS can be authorized in any environment where the deprivation of liberty is engaged, for example, care homes, hospitals, sheltered and supported accommodation, and also in a person's private residence.

Authorization Criteria

A responsible body (RB) may authorize arrangements if the following authorization conditions are met:

- the person lacks the capacity to consent to the arrangements;
- the person has a mental disorder within the meaning of section 1(2) of the *Mental Health Act 1983*; and
- the arrangements are necessary to prevent harm to the person and proportionate in relation to the likelihood and seriousness of harm to the person.

Consultation

The consultation process is essentially the same as the one in DoLS, although the Relevant Person's Representative role has now been replaced by 'any appropriate person'.

Pre-Authorization Review

The pre-authorization review is what provides the process with the required level of independence to be concordant with Article 5. This task can be undertaken by an Approved Mental Capacity Professional (AMCP) or another professional not involved in the person's care. It is expected that the Code of Practice and associated regulations will provide clarity as to who can undertake reviews, although it is possible that those BIAs who are not practising as AMCPs may fulfil this function. Where a referral has not been made to an AMCP, the independent reviewer must review the information and determine whether it is reasonable for the RB to conclude that the authorization conditions are met. A review can only be carried out by an individual who is not involved in day-to-day care, is not providing the person with any form of treatment, and does not have a proscribed connection with the care home.

AMCP Role

Where the individual is objecting to care arrangements or is being cared for in an independent hospital, or if the RB decides to refer the case to an AMCP and the AMCP accepts it, the AMCP will need to decide if the individual is objecting or not. Also, the RB will have to consider the views of the person and any relevant individual about the wishes of the person concerned. If an AMCP does become involved, then they will need to perform the following tasks:

- Meet with the person and anyone else involved in their care or an Independent Mental Capacity Advocate (IMCA) (if appropriate and practicable).
- Review all of the information and decide if the authorization conditions are met.

Arrangements cannot be authorized unless the pre-authorization review (and the AMCP) has confirmed that the authorization conditions are met or it is deemed to be reasonable for the RB to conclude that the authorization conditions are met (non-AMCP referrals).

Care Home Arrangements

Generally, care homes will now be able to undertake the relevant assessments themselves before submitting them to the RB for pre-authorization and authorization processes – this is a significant change in the LPS process in comparison with DoLS. If the care home proceeds to complete the process, then they will need to confirm via a statement that the person meets the relevant criteria while also providing copies of the assessments, evidence of their consultation, and a draft authorization record. Once the above information has been received, the RB will then decide whether to authorize the arrangements or not. This aspect of the LPS has attracted much criticism, with concerns being raised about the level of independence and also the potential lack of knowledge of the legislation amongst some care home providers.

Authorization Effect and Duration

A duly completed authorization will come into effect immediately or up to 28 days in advance, which is similar to the current DoLS legislation. Authorizations will initially last for up to 12 months and can then be renewed for a second period of 12 months, and then for a period of up to three years. With the new change, it has been suggested that a three-year authorization will only apply where the person's care arrangements and conditions are likely to remain stable and unlikely to require regular changes. As with DoLS, the authorization can cease at any time, with the criteria being similar to those which are currently *in situ*.

Renewals and Reviews

In contrast to DoLS, a RB can renew an authorization if it is satisfied that the person continues to meet the requirements and that they have followed the consultation process. Also, the RB must specify on the person's authorization record either the fixed date the reviews will be held or a prescribed timeframe as to when they will take place. Equally, reviews will have to be undertaken if there are any changes, if an interested person requests one, or if the person is made subject to the MHA 1983 or their condition/presentation changes.

Advocacy

IMCAs will continue to have a significant role to play in LPS, with the RB being required to appoint one if the person being assessed makes such a request or if they lack the capacity to consent to one being appointed. An IMCA does not have to be appointed if the RB believes that having support from an IMCA would not be in the person's best interests. An IMCA will not be required if there is an 'appropriate person' to represent the individual, although it should be noted that this person must consent to undertake the role. The person being assessed must also consent to the suggested appropriate person, or if they are unable to give consent, then the RB is required to make a best-interests decision. As with DoLS, the appropriate person is entitled to support from an IMCA.

Legal Appeals

Appeals against the LPS authorization can be made to the Court of Protection (section 21ZA). Such appeals can be made by the person concerned or others without the court's permission (the appropriate person and the IMCA). The powers of the court when it comes to LPS are similar to the powers granted under the DoLS.

MHA/LPS Interface

The interface between the MHA 1983 and LPS remains the same as the current DoLS legislation, which has been discussed earlier.

Conclusions

This judgment in the Supreme Court was a milestone in health and social care but nonetheless has provoked a measure of chaos. The test for deprivation of liberty is now clearer than before, although individuals will agonize over the wording. Inevitably, differences in the interpretation of 'continuous supervision and control' and 'free to leave' will persist. Despite this, clinicians must be able to recognize the circumstances when deprivation of liberty may arise and be sensitive to the distinction between restriction and deprivation of liberty, particularly in the context where restrictions are complete restrictions and a deprivation may arise within a short time frame.[21] Clinicians should be apprised of legal developments and know how to respond appropriately in order that care is lawfully delivered. Although there is statutory guidance in the form of the Codes of Practice it is likely that practice will be enhanced when supported by local policies and procedures.

However, one must not lose sight of the requirement to protect the most vulnerable of individuals given that decision-making can go badly wrong.[22, 23, 24] The shifting sands of the legal developments will continue to have a bearing on practice and resources in health and social care. Despite the clamour to replace the broken DoLS system, the new legislation is likely not without its flaws and it remains to be seen whether in practice the safeguards have been significantly watered down by the government.

Acknowledgement

For information, the original paper on which this chapter is based was:

Brindle N. The Supreme Court and deprivation of liberty: where are we now? *Adv Psychiatr Treat* 2015; 21: 417–424.

A related paper was: Brindle N, Branton T. Interface between the Mental Health Act and Mental Capacity Act: deprivation of liberty safeguards. *Adv Psychiatr Treat* 2010; 16: 430–437.

References

1. *P v Cheshire West and Chester Council and another and P and Q v Surrey County Council* [2014] UKSC 19.

2. *HL v United Kingdom* [2004] 40 EHRR 761.

3. Ministry of Justice. *Mental Capacity Act 2005: Deprivation of Liberty Safeguards. Code of Practice to Supplement the Main Mental Capacity Act 2005 Code of Practice.* TSO (The Stationery Office), 2008.

4. Cairns, R, Brown, P, Grant-Peterkin, H. et al. Judgements about deprivation of liberty made by various professionals:

comparison study. *Psychiatrist* 2011; **35**: 344–349.

5. Care Quality Commission (CQC). *Monitoring the Use of the Mental Capacity Act Deprivation of Liberty Safeguards 2013/2014.* CQC, 2015.

6. *Rochdale MBC v KW* [2014] EWCOP 45.

7. Care Quality Commission. *Mental Health Act – The Rise in the Use of the MHA to Detain People in England.* CQC, 2018.

8. Department of Health. *Code of Practice: Mental Health Act 1983.* TSO, 2015.

9. Welsh Assembly Government. *Mental Health Act 1983: Code of Practice for Wales.* TSO, 2016.

10. *AM v (1) South London & Maudsley NHS Foundation Trust and (2) The Secretary of State for Health* [2013] UKUT 0365 (AAC).

11. Brindle N. The Supreme Court and Deprivation of Liberty: where are we now? *Adv Psychiatr Treat* 2015; **21**: 417–424.

12. Directors of Adult Social Services (ADASS). *Number of DoLS referrals rise tenfold since Supreme Court ruling.* ADASS, 2014. Last accessed on 13 September 2019 via: www.adass.org.uk/number-of-dols-referrals-rise-tenfold-since-supreme-court-ruling-jun-14

13. Community Care. *Half of Deprivation of Liberty Safeguards cases breaching legal timescales.* Community Care, 2014. Last accessed on 13 September 2019 via: www.communitycare.co.uk/2014/10/01/50-deprivation-liberty-safeguards-cases-breaching-legal-timescales/

14. *AJ (Deprivation of Liberty Safeguards)* [2015] EWCOP 5

15. Law Society. *Identifying a Deprivation of Liberty: A Practical Guide.* Law Society, 2015. Last accessed on 13 September 2019 via: www.lawsociety.org.uk/support-services/advice/articles/deprivation-of-liberty/

16. *R (Ferreira) HM Senior Coroner for Inner South London and Others* [2017] EWCA Civ 3.

17. The House of Lords. *Mental Capacity Act 2005: Post Legislative Scrutiny.* TSO, 2014. Last accessed on 13 September 2019 via: www.publications.parliament.uk/pa/ld201314/ldselect/ldmentalcap/139/139.pdf

18. Brindle N, Branton T. Interface between the Mental Health Act and Mental Capacity Act: the deprivation of liberty safeguards. *Adv Psychiatr Treat* 2010; **16**: 430–437.

19. NHS Digital. *Mental Capacity Act (2005), Deprivation of Liberty Safeguards (England) 2017/18, Official Statistics.* Health and Social Care Information Centre, 2018. Last accessed on 13 September 2019 via: https://files.digital.nhs.uk/04/B15A3A/DoLS%201718%20Final%20Report.pdf

20. NHS Digital. *Deprivation of Liberty Safeguards (England) Annual Report, 2014–2015.* Health and Social Care Information Centre, 2015. Last accessed on 13 September 2019 via: https://files.digital.nhs.uk/publicationimport/pub18xxx/pub18577/dols-eng-1415-rep.pdf

21. *ZH (by his Litigation Friend) v Metropolitan Police Commissioner* [2012].

22. *Hillingdon v Steven Neary* [2011] EWHC 1377 (COP).

23. *Local Authority v Mrs D and Anor* [2013] EWHC B34 (COP).

24. *Essex County Council v RF & Ors* [2015] EWCOP 1.

Chapter 23

Residence Capacity
Its Nature and Assessment

Julian C Hughes, Marie Poole, Stephen J Louw, Helen Greener and Charlotte Emmett

Introduction

Residence capacity can be defined as the capacity someone requires to decide where to live. Its assessment is important in a variety of mental disorders. In this chapter we shall mainly focus on dementia, but the nature and requirements for assessment would largely be similar across all conditions. We shall also focus on the relevant law as it pertains to England and Wales, that is, the Mental Capacity Act (MCA), although, again, the nature of residence capacity and the principles for its assessment remain similar across jurisdictions.

Why Is Residence Capacity Important?

There are at least three reasons why residence capacity is important. First, we all love being at home. The place we call 'home' is usually surrounded by emotional resonances and is where we feel rooted and safe. The emotional importance of home was recognized by Mr Justice Baker in the Court of Protection when he said:

There is, truly, no place like home, and the emotional strength and succour which an elderly person derives from being at home, surrounded by familiar reminders of past life, must not be underestimated.[1]

Going further than this, the philosopher and clinician Wim Dekkers has argued that 'being human *is* to dwell'.[2] According to the philosopher Heidegger, for instance, we build 'because we dwell, that is, because we are *dwellers*'.[3] Thus, the notion of being at home is existential: it is part and parcel of what it is to be a human being in the world. So, assessing a person's capacity to make decisions about where to live has fundamental significance.

Second, if a person lacks residence capacity he or she is at increased risk of institutionalization. In people with dementia admitted to a medical ward, the finding of a lack of residence capacity is likely to lead to subsequent placement in a care home.[4]

Third, residence capacity is by no means as straightforward as some other capacities. This is because the nature of home – *the place where I dwell* – is complex. It means different things to different people. In weighing matters up, for instance, how much weight should be given to my insistence that this is the place I have lived with my spouse for 45 years, against your concern about my ability to cope and the risks I face? In connection with judgments about residence capacity, there is likely to be a variety of diverse and sometimes conflicting values at play.[5] The complexity around these value judgments means that the assessment of residence capacity is often not straightforward and can require considerable skill.

Background

Whereas some types of capacity, such as testamentary capacity, involve specific tests,[6] and whereas tools have been developed to assess other capacities,[7] residence capacity has been relatively ignored in the literature, despite its importance.[5]

Ripley et al. developed an algorithm to assess capacity to enter a care home that conforms with the principles outlined in the MCA,[8] but we need to turn to the Act itself, in combination with its principles, for best guidance. In England and Wales, the MCA established in statute law a definition of incapacity which leads to a two-stage test: first, the person must have an impairment or disturbance of the mind or brain; secondly, they must be unable (on account of the impairment or disturbance) to make the required decision, as shown by an inability to understand, retain, use or weigh the relevant information or to communicate the decision (see section 3 of the MCA). The principles in section 1 of the MCA (see Box 23.1) establish the legal context for judgments about residence capacity in England and Wales.

To return to the difficulties that stem from the need for evaluative decisions, it can be seen that my insistence on remaining in my spousal home, despite the risks that the professionals have highlighted, might be regarded as a failure to weigh things up adequately owing to my mental disorder (in which case I lack capacity), but might alternatively be regarded as simply an unwise decision. In the context of the MCA, therefore, we are immediately struck by the importance of values-based judgments.[9] But there is also relevant case law.

The Case of JB: Consent to Treatment

In *Heart of England NHS Foundation Trust v JB* [2014], Mr Justice Jackson considered the case of a 62-year-old lady named JB.[10] The decision concerned amputation of her lower leg because of gangrene. Her putative lack of capacity was said to stem from her diagnosis of chronic paranoid schizophrenia. Although the capacity under consideration was the capacity to consent to treatment, Justice Jackson made a number of comments pertinent to assessment of residence capacity.

For instance:

The temptation to base a judgement of a person's capacity upon whether they seem to have made a good or bad decision, and in particular upon whether they have accepted or rejected medical advice, is absolutely to be avoided. That would be to put the cart before the horse or . . . to allow the tail of welfare to wag the dog of capacity. Any tendency in this direction risks infringing the rights of that group of persons who, though vulnerable, are capable of making their own decisions.

Box 23.1 Section 1 of the *Mental Capacity Act 2005*: Some of the principles

. . .

(2) A person must be assumed to have capacity unless it is established that he lacks capacity.

(3) A person is not to be treated as unable to make a decision unless all practicable steps to help him to do so have been taken without success.

(4) A person is not to be treated as unable to make a decision merely because he makes an unwise decision.

. . .

Many who suffer from mental illness are well able to make decisions about their medical treatment, and it is important not to make unjustified assumptions to the contrary.[11]

Justice Jackson went on to make the following point, which is also relevant to residence capacity:

What is required here is a broad, general understanding of the kind that is expected from the population at large. JB is not required to understand every last piece of information about her situation and her options: even her doctors would not make that claim. It must also be remembered that common strategies for dealing with unpalatable dilemmas – for example indecision, avoidance or vacillation – are not to be confused with incapacity. We should not ask more of people whose capacity is questioned than of those whose capacity is undoubted.[12]

So, too, decisions about change of residence in connection with dementia often invite avoidance and vacillation because the thought of moving into care is unpalatable. Later, the judge said of JB:

Her tendency at times to be uncommunicative or avoidant and to minimise the risks of inaction are understandable human ways of dealing with her predicament and do not amount to incapacity.[13]

Again, people with dementia or an intellectual disability (learning disability) might well, on account of their mental difficulties, be less than communicative and might minimize risks. However, these traits do not in themselves prove that they lack the requisite capacity and the burden of proof lies with those who wish to say that they do; otherwise capacity must be assumed (see Box 23.1). The case of JB, therefore, offers pertinent guidance in relation to residence capacity assessments.

PC & NC v City of York Council [2013]

This case concerned a 48-year-old married woman (PC) with a significant learning disability and whether or not she had the capacity to decide to go to live with her husband (NC).[14] An important issue was that NC had been imprisoned for 13 years for serious sexual offences (which he denied), although there was no evidence that PC had ever suffered serious harm from NC, who was now released from prison on licence. The case raised a number of interesting legal questions to do with the assessment of capacity, but perhaps the key issue for our purposes was to do with the 'causative nexus'.

Section 2(1) of the MCA provides a definition of what it is for a person to lack capacity:

For the purposes of this Act, a person lacks capacity in relation to a matter if at the material time he is unable to make a decision for himself in relation to the matter because of an impairment of, or a disturbance in the functioning of, the mind or brain.

In *PC & NC v City of York Council* [2013], Lord Justice McFarlane made this comment on section 2(1):

...for the Court to have jurisdiction to make a best interests determination, the statute requires there to be a clear causative nexus between mental impairment and any lack of capacity that may be found to exist.[15]

Later he made this point:

The danger is that the strength of the causative nexus between mental impairment and inability to decide is watered down. That sequence – 'mental impairment' and then 'inability to make a decision' – is the reverse of that in s 2(1) – 'unable to make a decision . . . *because of* an impairment of, or a disturbance in the functioning of, the mind or brain' [emphasis added].[16]

It was not good enough, on his view, to say that the person's inability to make a decision was merely 'referable to' or 'significantly related to' the impairment or disturbance in the functioning of the mind or brain. There had to be a *causal connection* (nexus) between the impairment or disturbance and the inability to decide. This builds on the point that diagnoses of dementia or intellectual disability in themselves do not render a person lacking in capacity; indeed, what has to be established is that the person cannot decide *because* he or she has such-and-such a diagnosis.

The House of Lords and the Supreme Court

Residence capacity is important because of its implications for human rights. A Select Committee of the House of Lords reported on the Mental Capacity Act in 2014. While celebrating the innovative nature of the Act and noting its potential 'to transform the lives of many',[17] they went on to say that the implementation of the Act had not met expectations. In particular, '. . .the prevailing cultures of paternalism (in health) and risk-aversion (in social care) have prevented the Act from becoming widely known or embedded'.[17]

The Select Committee's report was published on the 13 March 2014 and on 19 March 2014 the Supreme Court handed down its judgment on *P (by his litigation friend the Official Solicitor) v Cheshire West and Chester Council & Anor* [2014].[18] This concerned the criteria for judging whether or not the living arrangements made for a person who lacked capacity amounted to a deprivation of liberty. (For further discussion see Chapter 22.) The judgment has had significant repercussions mainly because it establishes, in paragraph 49, an 'acid test' for deprivation of liberty, namely that the person is *under continuous supervision and control and is not free to leave*. The stringency of this test means that many people with dementia who lack residence capacity and are moved into residential care may well thereby be deprived of their liberty. The same holds true of people with learning disabilities who live in a variety of institutional settings. Hence, as with any type of capacity, residence capacity is important because human rights are at stake; and, as the Supreme Court's judgment shows, there is a real chance that the right to liberty will be compromised as a consequence of an assessment of residence capacity.

Case Vignettes (see Box 23.2)

Mr Jones and Mrs Jarvis are not unique. From the information presented it is not possible to say with any certainty whether or not they have residence capacity. Careful assessments would be required to determine whether they do or not.

Where assessments of residence capacity have to be made on acute medical and surgical wards, as for Mr Jones, issues around time and timing become important.[4] Assessing the person's residence capacity in the context of delirium is usually a waste of time: the assessment needs to be undertaken when the person's cognitive function is as optimal as it is likely to be. This poses a significant problem for acute units, with pressure on beds, which cannot always afford to wait. Step-down or rehabilitation units provide a better setting for such assessments, but they are not always available. Still, some social service departments in the UK have designated resources for beds in residential homes which they

Box 23.2 Case histories*

Mr Jones in hospital

Mr Jones, who is 82 years old, was found on the floor of his kitchen by a neighbour. In hospital a urinary tract infection was diagnosed. But his neighbour, and subsequently his daughter, confirmed that he had had memory problems for some while. He remained confused, even when the infection was treated. An occupational therapy assessment in the ward kitchen showed that he was unsafe making a pot of tea. He had lived alone since the death of his wife and his house is now described as chaotic and squalid. Questions are raised about whether or not Mr Jones should be allowed to go home. He says he wishes to go home, but he thinks he does his own shopping, whereas his neighbour does this for him. His daughter feels he would be safer in a care home.

Mrs Jarvis at home

Mrs Jarvis is 79 years old and since her husband died four years ago, has lived alone in their marital home of over 50 years. She has moderately severe vascular dementia and has had a number of falls, for which she has a telecare alarm service to summon help. She continues to fall and will sometimes activate the Care-call system, but sometimes does not. At other times she rings Care-call just because she is lonely. She sometimes wanders out of her house. This has been happening more often, including at night, and sometimes involves the police. Her family are very worried about her. Home care visit three times a day to make sure she is washed and to provide food. But she will not always eat the food, which is later found discarded in various places in the house. Occasionally, she does not, despite being prompted, accept her medication. Family and professionals are putting pressure on Mrs Jarvis to accept a move into a residential care home. But she steadfastly refuses to consider this option.

*Both Mr Jones and Mrs Jarvis are fictitious characters.

call 'time to think beds', which seems very helpful particularly because, indeed, the assessment of residence capacity inevitably takes time (see Box 23.3).

A lot of information (see subsequently) is required before the assessment can even be undertaken. It must occur in circumstances that are optimal for the person. He or she must be able to hear and see adequately; if special means of communication are required they should be available; and so on. In keeping with the principles of the MCA (Box 23.1), 'all practicable steps' must be taken to help the person make a decision.

Approaches to Assessment: Functional versus Outcome

There are three approaches to the assessment of capacity (see Box 23.4). Professionals are mostly aware that assessments based on status should be avoided because they are unfairly discriminatory: a person should not be assumed to lack capacity just because he or she has dementia or an intellectual disability.

However, clinicians and others tend to conflate the outcome and functional approaches.[20] The MCA requires that a functional approach is pursued. Despite this, people who have to make decisions for others tend to be protective of them and this tendency influences judgments about capacity.

In *CC v KK and STCC* [2012], Mr Justice Baker made just this point in his ruling:

Box 23.3 Delirium, time and the UN convention

In acute medical settings, delirium and dementia frequently present together. In these people it is impossible to be certain what the person's level of cognitive functioning will be once the delirium is treated. In addition, not all deliriums resolve quickly. In which case, time becomes a key issue. Not only will assessments take time, they will also need to be carried out at the appropriate time.[4] Providing a setting in which this can occur is a challenge. But the *UN Convention on the Rights of Persons with Disabilities* (UN CRPD) makes it plain in Article 12 (2) that states 'shall recognize that persons with disabilities enjoy legal capacity on an equal basis with others in all aspects of life'.[19] And then, in Article 12 (3), the Convention stipulates that states must provide the support they may require to exercise their legal capacity. Countries, such as the UK, which have signed the Convention, might thereby be considered bound to the paradigm of supported decision-making commended by the Convention, despite the time and other resources required.

Box 23.4 Approaches to the assessment of capacity

STATUS: capacity is determined by the person's status as someone who is old, has an intellectual disability or dementia, has speech problems, has suffered a stroke, etc.

OUTCOME: capacity is determined by what is likely to be a good outcome for the person as judged by others and by the person's tendency to pursue that good outcome.

FUNCTIONAL: capacity is determined by a test of the person's functional ability (as judged in the MCA by their ability to understand, retain, weigh, and communicate) to make a decision on the basis of the information available.

... in cases of vulnerable adults, there is a risk that all professionals involved with treating and helping that person – including, of course, a judge in the Court of Protection – may feel drawn towards an outcome that is more protective of the adult and thus, in certain circumstances, fail to carry out an assessment of capacity that is detached and objective. On the other hand, the court must be equally careful not to be influenced by sympathy for a person's wholly understandable wish to return home.[21]

The case concerned an 82-year-old lady, *KK*, who was hemiplegic and had Parkinson's disease and vascular dementia. She was totally dependent on others for her personal care, frequently sought help by the use of a telecare alarm service and showed considerable anxiety. Finally, she was admitted to a nursing home with dehydration and a urinary tract infection. But she wanted to return home. Her case involved a number of professionals assessing her capacity on a number of occasions. They all found that she lacked residence capacity, but Mr Justice Baker determined otherwise. He reiterated the point about the importance of the objective test of capacity being made *without* reference to what might be best for the person and emphasized again the saliency of home:

There is, I perceive, a danger that professionals, including judges, may objectively conflate a capacity assessment with a best interests analysis and conclude that the person under review should attach greater weight to the physical security and comfort of a residential home and less importance to the emotional security and comfort that the person derives from being in their own home.[22]

The issues that weigh on the minds of professionals are often those of safety and risk, but Mr Justice Baker was keen to cite a lecture delivered by Lord Justice Munby, in which he made this powerful statement:

The State must be careful to ensure that in rescuing a vulnerable adult from one type of abuse it does not expose her to the risk of treatment at the hands of the State which, however well intentioned, can itself end up being abusive of her dignity, her happiness and indeed of her human rights. *What good is it making someone safer if it merely makes them miserable?* None at all! And if this is where safeguarding takes us, then is it not, in truth, another form of abuse – and, moreover, abuse at the hands of the State?[23]

Unusually, in cases where capacity is in doubt, *KK* actually appeared in court to give evidence and when pushed about the possibility that she might fall ill, she made the arresting assertion: 'If I die on the floor, I die on the floor. I'd rather die in my own bungalow, I really would.'[24] The judge felt that this demonstrated her ability to weigh things up. As he opined,

I venture to think that many and probably most people in her position would take a similar view. It is not an unreasonable view to hold. It does not show that [sic] a lack of capacity to weigh up information. Rather it is an example of how different individuals may give different weight to different factors.[25]

This is a helpful demonstration of how legal minds consider these matters, but it also reveals a tension. On the one hand there is the requirement to test capacity in an objective and functional manner; on the other hand, it shows that evaluative judgments are still required. We should, however, recall the advice of Justice Jackson in the *JB* case: 'We should not ask more of people whose capacity is questioned than of those whose capacity is undoubted.' Tests of capacity *are* tests, but they should not be unreasonable tests. And there is evidence that there are strategies which can improve the likelihood of a person being found to have capacity, for instance by attending to the physical environment: it should be quiet and private. 'A well-conducted capacity assessment can . . . become a therapeutic intervention.'[26]

Still, practitioners have to be on their guard against the possibility of conflating their wishes for a good outcome with a functional assessment of capacity. Even for experts it is easy to make the mistake of such a conflation. In *FX, Re* [2017], for instance, which concerned whether FX, a 32-year-old man with Prader–Willi Syndrome, had the capacity to make decisions in relation to residence and care, it was difficult for the expert witness, who saw FX twice, to engage with him.[27] The judge was 'cautious' about the evidence of the expert witness who had 'conflated best interests with capacity'.[28] The expert had set the bar quite high in terms of the information that FX might be reasonably expected to retain, understand and weigh precisely because he was concerned about the outcome for FX. In doing so, he had not considered that FX might simply be making an unwise decision, which of course FX should be – like everyone else – free to do (see Box 23.1). The case also raises an issue about how much information a person has to be able to hold in mind in making a decision.

Information

In order to have capacity, the person must be assessed as able to understand, retain and weigh the relevant information before communicating a decision. But what information? It seems important to try to pin down the key elements that need to be tested when a question about residence capacity has been raised.

Manuela Sykes was an 89-year-old lady with dementia whose case was heard in the Court of Protection.[29] The judgment mainly concerned a detailed assessment of Manuela Sykes's best interests. Her lack of capacity was not at issue. But District Judge Eldergill usefully set out the grounds for reaching this conclusion. He said:

... she cannot recall the circumstances and behaviour that caused others to remove her from her own home to hospital and to transfer her to residential care. Lacking this information, she does not accept that she had significant problems at home, nor therefore that she requires a significant package of care and support. Nor can she appreciate that, without additional care, it is likely that the problems will be the same as before, because the situation is the same as before.[30]

A good example of the level of detail required in order for a person to have capacity is provided in the judgment of Mrs Justice Theis in a long-running case concerning, amongst other things, residence capacity for a man (L) of 29 years with intellectual disabilities.[31] Some of the relevant considerations for residence capacity included there being two options open to L, what they were, the sort of facilities the places had, the difference between living somewhere and merely visiting it, the sort of area they were in, specific known risks, what activities L would be able to do if he lived in each place, how easy access by family and friends might be, the financial considerations, who he would be living with, what sort of care he would receive, and the risk that some family members might choose not to visit a certain location. But L had to understand these things only 'in broad terms'.

Avoiding 'Silos': Taking Account of All the Information

In *B (by her litigation friend, the Official Solicitor) v A Local Authority* [2019], the findings of Justice Cobb sitting in the Court of Protection were scrutinized by the Court of Appeal.[32] The case concerned B, a 31-year-old woman with intellectual difficulties and considerable social care needs, who wished to live with Mr C, a man in his seventies who had been convicted of multiple sexual offences and was subject to a Sexual Harm Prevention Order. She had stated that she wished to have Mr C's babies. Justice Cobb had applied Mrs Justice Theis's list, as described earlier, concerning which the Court of Appeal stated:

We see no principled problem with the list provided that it is treated and applied as no more than guidance to be expanded or contracted or otherwise adapted to the facts of the particular case.[33]

The justices were critical, however, of Justice Cobb's ruling about B's capacity to make decisions concerning place of residence. They agreed with the Local Authority that the ruling in the lower court '... was fundamentally flawed' in that it did not take into account information relevant to the other decisions presented to the court; it produced a situation in which there was an 'irreconcilable conflict' between the judgments about B's decision-making capacity which would make care for and treatment of B 'practically impossible'.[34] The Local Authority,

... submitted that the Judge's flawed conclusion followed from his approach in analysing B's capacity in respect of different decisions as self-contained 'silos' without regard to the overlap between them (paragraph 63).[34]

Thus, Justice Cobb had placed the risks associated with living with Mr C in with decisions about care and contact. The judge said both that B understood in broad terms about the care she would receive living with Mr C, but later that she lacked the capacity to make decisions about care.[35] Further, in connection with capacity to decide whether or not to move to live with Mr C, Justice Cobb ruled that B did not have capacity to make a decision as to the persons with whom she had contact.

But that conflicted directly with the Judge's conclusion that B had capacity to decide to move to live with Mr C. The point is reinforced by the fact that [Justice Cobb] had already granted an interim injunction prohibiting Mr C from having any contact with B. Permitting B to move to live with Mr C would presumably have placed both him and B in contempt of court for breach of the injunction.[36]

They went on to note that Justice Cobb had made an interim declaration that B did not have capacity to consent to sexual relations, and yet,

One of B's explicit motivations for moving to live with Mr C is to have sexual relations with him and, it would seem, to have his baby. Again, there is a direct conflict with the Judge's interim finding that B has capacity to decide to live with Mr C in his home.[37]

The point made by the local authority's barrister, therefore, about 'silos' seems appropriate; and it is underpinned by deeper philosophical, psychological and sociological observations that we should be seen as wholes and not as separate parts.

A similar point arises in connection with people with dementia in connection with frequent bouts of delirium. It may be that the patient fails to grasp the gravity of their condition at times when they have delirium. Under these circumstances an holistic assessment is required. Patients will often not recall the full effects of a delirium, even though at the time the experience might be very frightening (if psychotic experiences are involved) and may be life-threatening. The episodes of delirium might be both frequent and very distressing. Yet the patient may not be able to appreciate the concerns of the relatives, neighbours, carers, medical and social professionals involved. This common scenario also requires both an holistic overview, which the patient will need to understand (at least to some extent), and that judgments are not made in silos.

The Causal Nexus

It remains important that the actual capacity being assessed is specific, so that the information required can be suitably specific. In *London Borough of Hackney v SJF (through her Litigation Friend the Official Solicitor), JJF* [2019], the case concerned the care and residence of a 56 year old woman with significant physical health problems, schizophrenia and an intellectual disability.[38] She had lived for many years with her son (JJF) who had special educational needs whilst growing up and had been in prison including for assaulting his mother (SJF). Health professionals were scared for their own safety on account of threats by SJF's son, which led to her being moved urgently to a care home. Despite such problems, SJF wished to return to live with her son.

The key issue was whether SJF was unable to understand or weigh information about the risk to her health of living with her son, given this would make it difficult for health care professionals to visit because of their fear of her son. In this case, expert evidence helped to decide matters, both because it established a causal nexus between SF's intellectual disability and her difficulties making the particular decision and because it was shown that she failed to grasp the specific bits of information relevant to the decision she had to make.

It was noted that she had the natural belief as a mother that her son's behaviour would improve, but her intellectual disability had a direct impact on her ability to understand the consequences of living with JJF and, therefore, to appreciate the risks of not having appropriate care. She could also not come up with other possibilities for her son. It was felt she lacked the requisite capacity to make a decision about where she lived *because* she failed to understand the risks to her health (*because* of the risks posed by her son to healthcare workers) and this in turn was *because* of her intellectual disability and not simply because she was unwise. Over time, the importance of establishing the causal nexus between the impairment of the mind or brain and the functional inability in terms of decision-making has been increasingly recognized in England and Wales by the Court of Protection.[39]

A Test of Residence Capacity

In Box 23.5 we have set out some potential items of information that might form the basis of the test of residence capacity. We have proposed similar items elsewhere,[20] but here they are developed and generalized to fit different circumstances. Of course, residence capacity will only be an issue when it is felt a change of residence might be beneficial. So the information required to be known will be specific, even if there are various options open to the person.

Thus, to return to the cases in Box 23.2, the information to be put to Mr Jones might be (1) there are concerns he had a fall because he was unwell and worries that his memory problems might mean he is not able to cope at home on his own; so (2) it is being suggested he should go into a care home; but (3) an alternative would be for him to go home with professional carers coming in to see him several times a day; and (4) he should understand that if he goes into a care home it might well become the place he lives permanently and, alternatively, if he goes home and accepts the care package it cannot be guaranteed that he will not run into similar problems again in the future. Mrs Jarvis, meanwhile, must understand that (1) there is a lot of concern about her safety at home because of the problems being caused by her dementia; so (2) it is being suggested that she should live in a care home; alternatively, (3) attempts could be made to enhance the care she receives at home; but (4) if she goes home, and especially if she does not accept the care, she will be putting herself at risk in a variety of ways, which would be lessened in a care home, albeit she would lose her independence and might still have falls.

This information would need to be presented to Mrs Jarvis and to Mr Jones under the appropriate circumstances, with enough time in a quiet and comfortable environment. They are allowed to make unwise decisions (see Box 23.1), but then the assessor must be able to indicate why the decision seemed unwise rather than incapacitated; and we should recall Justice Jackson stating in the case of *JB*: 'We should not ask more of people whose capacity is

---

Box 23.5 Information necessary for residence capacity

1. The person should know **why** a change of residence is being proposed: what have the problems been that have caused a concern (e.g. they should know why they had to come into hospital or what has caused a worry in the community)?
2. The person should know **what** is being proposed (e.g. they should know that it is being suggested they should move into a care home).
3. The person should be informed if there are **other options** (e.g. that they could go home but extra help is recommended because of the risks identified).
4. The person should understand the **likely consequences** of making any particular decision, including a decision not to follow the advice being given, as well as the consequences of making no decision at all.

questioned than of those whose capacity is undoubted'. Having been presented with this information, the decision-maker must determine whether or not Mr Jones and Mrs Jarvis can understand, retain and weigh it up before communicating their decisions.[26] If, on balance, they can do this, they have residence capacity; if they cannot, they lack this capacity because the presumption of capacity has been rebutted.

Conclusion

Residence capacity is an important decision-making capacity which needs to be assessed commonly and should be assessed with considerable care given its implications for the person and for human rights. It will often involve evaluative decisions, but it should be based on a functional assessment of the person's capacity. We have suggested some basic information that should be conveyed to the person faced by the prospect of a change of residence where there is a doubt about capacity. If the person lacks capacity, then a decision will have to be made in the person's best interests, which must also be assessed fairly and fully.[40]

Acknowledgement

For information, the original paper on which this chapter is based was:

Hughes JC, Poole M, Louw SJ, Greener H, Emmett C. Residence capacity: its nature and assessment. *BJPsych Adv* 2015; 21: 307–312.

The work stemmed from independent research funded by the National Institute for Health Research (NIHR) under its Research for Patient Benefit programme (PB-PG-0906-11122). The views expressed in this paper are those of the authors and not necessarily those of the NHS, the NIHR or the Department of Health.

References

1. *CC v KK and STCC* [2012] EWHC 2136, (COP); paragraph 70.

2. Dekkers W. Dwelling, house and home: towards a home-led perspective on dementia care. *Med Health Care Philos* 2011; **14**: 291–300. DOI:10.1007/s11019-011-9307-2

3. Heidegger M. Building dwelling thinking. In *Poetry, Language, Thought* (ed. M Heidegger; trans A Hofstadter): 145–161. Harper & Row, 1971.

4. Poole M, Bond J, Emmett C, et al. Going home? An ethnographic study of assessment of capacity and best interests in people with dementia being discharged from hospital. *BMC Geriatr* 2014; **14**: 56.

5. Greener H, Poole M, Emmett C, et al. Value judgements and conceptual tensions: decision-making in relation to hospital discharge for people with dementia. *Clin Ethics* 2012; 7: 166–174.

6. Jacoby R. Testamentary capacity. In *Oxford Textbook of Old Age Psychiatry* (2nd edition) (eds. T Dening, A Thomas): 797–804. Oxford University Press, 2013.

7. Vellinga A, Smit JH, van Leeuwen E, van Tilburg W, Jonker C. Instruments to assess decision-making capacity: an overview. *Int Psychogeriatr* 2004; **16**: 397–419.

8. Ripley S, Jones S, Macdonald A. Capacity assessments on medical in-patients referred to social workers for care home placement. *Psychiatr Bull* 2008; **32**: 56–59.

9. Hughes JC, Williamson T. *The Dementia Manifesto: Putting Values-Based Practice to Work*. Cambridge University Press, 2019.

10. *Heart of England NHS Foundation Trust v JB* [2014] EWCOP 342.

11. See reference [10] paragraph 7.

12. See reference [10] paragraph 26.

13. See reference [10] paragraph 39.

14. *PC & NC v City of York Council* [2013] EWCA Civ 478.

15. See reference [14] paragraph 52.

16. See reference [14] paragraph 58.

17. House of Lords Select Committee on the Mental Capacity Act 2005. *Mental Capacity Act 2005: Post-Legislative Scrutiny*. The Stationery Office, 2014; page 6. Last accessed on 30 September 2019 via: www .publications.parliament.uk/pa/ld201314/l dselect/ldmentalcap/139/13902.htm.

18. *P (by his litigation friend the Official Solicitor) v Cheshire West and Chester Council & Anor* [2014] UKSC 19.

19. United Nations (2006) *Convention on the Rights of Persons with Disabilities and its Optional Protocol* (A/RES/61/106). Last accessed on 30 September 2019 via: www .un.org/development/desa/disabilities/con vention-on-the-rights-of-persons-with-disabilities.html.

20. Emmett C, Poole M, Bond J, Hughes JC. Homeward bound or bound for a home? Assessing the capacity of dementia patients to make decisions about hospital discharge: comparing practice with legal standards. *Int J Law Psychiatry* 2013; **36**: 73–82.

21. See reference [1], paragraph 25.

22. See reference [1], paragraph 65.

23. Cited in reference [1], paragraph 66.

24. See reference [1], paragraph 50.

25. See reference [1], paragraph 73.

26. Spencer B, Hotopf M. The assessment of mental capacity. In *Mental Capacity Legislation: Principles and Practice* (2nd edition) (eds. R Jacob, M Gunn, A Holland): 13–33. Cambridge University Press, 2019.

27. *FX, Re* [2017] EWCOP 36.

28. See reference [27] paragraph 43.

29. *Westminster City Council v Manuela Sykes* [2014] EWHC B9 (COP), [2014] EWCOP B9.

30. See reference [29] paragraph 7.

31. *LBX v K, L and M* [2013] EWHC 3230 (Fam), [2013] MHLO 148.

32. *B (by her litigation friend, the Official Solicitor) v A Local Authority* [2019] EWCOP 3.

33. See reference [32] paragraph 62.

34. See reference [32] paragraph 63.

35. See reference [32] paragraph 64.

36. See reference [32] paragraph 65.

37. See reference [32] paragraph 66.

38. *London Borough of Hackney v SJF (through her Litigation Friend the Official Solicitor), JJF* [2019] EWCOP 8.

39. Keene AR, Kane NB, Kim SYH, Owen GS. Taking capacity seriously? Ten years of mental capacity disputes before England's Court of Protection. *Int J Law Psychiatry* 2019; **62**: 56–76.

40. Emmett C, Hughes JC. Best interests. In *Mental Capacity Legislation: Principles and Practice* (2nd edition) (eds. R Jacob, M Gunn, A Holland): 34–55. Cambridge University Press, 2019.

Chapter 24

Understanding the Person with Dementia

A Clinico-Philosophical Case Discussion

Julian C Hughes and Aileen Beatty

Introduction

This chapter considers the notion of personhood and shows how it offers a robust conceptual underpinning to person-centred care. We use a fictitious case vignette to clarify the nature of personhood. Although the vignette is fictional, it is based on an amalgam of real and made-up cases. We believe it would seem a familiar story to most people who know or care for people with dementia. We contend that we need a broad view of personhood, which we feel is best captured by regarding the person as a situated embodied agent (SEA), which will be explained. Using this characterization, we aim to demonstrate how it can underpin the notion of person-centred care and show the practical implications of this in connection with our fictitious case. The broad view supports a specific approach to people with dementia, but also shows the challenges that face the implementation of good-quality dementia care. Discussion of this case shows both the relevance of philosophy for clinical practice and the ways in which clinical practice can enrich the debates of philosophy.

As is well known, the prevalence of dementia is set to rise inextricably with the ageing of the population.[1] Person-centred care is the watchword of dementia services.[2, 3] But it is rarely the reality.[4] Indeed, in an Afterword to the second edition of Kitwood's seminal book on personhood, now called *Dementia Reconsidered, Revisited: The Person Still Comes First*, Kate Swaffer, an Australian dementia activist, who lives with a diagnosis of dementia, states: 'I believe Kitwood's Person Centred Care has not generally been translated into practice, and instead has mostly been a tick-box in an organization's paperwork.'[5] Furthermore, despite the alleged ubiquity of person-centredness, we continue to see a variety of scandals affecting people with dementia, especially those in long-term care.[6, 7] One researcher, Dr Penny Rapaport, was quoted as saying, in response to findings which suggested that abuse was taking place in 99% of care homes,[8] 'Carers can't just be told that care should be person-centred – they need to be given the support and training that will enable them to deliver it.'[7]

The question is sometimes raised, therefore, as to whether the mantra of person-centred care is empty. Alternatives to person-centred care, such as relationship-centred care, have been suggested.[9] However, the extent to which these alternatives represent substantial conceptual differences can be questioned.[10] It may be that the problems in terms of realizing person-centred care in practice reflect deeply conceptual issues, which we hope to gesture at in this chapter.

Our aim is to unpack the notion of personhood and show how it does indeed offer a robust conceptual underpinning to person-centred care. But, in doing so, we also show why, despite its acceptance at the level of policy,[11, 12, 13] the radical change suggested by person-centred care means that its successful implementation cannot be achieved in a facile manner. Our aim is, by using a fictitious case vignette, to clarify the nature of personhood in order to show that it:

- underpins the notion of person-centred care;
- demonstrates practical implications of this;
- supports a specific approach to people with dementia;
- shows the radical challenges which face the implementation of good-quality dementia care.

We shall initially outline a characterization of personhood, which we shall then use to comment, first, on the story provided by a case vignette and, secondly, on the interventions devised to manage the behaviour of the fictitious patient. Finally, we shall discuss some of the broader implications of this way of thinking of people living with a diagnosis of dementia.

The SEA View of the Person

In this section we introduce the notion of the person as a situated embodied agent.[14] This way of characterizing what it is to be a person (i.e. personhood) was a reaction to more limited views according to which the key characteristic of the person is that he or she is consciously able to remember (see Box 24.1).

Locke is probably the best example of this approach, although the interpretation of what he said can be questioned.[18, 19] But he says: 'as far as . . . consciousness can be extended backwards to any past action or thought, so far reaches the identity of that person.'[20] Similarly, Parfit (see Box 24.1) has put forward the view that when we speak of persons we are simply speaking of continuing and connected psychological states.[21] The key thing for Parfit is 'psychological connectedness', which involved 'psychological continuity', which is 'the holding of overlapping chains of *strong* connectedness'.[22]

Box 24.1 Some philosophers on being a person

John Locke (1632–1704), regarded as the first of the British empiricists (who argued that knowledge comes from the five senses, rather than from reason alone), famously described the person as: '. . . a thinking intelligent being, that has reason and reflection, and can consider itself as itself, the same thinking thing, in different times and places; which it does only by that consciousness which is inseparable from thinking, and . . . essential to it.'[15]

David Hume (1711–1776), a Scottish philosopher who continued the tradition of Locke, has been called a 'bundle theorist' because he wrote that when he attempted to find *himself*, he found 'nothing but a bundle or collection of different perceptions'.[16] He wrote: 'Had we no memory, we never should have any notion of causation, nor consequently of that chain of causes and effects, which constitute our self or person.'[16]

Derek Parfit (1942–2017) was a contemporary Oxford philosopher, who also admitted to being a bundle theorist: '. . . we can't explain either the unity of consciousness at any time, or the unity of a whole life, by referring to a person. Instead we must claim that there are long series of different mental states and events – thoughts, sensations, and the like – each series is unified by various kinds of causal relation, such as the relations that hold between experiences and later memories of them.'[17]

The worry about this sort of view, as far as thinking about people with dementia is concerned, is that it can readily seem to suggest that personhood is lost in severe dementia. In dementia, that is, the 'chains of strong connectedness' between conscious states of remembering are increasingly loosened. Thus, we find Dan Brock writing:

I believe that the severely demented, while of course remaining members of the human species, approach more closely the condition of animals than normal adult humans in their psychological capacities. In some respects the severely demented are even worse off than animals such as dogs and horses who have a capacity for integrated and goal directed behavior that the severely demented substantially lack. The dementia that destroys memory in the severely demented destroys their psychological capacities to forge links across time that establish a sense of personal identity across time and hence they lack personhood.[23]

In response to this rather narrow view of what it is to be a person, the SEA view offers a broader perspective. Whether as embodied beings or as agents, we are always situated or embedded in a context, which is always unique and multifaceted and which itself provides strong scaffolding for the preservation of personhood.

We are situated in our personal histories, which themselves have biological, psychological, social, and spiritual aspects; but we are also situated in particular families, cultures, and historical and geographical settings, and we have our uniquely evolved legal and moral codes, and so forth. Our bodies, too, contribute in an important way to our standing *as* human persons; and, of course, as persons we act in and on the world in which we live. But we are neither *just* bodies, nor are we agents *simply* in the sense that we wish to live autonomous lives. The notion that we are autonomous runs up against our deep rootedness (or embeddedness) in a world of other agents with whom we must interact and interconnect, and with whom we are – we have been and always will be – mutually dependent. Hence, the notion of 'relational' autonomy seems more apt.[24] But the idea of being embodied is also layered. Thus, the Canadian philosopher Charles Taylor (born 1931) spells out that:

Our body is not just the executant of the goals we frame, . . . Our understanding is itself embodied. That is, our bodily know-how, and the way we act and move, can encode components of our understanding of self and world. . . . My sense of myself, of the footing I am on with others, is in large part also embodied.[25]

Indeed, for Taylor, rather than particular internal mental states, crucial to our understanding of ourselves are the notions of 'embodied agency and social embedding'.[26] These thoughts draw on the work of thinkers such as Wittgenstein, Heidegger, and Merleau-Ponty (see Box 24.2).

Taylor emphasizes that the person must be seen as 'engaged in practices, as a being who acts in and on a world'.[31] The point to note is that, according to this way of thinking, being engaged with the world is not a mere empirical feature of personhood, that is, it is not that persons just happen to act like this; it is rather that, at a conceptual level, it is constitutive of persons that they must act 'in and on a world'.

A conception of persons that left out this aspect of our lives would not simply be thin, it would be missing a constitutive feature. That is, our situated embodied agency – our Being-with others, our bodily engagement in and with the world – is not a matter of contingency (see Box 24.3). This is what it *is* to be a human being: it is precisely to be a person with a certain sort of standing (as a situated embodied agent) with others in the totality of the world.

If we are giving a constitutive account of what it is to be a person, then person-centred care, if it is to reflect such an account, must engage at this level. As Heidegger might have

---

Box 24.2 Some philosophers on being human in the world

Ludwig Wittgenstein (1889–1951) emphasized that language is an activity or practice in which we are engaged as a 'form of life'.[27] Our very understanding, according to Wittgenstein, is only possible in a human worldly context: 'Only in the stream of thought and life do words have meaning' (Wittgenstein 1981, §173).[28]

Martin Heidegger (1889–1976), in his seminal work *Being and Time*, set out how the nature of a human being is precisely that he or she is a 'Being-in-the-world'. Moreover, a human being is not a disconnected observer of the world, but one whose nature is typified in terms of 'Being-with'. Heidegger accepts human beings can be *indifferent* to one another, but from the point of view of being a human being *as such*, '. . . there is an essential distinction between the "indifferent" way in which Things at random occur together and the way in which entities who are with one another do not "matter" to one another'.[29]

Maurice Merleau-Ponty (1908–1961) was (like Heidegger) another existentialist who characterized our being as 'Being-in-the-world', but considered the special role that our bodies play in presenting us to the world. His philosophy is sometimes summed up by the use of the phrase 'body-subject', which suggests both how our subjectivity is embodied and how our bodies are the means by which we gain a subjective purchase on the world: 'The body is our general medium for having a world.'[30]

Box 24.3 Contingent and constitutive accounts

The difference between these sorts of account is crucial. A contingent account of what it is to be a person might have been otherwise. It is contingently true that one of the authors of this chapter was born in London and one was born in Whitehaven. But these facts could have been otherwise. A constitutive account, alternatively, sets out what constitutes being a person: what it is to be a person *as such*, whatever one's life history.

---

said (see Box 24.2), if you are indifferent to me, which you can be, if you treat me as a *mere* object (not as a 'body-subject' to use the expression derived from Merleau-Ponty), it is nevertheless a matter of being indifferent and uncaring in the face of our nature as human beings who are, constitutively, mutually engaged, inter-connected, and inter-dependent. It is a contingent fact that you can ignore me or not, but there is no getting around the fact that our situated nature as beings of this sort means that our characteristic response to one another should be that of (what Heidegger called) solicitude.

The SEA View in Practice

So far we have sketched a characterization of personhood. In the next section we shall show how this broad view underpins our understanding of real people, including those with dementia.

Case Vignette: Mr Walker (Part 1)

Life Story

Mr Walker was one of seven children. He had a poor relationship with his father who would frequently drink and become violent. When, as a child, Mr Walker wet the bed his father would become very angry, sometimes hosing him down in the backyard, which was very frightening and humiliating. He adored his mother, however, and was devastated when she died relatively young. He left school when he was 15 years old and worked in the building trade. He progressed to supervisory roles and was known as a tough but fair boss. He married Margaret and they had three children. His family describe him as strict and quick to temper: he was frequently intolerant of his own children, but in later life enjoyed spending time with his grandchildren. He also enjoyed being outdoors, working on his allotment.

Personality

Mr Walker was a very private man and disliked visitors in the house. Nevertheless, he spent three or four evenings a week at the local social club where he, too, drank quite heavily. He was quick-tempered but rarely violent physically. He was quite possessive and jealous, but also loved his wife dearly. His family describe a mellowing in later years and attribute his parenting style to his own tough upbringing. Alcohol brought out the worst in him. He was normally well mannered in public, disliked bad language in front of women and valued hard work and discipline.

Cognitive Health

Mr Walker began displaying signs of memory impairment in 2007, when he was 76 years old. He was initially thought to be depressed and was treated with an antidepressant. He was eventually diagnosed in 2009 with mixed vascular and Alzheimer's dementia, with frontal lobe involvement. His deteriorating behaviour and aggression led to his admission to long-term care. He can be sexually disinhibited and has paranoid ideas about his family spending money, his wife having affairs, or people trying to steal his job. He can become more agitated during periods of high activity and staff changeover. He sometimes tries to follow staff out of the door, either to go home or to get to work.

Physical Health

Mr Walker suffers from arthritis in his hands and knees, which can cause pain. He is prone to chest infections and urinary tract infections. He is otherwise physically well and his mobility is generally good. Mr Walker has a reasonable appetite but is not always keen to eat in the company of others. He suffers from urinary incontinence at times and becomes very embarrassed and anxious when this happens.

Understanding Mr Walker

The story of Mr Walker immediately allows us to understand something about him. The more details we have, the greater our understanding. This seems obvious. But we wish to make two points. First, in understanding his narrative, which we might hear from him or from others, we understand him precisely *as a person*. Second, the understanding we gain from his narrative is not an understanding solely of his conscious mental states, albeit we learn something about his mental states; rather, inasmuch as it is an understanding of him *as a person*, it is an understanding of a whole lot of things which make up his surround,[32] which will maintain his standing as a person even if the 'chains of strong connectedness' between his psychological states start to loosen.

Situation

Let us briefly consider how we can characterize Mr Walker as a person using the SEA view. His history situates him. But it does more than this, because without it we understand nothing. His behaviour as an adult stems from his experience of the world as a child. His whole way of being-in-the-world reflects his embedding in a particular time and culture: the inner city, Newcastle upon Tyne, in the 1930s. But Mr Walker's situated narrative is not just a social or cultural phenomenon, it is embodied in this man in particular ways which reflect his unique experience of, for instance, his father and his mother. Part of that experience is itself embodied in genetic predispositions, to drink alcohol perhaps, and embodied too in the automatic reactions and thoughts he might have as a consequence of his life experiences. These reactions and ways of thinking are themselves bodily manifestations of psychosocial influences, which have imprinted themselves on Mr Walker's character. There are characterological traits which predispose him to depression, anger, or paranoia under particular circumstances.

Embodiment

Meanwhile, his embodiment shows itself in terms of his arthritic pain, his frontal lobe brain dysfunction, and his urinary incontinence. But these are not simply bodily happenings. They are real occurrences in the life of this man right now and their consequences are, at one and the same time as being biological, also psychological and social. His embodiment is situated in his present context, but it has consequences in terms of his actions.

Agency

Mr Walker's agentive being, his need to be in control and to feel usefully employed, is compromised by his whole situation. But rather than this undermining his standing as a person, it should point us in the direction of how we might help to maintain his personhood.

The Sum: A Situated Embodied Agent

These sorts of consideration, which show a deepening of understanding of Mr Walker, also establish the points we wish to make. First, his narrative, which has to be regarded as something situated – it cannot float free from its multifarious surroundings – reveals to us Mr Walker, neither as an abstract nor disengaged entity, but as a human person embedded in his own, unique, multilayered context. Furthermore, part of the appeal of this view of the person is that it is not circumscribed: for any individual, we cannot stipulate in advance what it is that will constitute his or her unique field. Second, because of the way in which the surround or context is constitutive for the individual person, it provides a means by which the individual's personhood can be maintained even in the face of worsening dementia.[33] This stands over against the narrower view of the person according to which personhood is undermined by loss of memory. In which case, the broader view should support any approach that seeks to maintain the person's standing by attention to his or her surroundings: psychosocial, cultural, spiritual, environmental. The list of factors that might be important is, in principle, uncircumscribable.

In the next section, therefore, we shall consider Mr Walker's needs and how they might be met.

Case Vignette: Mr Walker (Part 2)

Current Environment

Mr Walker now lives in an all-male care home. He has good relationships with staff and other residents, although he can also react badly to the behaviour of others. He can be very sociable and witty and often enjoys group activities, such as bingo, or listening to music. But he gets very bored at times and he can become restless, pacing, and looking somewhat lost. Mr Walker gets little opportunity to go outdoors, which he used to enjoy so much. His wife and children visit weekly.

Behaviour Support Plan

Target Behaviours

Staff have identified the following behaviours as causing them and Mr Walker the most distress:

- Agitation and aggression, swearing at staff and residents, demanding they leave his home, telling them to get to work and stop being lazy.
- Embarrassment and distress following urinary incontinence, which can turn to aggression.
- Agitation and aggression when trying to follow staff out of the building when he thinks he should be going to work or home.

During these episodes Mr Walker can appear angry, frightened, and frustrated. Staff have identified that Mr Walker has a need for purpose, independence, and to feel safe and secure.

Interventions

- Mr Walker misidentifies other people as being family members, old work colleagues, or his wife. He can become angry and threatening towards those he is targeting. Staff should attempt to distract Mr Walker with a short walk or a cup of tea and take him to a less stimulating environment. He can respond badly if his beliefs are challenged so it is best not to do this directly. He can respond well to empathy about how upsetting he must be finding things. He responds better to male staff (he has been described as 'a man's man'). Personalizing his room and making him feel more at home might lead to Mr Walker viewing his room as a place of safety away from others. It might be useful to consider a trial of anti-dementia medication.
- Following urinary incontinence, Mr Walker sometimes tries to disguise what has happened and can be sheepish, embarrassed, and fearful of the possible consequences. He was always very private so the combination of this and the fear of repercussions can cause him to react violently. Staff must deal with these episodes as discreetly as possible with a minimum of fuss and a maximum of sensitivity. Mr Walker does not mind female staff helping him at these times and responds well to reassurance. He may sometimes deny that he has been incontinent, in which case it may be better to wonder whether there has been some other form of accident, such as some spilt tea, rather than confronting him and drawing attention to what has occurred. This might encourage him to change whilst avoiding embarrassment. It can help to compliment him too about how smart he always is.

- Periods of high activity and staff changeovers are difficult for Mr Walker. Mealtimes are a known trigger, so one tactic is to offer him meals in a quiet environment where staff can come and go quietly. Staff should also avoid wearing coats in residents' communal areas and shouting goodbye to one another. Sometimes taking time to disengage from Mr Walker can help, with the new staff member sitting for a few minutes with him before the other staff member leaves. Providing meaningful occupation is important. Mr Walker gets bored easily, so it is very natural that he feels the need to go elsewhere in search of something to do.

Therapeutic Engagement

We have described Mr Walker's current circumstances and set out the behaviours that can seem challenging. In addition, we have outlined a behaviour support plan which attempts to identify target behaviours and interventions which might meet the needs that drive the behaviours.[34] In this section we wish to stress the ways in which the broader (SEA) view of the person supports the holistic presuppositions of the sort of model we have used. Indeed, the SEA view suggests that such a model is inevitable, since anything less would, by implication, overlook some aspect or other of the individual's standing as a person.

To put this another way, the sort of behavioural model captured above takes seriously every aspect of Mr Walker's life. If, clinically, we are trying to understand his behaviours, then from the perspective of the SEA view we need to think as broadly as possible. To put it all down to his brain pathology, which is then best treated by altering neurochemicals using psychotropic medication, ignores the profound effects of his early life history. To try to explain his actions simply as deeply ingrained patterns of behaviour and to ignore the effects of his current environment and of the pain he now experiences from his knees seems too crass. To understand the paranoia and anger that accompanies his misidentification of others purely in social constructionist terms (i.e. to look solely for the social causes of his distress) is potentially to ignore the possibility that medication might help him. To deal with his urinary incontinence as if it were simply a physical problem would be to ignore his whole psychosocial history.

Not only does the SEA view support the broadest possible understanding of Mr Walker, which will help in our understanding of his needs and his behaviours, it also points in the direction of how we might intervene to help him. Providing him with privacy in a space which feels to him to be his own, taking him seriously, these are ways of showing him true respect on the basis of our understanding of his life history, in which his current state is after all embedded. His situated being in the world as a man of this sort (biologically, psychologically, socially, and spiritually) means that we should take him seriously on these grounds. His embodied nature means that we must look after him bodily; but through our bodily encounters with him we can still show our concern and understanding. Mr Walker remains an agent, someone to whom meaningful activity and human interactions are important.

Discussion

In this chapter our aim was to clarify the nature of personhood. Once we consider real people, such as Mr Walker, the view of what it is to be a person inevitably broadens. Mr Walker's being-in-the-world is inevitably multifaceted. Moreover, it reaches out and, as a constitutive feature, his situated narrative engages with the world around him in ways that might either sustain or undermine his standing as a self.[35] Mr Walker's own understanding of the world, even when he cannot articulate it well, is also an embodied understanding: his understanding is shown by his bodily responses and gestures, and will continue to be shown in these ways even when his cognitive skills have significantly deteriorated.[36] He remains a situated agent: a being-with-others who interacts 'in and on a world'. So the philosophy supports clinical practice; but we also see how clinical practice informs the philosophical discussion. In summary, the lessons we might learn from Mr Walker's story are the following:

- What it is to be a person – personhood – cannot be circumscribed; that is, it cannot be narrowed down to one or other facet of our human lives: we are complex biological, psychological, social, and spiritual creatures.
- We can characterize the person as a situated embodied agent. This characterization is useful in terms of contingent matters, but also gives us a constitutive account of personhood.
- Where there is behaviour that is challenging, taking the broadest possible view of personhood, which encourages a fuller understanding of our patients' narratives, is likely to enable us to comprehend their unmet needs.
- This broad-view approach is in keeping with and should encourage person-centred dementia care.

The role of the SEA view of the person is at two levels. First, it encourages a truly holistic person-centred approach. But this is a contingent level in the sense that things might have been different for Mr Walker and will be different for other people. At a deeper level, the SEA view of personhood presents us with a constitutive account according to which we must try to engage with him in this broad manner because this is intrinsic to our nature as human beings. We can treat him badly or just in a mediocre fashion; but we cannot then claim that this is person-centred care.

Conclusions

We hope to have shown that our view of what it is to be a person underpins the notion of person-centred care. Given a broad notion of personhood, person-centred care must be understood broadly too. There are practical implications, summed up by saying that nothing (from aromatherapy to dolls, from antidepressants to dance) should be ruled out when it comes to seeking ways to help people with dementia. When it comes to behaviours that challenge, the SEA view also supports the use of a broad formulation in order to encourage our understanding of needs which will have to be met in order to help the person with dementia. Moreover, the constitutive nature of the account we have given of personhood means that person-centred care is not a matter of getting things right according to a contingent protocol. It is to do with our deep engagements as people.[37] This is, therefore, also the challenge to implementing person-centred care. Nonetheless, the challenge cannot be shirked because our situated nature as mutually dependent human beings suggests the need for solidarity, which is: 'The need to recognize the citizenship of people with dementia, and to acknowledge our mutual interdependence and responsibility to support people with dementia, both within families and in society as a whole.'[38]

Acknowledgement

We should like to thank the two anonymous reviewers whose comments improved the original paper from which this chapter is derived; its deficiencies remain our own.

For information, the original paper on which this chapter is based was:

Hughes J, Beatty A. Understanding the person with dementia: a clinicophilosophical case discussion. *Adv Psychiatr Treat* 2013; 19: 337–343.

References

1. Hughes JC. *Alzheimer's and Other Dementias.* Oxford University Press, 2011.

2. Kitwood T. *Dementia Reconsidered: The Person Comes First.* Open University Press, 1997.

3. Brooker D. What is person centred care? *Rev Clin Gerontol* 2004; **13**: 215–222.

4. Kirkley C, Bamford C, Poole M, et al. The impact of organisational culture on the delivery of person-centred care in services providing respite care and short breaks for people with dementia. *Health Soc Care Community* 2011; **19**: 438–448.

5. Swaffer K. Afterword. In *Dementia Reconsidered, Revisited: The Person Still Comes First* (Second Edition) (ed. D Brooker): 178–180. Open University Press, 2019 (page 180).

6. Parson K. Panorama documentary highlights why elderly people in care need a voice. *Guardian Professional*, 2012 (24 April). Accessed last on 14 September 2019 via: www.guardian.co.uk /social-care-network/2012/apr/24/panor ama-documentary-elderly-people-care

7. Bulman, M. Abuse taking place in 99% of care homes amid 'chronic' underfunding, survey shows. *Independent*, 2018 (22 March). Last accessed on 14 September 2019 via: www .independent.co.uk/news/uk/home-news/ca re-homes-abuse-residents-funding-staff-uk-elderly-protection-a8266936.html

8. Cooper C, Marston L, Barber J et al. Do care homes deliver person-centred care? A cross-sectional survey of staff-reported abusive and positive behaviours towards residents from the MARQUE (Managing Agitation and Raising Quality of Life) English national care home survey. *Plos One*, 2018. Last accessed on 14th September 2019 via: https://doi.org/10 .1371/journal.pone.0193399

9. Nolan MR, Davies S, Brown J, Keady J, Nolan J. Beyond person-centred care: a new vision for gerontological nursing. *J Clin Nurs* 2004; **13**: 45–53.

10. Hughes JC, Bamford C, May C. Types of centredness in health care: themes and concepts. *Med Health Care Philos* 2008; **11**: 455–463.

11. Department of Health. *National Service Framework for Older People.* Department of Health, 2001.

12. National Institute for Health and Clinical Excellence and Social Care Institute for Excellence (NICE-SCIE). *A NICE-SCIE Guideline on Supporting People with Dementia and their Carers in Health and Social Care. National Clinical Practice Guideline Number 42.* Leicester and London: The British Psychological Society and Gaskill (The Royal College of Psychiatrists), 2007.

13. Department of Health. *Living Well with Dementia: A National Dementia Strategy.* Department of Health, 2009.

14. Hughes JC. Views of the person with dementia. *J Med Ethics* 2001; **27**: 86–91.

15. Locke J. *An Essay Concerning Human Understanding* (edited and abridged by AD Woozley) II. xxvii. 9. William Collins/ Fount Paperbacks, 1964 (first published in 1690) (page 211).

16. Hume D. *A Treatise of Human Nature* (Book One) (ed. DGC Macnabb) I. iv. section vi. Glasgow: Fontana/Collins. 1962 (first published in 1739) (page 302).

17. Parfit D. Divided minds and the nature of persons. In *Mind Waves: Thoughts on Intelligence, Identity and Consciousness* (eds. C Blakemore, S Greenfield): 19–26. Blackwell, 1987 (page 20).

18. Gillett G. *Subjectivity and Being Somebody: Human Identity and Neuroethics.* Imprint Academic, 2008 (page 14).

19. Hughes JC. *Thinking Through Dementia.* Oxford University Press, 2011 (page 35).

20. Locke J. *An Essay Concerning Human Understanding* (edited and abridged by AD Woozley) II. xxvii. 9. William Collins/Fount Paperbacks, 1964 (first published in1690) (page 212).

21. Parfit D. *Reasons and Persons.* Oxford University Press, 1984.

22. See reference [21], (page 206).

23. Brock DW. Justice and the severely demented elderly. *J Med Philos* 1988; **13**: 73–99.

24. Nuffield Council on Bioethics. *Dementia: Ethical Issues.* Nuffield Council on Bioethics, 2009.

25. Taylor C. *Philosophical Arguments.* Harvard University Press, 1995 (pages 170–171).

26. See reference [25], (page 169).

27. Wittgenstein L. *Philosophical Investigations* (eds. GEM Anscombe, R Rhees; trans GEM Anscombe). Blackwell, 1968 (First edition 1953; second edition 1958; third edition 1967); §23.

28. Wittgenstein L. *Zettel* (eds. GEM Anscombe, GH von Wright; trans GEM Anscombe). Blackwell, 1981; §173.

29. Heidegger M. *Being and Time* (trans. J Macquarrie, E Robinson). Blackwell, 1962; p. 158. (Originally published as *Sein und Zeit* in 1927.)

30. Merleau-Ponty M. *Phenomenology of Perception* (trans. C Smith). Routledge, 1962; p. 169. (Originally published as *Phénomènologie de la Perception* by Gallimard, Paris (1945).)

31. See reference [25], (page 170).

32. See reference [19], (pages 3–4; 9–12; 33–34).

33. Aquilina C, Hughes JC. The return of the living dead: agency lost and found? In *Dementia: Mind, Meaning, and the Person* (eds. JC Hughes, SJ Louw, SR Sabat): 143–61. Oxford University Press, 2006.

34. James IA, Jackman L. *Understanding Behaviour in Dementia that Challenges: A guide to Assessment and Treatment* (2nd edition). Jessica Kingsley, 2017.

35. Sabat SR. *The Experience of Alzheimer's Disease: Life Through a Tangled Veil.* Blackwell, 2001.

36. Dekkers W. Persons with severe dementia and the notion of bodily autonomy. In *Supportive Care for the Person with Dementia* (eds. JC Hughes, M Lloyd-Williams, GA Sachs): 253–261. Oxford University Press, 2010.

37. See reference [19], (pages 232–236).

38. See reference [24], (Box 2.1).

Concluding Reflections

Philippa Lilford

It is no accident that Julian C. Hughes, who is coming to the end of an extremely distinguished career, introduces this book and I, a psychiatry trainee drawing ever closer to my first consultant job, write the conclusion. Before looking to the future of old age psychiatry, I want to say something about Julian C. Hughes.

He is the reason for this book. With his craft for communicating ideas and with people, he built and shaped this book into what we hoped it would become. He has encouraged, inspired, and led the editing not only of this book, but also my relationship with old age psychiatry. If Julian is the face of old age psychiatry, with his intelligence, humour, and wisdom, we budding psychiatrists have an enormous mantle to assume, and one exceptional role model to follow.

Looking forward then, what strikes me when reading these chapters is how much will change during my career, but also how much should stay the same. Advances in neuroscience and genetic epidemiology will shine a light on the aetiology of common neuropsychiatric conditions such as Alzheimer's disease and lead to the development of new treatments. Imagine a 70-year-old gentleman who is referred to my clinic in 15 years' time with a subjective report of memory decline. First, he may have a genetic risk score to help me understand his risk of developing Alzheimer's, with all the uncertainties and ethical conundrums which are associated with this. Second, how a diagnosis of Alzheimer's disease is made may be quite different. Perhaps, for example, I shall be performing lumbar punctures and using Alzheimer's disease biomarkers routinely (or referring these patients to my neurology colleagues!). Finally, what treatment I can offer may be different, for example with the development of disease-modifying drugs. As we understand more about the genetic and environmental risk factors for Alzheimer's disease more drug treatments are likely to become available, perhaps with no single drug as a cure, but with primary and secondary prevention medications alongside immune-modulating drugs, which may alter the pathological cascade that is presumed to result in Alzheimer's dementia.

However, even as developments in neuroscience enhance our understanding of mental illness, they do not help to capture the person as a whole. The unique position of the old age psychiatrist appears to be the privileged opportunity to try to understand the person, share the stories of their lives, and offer an holistic assessment and treatment model.

I first considered a career in old age psychiatry during my second year as a junior doctor working on a vascular surgery ward. I clerked an elderly gentleman who was an elective admission for an aortic aneurysm repair. I remarked on his extremely handsome and dilapidated leather suitcase. 'It travelled with me as an evacuated child during the Second World War', he told me. He subsequently suffered numerous complications of his surgery and left the hospital with a new diagnosis of bowel cancer and feeling ten years older in his body. His mind, however, still raced with his glorious anecdotes, humour, and stoicism. He told me he concentrated on the aphorism of 'adding life to years, rather than years to life'. The wealth of experience he had accumulated during his lifetime, including the ordeal he had been through with his trusty suitcase when evacuated and separated from his family in the Second World War, served as a platform not only to understand him as a person, but for him to cope in incredibly difficult circumstances.

Whilst editing this book I thought often of this gentleman who sparked in me the desire to become a psychiatrist. Mental illnesses are common in older people and carry significant morbidity and mortality. Assessments are holistic and personal, and treatments often include making best-interest decisions for that person. This is a unique and privileged position to hold and one which has the potential to continue to add life to the years of our ageing population. Our hope is that this book sparks in our readers something similar; that it will inspire and encourage the reader in some way for the good of our specialty and for the good of the patients we serve.

Index

Printed in the United States
by Baker & Taylor Publisher Services